Endemic Cretinism

John Dennison • Charles Oxnard • Peter Obendorf

Endemic Cretinism

Springer

Authors
John Dennison, M.Sc., B.A.
Department of Anatomy
Otago School of Medical Sciences
Dunedin, New Zealand
john.dennison@stonebow.otago.ac.nz

Peter Obendorf, B.Sc (Hons), Ph.D., M.Litt.
RMIT University
School of Applied Sciences
Melbourne, VIC, Australia
peter.obendorf@rmit.edu.au

Charles Oxnard, MBChB, Ph.D., D.Sc.
University of Western Australia
School of Anatomy and Human Biology
and in the Forensic Science Centre
Crawley, WA, Australia
charles.oxnard@uwa.edu.au

ISBN 978-1-4899-9782-1 ISBN 978-1-4614-0281-7 (eBook)
DOI 10.1007/978-1-4614-0281-7
Springer New York Dordrecht Heidelberg London

Printed on acid-free paper

Springer is part of Springer Science+Business Media (www.springer.com)

Foreword

I am honoured to contribute this update as recognition of the pioneering work of Professors F. De Quervain and C. Wegelin in their classic book on endemic cretinism published in 1936. Their book, which provides a remarkable coverage of the literature on cretinism over hundreds of years, is now available for the first time in English.

We are indebted to John Dennison of Otago University, New Zealand for this expert translation from the original German Text.

I include also reference to the current status of the problem, its scientific understanding and the significant activities which have developed over the past 25 years to control what has been a substantial global scourge. Iodine deficiency is now recognised by the World Health Organization as the most common preventable cause of brain damage in the world today.

The Appendix is based on a longer paper entitled 'Cretinism Revisited' by my colleague Professor Chen Zu Pei (Tianjin Medical University, China) and myself and published in *Best Practice & Research Clinical Endocrinology & Metabolism* 24: (2010) 39–50.

Basil Hetzel A.C., M.D., F.R.A.C.P.
Former Executive Director and then Chairman of the International Council
for Control of Iodine Deficiency Disorders (ICCIDD)
Michell Building
Women's & Children's Hospital
72 King William Road
North Adelaide SA 5006
Australia

Preface

On 26 September 1936 the *British Medical Journal* reported: "The house of J. Springer, Berlin, notable for its scientific publications, issues the seventh volume of a series of monographs on topics of special interest to clinicians and pathologists… This little book is a valuable compendium of the latest views on a difficult subject."

On 3 October 1936 *The Journal of the American Medical Association* wrote: "Professor de Quervain is chief of the surgical clinic at the University of Bern, Switzerland, and received his early training under Professor Kocher. Prof. Carl Wegelin is director of the institute of pathologic anatomy of the University of Bern. Both de Quervain and Wegelin have been intensely interested in the goiter problem, situated as they are in Bern near the center of the endemic goiter belt of Switzerland, where unfortunately a large proportion of the population is affected by a "goiter noxia" which results in cretinism. This monograph summarizes their lifelong study of the problem and presents in an authoritative manner the various clinical types of cretinism, the pathologic anatomy and histology, the pathologic physiology, the pathogenesis and the accepted methods of prophylaxis and treatment."

Those quotations may set the scene for a "nice little historical read". However, in the World Health Organization/UNICEF Report (2007) *Iodine deficiency in Europe: A continuing public health problem*, this work of de Quervain and Wegelin is still cited for its value, among 217 references. In 1993 Steven Boyages and Jean-Pierre Halpern, writing in *Thyroid*, described this work as "their classic monograph", while a two-page 1936 review that was republished online in *The Journal of Pathology and Bacteriology* (2005 DOI/10.1002/path.1700430224/pdf) concluded: "Since cretinism is unknown in the sites of endemic goitre in Britain this monograph should be welcome to British pathologists interested in endocrine disturbances."

All these comments describe a text that has, to our knowledge, never been published in English!

As an anatomist at the University of Otago, Dunedin, New Zealand, and a published translator of similar books, I was contacted and invited to undertake this translation by Dr. Peter Obendorf (School of Applied Sciences, RMIT University, Melbourne, Victoria, Australia), and Prof. Charles Oxnard (School of Anatomy and

Human Biology and Forensic Science Centre, University of Western Australia, Crawley, Western Australia), who point out that there is so little detailed knowledge or numerical data on cretinism available in the English-speaking world.

Professor Basil S. Hetzel, recently-retired WHO Chairman of the International Council for Control of Iodine Deficiency Disorders, suggested that Springer-Verlag, as publisher of the 1936 book, would be the appropriate publisher of "this valuable work", especially given the current re-emergence of iodine deficiency around the world. Basil Hetzel has recently published (end 2009) with Dr. Chen Zu-pei on the resurgence of iodine deficiency in China. Charles Oxnard has this year been invited by the Government agency to participate in an iodine survey of Timor Leste where 26% of school-age children are iodine-deficient (Ministry of Health National Nutrition Strategy, 2004). Australia has now made it mandatory for most bread to contain iodized salt in place of ordinary salt.

The aim of this project, therefore, is to make this much-cited work, "... which remains the most authoritative and comprehensive account of this condition" (*British Medical Bulletin*, 1960) available to English-speaking researchers.

My wife, Ann, spent many long hours correcting, and rechecking my initial draft. I am most grateful for her meaningful discussions.

Professor Oxnard and Dr. Obendorf have joined with me, the translator, to edit this work.

Dunedin, New Zealand Kenneth John Dennison

Contents

Introduction

Monographs on cretinism have appeared from time to time over the last 150 years. These sometimes included a discussion of endemic goitre; at other times they gave a presentation on hypothyroid conditions, congenital myxoedema, and acquired myxoedema. In reviewing these studies, we become aware that quite varied reflections have awakened interest in the characteristic clinical picture of cretinous degeneration. At the forefront, for the whole of the last century, were the humanitarian and economic aspects of the problem. People felt the urgency for a remedy, and, in a systematic manner, sought out the causes of this assault on public health. Anthropology, epidemiology, and pathological anatomy were all taken into consideration to solve the dual puzzle of the origin of goitre and the relationship between cretinism and goitre. There was a fair share of natural philosophical speculation alongside detailed scientific observation. However, from a merely cursory glance, the importance of an investigation into cretinism as a scientific problem gained full recognition only when the physiology of the thyroid gland became understood. In anticipation of this, in 1830 Troxler, in Berne, expressed the idea.that the function of the thyroid gland could be clarified only by studying cretinism. However, another 50 years passed before this idea took shape through the investigations of Horsley, Kocher, Bruns, and others. Nevertheless, it should not be thought that the purely human and economic side of the question had receded into the background. Scientific interest supervened, raising cretinism from a series of disease processes of purely local interest to one of general physiological enquiry. We have dedicated several years of particular interest in this aspect of the problem, continuing the fundamental research of our teachers and predecessors in office, Theodor Kocher and Theodor Langhans, which would likewise guide our further analyses. We have also been able to rely on the constant support of physiologists like Asher and Abelin. Our study was further assisted by the availability of a large observational sample. The almshouses of Berne canton, especially those of Riggisberg, Frienisberg, Utzigen, Worben, and Langnau, which through the courtesy of their medical and administrative leadership had always been forthcoming, care for some several hundred cretins of every type, from puberty right through to old age. We were always able to observe any typical case or any specially noteworthy case from among these people, in a clinical setting. We found younger cretins, from school-age onward, in institutions for the feeble-minded and for deaf-mutes, and we were also able to observe them in the clinic when necessary. We thus had access to a sample that probably had never been so localised. One of us acquired extremely grateful, devoted patients from among the numerous cretins who became free from severe goitre in the clinic, and was given ample opportunity of examining their physical and mental behaviour. The only regret is that up till now it has not been possible to undertake an autopsy of those cretins who had died in institutions. Up until now the administration has not granted permission for this. Accordingly our anatomical material is relatively small, being restricted to those individuals who had died in the *Inselspital* [the Berne University Hospital] and in asylums for the insane.

We hesitated to undertake the present exposition, already long-overdue, after Eggenberger (1927) in the *Handbuch der inneren Sekretion*, and Gamper and Scharfetter (1932) in the *Handbuch der Geisteskrankheiten* had compiled the current wisdom and their own observations into first-class presentations. However, once we had resolved, at the behest of the publisher, to set down these pages, it was not done with the intention of reaffirming what has been known for a long time, but from a perceived, over-arching need to bring to light the problem of cretinism, from our own study and observations, as being not only an epidemiological problem but also a pathological-anatomical and pathological-physiological problem. It is in the nature of things that we will come into constant contact with the pathology and the clinical aspect of endemic goitre. Cretinism and goitre behave like two circles with a common centre – the inner circle has dropped out to a greater or lesser extent depending on the demarcation of cretinism. A sharp boundary occurs just as rarely as in most other natural processes, and the dividing line between the man who appears normal apart from his goitre, and the cretinous goitre-sufferer, is, to some extent, hidden by subjective experiences. Nevertheless it cannot be our mission to bring forth a definitive presentation on the problem of endemic goitre. We must simply be satisfied with pointing out the tip of the iceberg, whose surfaces become blurred whenever we are able to introduce a comparison from a country where goitre is at a low level.

Chapter 1
Etymology of the Word 'Cretin'

Until quite recently a kind of uncertainty has predominated as to the origin and original meaning of the word 'cretin'. It is acknowledged that it emerged only in the eighteenth century, and was mentioned for the first time in the French encyclopaedia of 1754. The word belongs among the dialects of south-eastern France.

By far the most likely derivation is from 'Christianus', from which the word 'Cretin' has evolved via 'Crestin'. Salvioni states that 50 years earlier at Lake Maggiore the word 'Christian' was used to designate a cretin. The relationship with the word *Chrétien* is therefore at hand. The change in meaning has perhaps been brought about in such a way that the cretin was, to begin with, labelled as *pauvre chrétien* out of sympathy. According to another explanation, said to have come from Fodéré, the cretin, because of his limited intellect and harmlessness, might have appeared as *bon chrétien*, which would agree with the fact that in certain areas of the French Alps the cretins were also called *beats* or *innocents*. However, as Virchow has already pointed out, such references cannot be found in the original text of Fodéré's work.

Tracing the word 'cretin' back to 'cretira' (*cretura*) is highly unlikely. Ackermann states that around Ilanz in the canton of Graubünden the designation *cretira*, which belongs in the Rhæto-Romanic language, is used for 'wretched creature, rascal' and that is how the expression 'cretin' arose.

The derivation from *creta* (chalk) is equally unsatisfactory. It is based on Rösch's comment that young cretins are said to have a chalky-white appearance, which is certainly not always accurate and has already been refuted by the brown skin tone of many cretins having led to their being called 'marrons'. Also, as my colleague Prof. Jaberg, Professor of Romance Philology in Berne, has assured me, the word 'cretin' could not have been derived etymologically from *creta*.

Finally, Finkbeiner believes that he has found the explanation in the Swiss dialect word *Krätti*, which means 'pannier', and is used for both the carrier of the basket and for hunch-backed and misshapen. 'Cretin' might then be nothing other than the French dialect form of the Swiss-German *Krätti*. This deduction however appears totally erroneous since cretins due to their physical weakness usually do not carry

J. Dennison et al., *Endemic Cretinism*,
DOI 10.1007/978-1-4614-0281-7_1, © Springer Science+Business Media, LLC 2011

panniers, nor do they suffer kyphosis, nor can it be assumed that the Swiss-German dialectic word would have penetrated as far as Piemont and Savoie.[1]

It is certain that the term 'cretin', which has found entry today not only into the medical nomenclature but also into the common language of every country, had been limited originally to quite a small region, and was used only in Savoie, the Aosta Valley, and the French portion of Valais. Other countries had their own names – actually, in the German language a whole heap of labels has been coined for cretins according to local region, for example *Fexe* in Salzburg, *Trottel* in Steiermark, *Gauche* in German Wallis. Today all these names have only historical and folkloristic value. Therefore we refer here to the older works of Rösch and Iphofen, which introduce the expressions occurring in the various dialects. They give a looking-glass picture of cretinism in the whole richness of its shades and nuances. It should also be mentioned that in certain areas of France it was customary to use the word *Cagots*.

[1]I express my deepest gratitude to Professor Jaberg, who most willingly advised me on these etymological questions.

Chapter 2
Definition

More far-reaching than the label question is the problem of *defining* cretinism. Setting aside all theories for the time being, when we simply ask ourselves which physical and intellectual defects have been designated by the name 'Cretinism' over the course of time, we come to the conclusion that it is a localised physical and intellectual limitation of development and an inferiority that is distinguished in popular perception from forms of feeble-mindedness and dementia common to all countries and all peoples. A second statement from time immemorial is that cretinism is found only where endemic goitre also occurs to a pronounced degree. We must acknowledge these two 'historical' attributes if we do not want to lose ourselves in the infinity of universal intellectual and physical insufficiency – the so-called international imbecility and nonsense.

Research, as we shall see, has so far indicated the justification for such a demarcation, both in terms of localization and in relationship with endemic goitre. Comparative geographical-pathological investigation reveals more and more that there is actually a condition of physical and intellectual retardation of development that is not influenced by 'race', and occurs in all parts of the world where endemic goitre is deeply entrenched, i.e., the centre of endemic zones, and is bound to these zones. We combined these statements in the definition of cretinism that we proposed in 1923.

> Cretinism is an endemic complex of somatic and mental disorders occurring in centres of severe, endemic goitre, appearing mainly on the skeleton, skin, and nervous system, in which retardation of developmental processes and vital functions play a principal role, and which cannot be traced back to either some other congenital or acquired cerebral illness (encephalitis etc.), or to a well-defined skeletal disease that is independent of endemic goitre, such as rachitis, chondrodystrophy etc.

When we utter this sentence we must immediately identify two groups of cases that have often caused confusion in the literature by obscuring and preventing a clear recognition of the picture of cretinism.

The first of these, occurring in every country independently of any endemic goitre, are cases of teratological errors of the thyroid gland – *thyroaplasia*. This is purely a malformation, with the thyroid gland absent or limited to a rudiment in the tongue region (Thomas' 'dystopic hypoplasia'), while the parathyroid glands are

J. Dennison et al., *Endemic Cretinism*,
DOI 10.1007/978-1-4614-0281-7_2, © Springer Science+Business Media, LLC 2011

still present. This malformation, which can present widely variable clinical degrees of hypothyroidism depending on the level of function of the tongue–thyroid gland rudiment, has nothing to do with endemic thyropathy and, as Pineles emphasised back in 1902, it causes only confusion when Gull's original diagnosis of 'sporadic cretinism' continues to be used for such cases. Whether in individual cases thyroid gland failure can be traced back to an intrauterine inflammatory lesion as Siegert surmises, rather than a teratological process, must be left unresolved. As yet, there is no anatomical evidence for this. On the other hand, the distinction between teratological-, congenital-, and early-childhood-acquired myxœdema among the following group is blurred in that the congenital thyroaplasia is often incomplete so that its clinical *sequelae* do not begin to be expressed immediately after birth but only after infancy.

The second world-wide group of thyroid gland disorders causing confusion is *acquired, infantile myxœdema*. This is based on a lesion of the thyroid gland (acute infectious disease), probably almost always inflammatory, acquired postnatally and leading to a cretin-like appearance while not being aetiologically related to endemic cretinism. These cases too would earn the term 'sporadic cretinism'. Their only common feature with genuine cretinism is thyroid malignancy, but this is not the cause. In 1923 Wieland did splendid work on this topic both historically and clinically, in particular pointing out the importance of radiology for all thyrogenic disorders. Progress in defining the *underlying clinical picture* can be brought about only through careful pathological investigation of cases of illness accurately observed in a clinical setting. We undertook this monitoring during therapeutic implantations in several cases that could be clarified only in this manner.[1]

In addition to the thyroid disorders not attributable to endemic cretinism, in the endemic arena, just as anywhere else, we find the most varied forms of congenital and acquired primary mental deficiency. We also find growth disorders and systemic diseases of the skeleton which have nothing to do with the thyroid gland, such as hereditary dwarfism, chondrodystrophy, osteogenesis imperfecta, etc. All of these pathologies have been preferentially ascribed to the thyroid gland by physicians inexperienced in this field, especially when the patient is somewhat goitrous. Given the current state of our knowledge, to throw every chance-event in the endemic arena into a big pot together with endemic cretinism is no longer justifiable as a means of circumventing certain diagnostic difficulties and easing the attainment of a solution to pathogenetic problems. We will make an advancement in our knowledge of individual forms of physical and mental developmental errors only when we try to trace them back to their *origins* and clearly differentiate the various possible causes. By using blurred concepts we drop back a whole century. The discussion on pathogenesis will give us the opportunity of returning to this argument.

A particular difficulty in the definition of cretinism is the *multi-faceted nature of the clinical picture*, both from a somatic and a psychological point of view.

---

[1] It is noted here that the case introduced in Wydler's series as No.111 is not to be regarded as a full cretin, but as a case of thyroaplasia. In error, it was not excluded.

Finally, the dissociation of cretinism from the normal state is made more difficult by our having to deal with *fleeting transitions*. We find certain psychological *stigmata* of cretinism suggested also among individuals who earn their living well or poorly, keep up their civil duties and perhaps even serve in a minor post. You could even say that endemic thyropathy puts its stamp on the entire population of certain regions. Extensive personal observation of a great amount of material is obligatory in order to review all these demarcation problems. This cannot be substituted by studying books. It alone gives an overview and critique, and offers a safeguard against hasty conclusions.

Maffei, who devoted his 1813 dissertation to cretinism, stated in 1844 when he was working again in that field that the subject became steadily clearer and more understandable to him during the first 15 years, but in the subsequent years it seemed to diminish in clarity once more because, with greater experience, that which had seemed positive and correct steadily collapsed in on itself. He is not the only one to have experienced this.

Chapter 3
Historical

In spite of cretinism's very probably having been indigenous to certain countries over many centuries, we have had scientific information of its occurrence only for a relatively short time. That it is not mentioned anywhere by the physicians of ancient times is all the more remarkable, since even non-medical writers of Roman times (Pliny, Vitruvius, Juvenal, Ulpian) have drawn attention to goitre endemic to the Alps. For the first definite account of the occurrence of cretinism we are indebted to Paracelsus (1493–1531) who, as an outstanding observer, recognised immediately the connection between goitre and cretinism. I shall quote several examples demonstrating this in all its clarity (cited in part from Damerow):

> "The lunatics that the animal spirits have given birth to, are ill-bred through weakness; belong among reasonable cattle; probably carry a misgrowth, an outgrowth such as goitre and the like on their body, and even though this is not *proprium stultorum* [the stuff of fools] but is something else, this applies most often." According to Paracelsus the origin lies in that "not only is reason shredded, but the body also."

Further accounts came from Felix Platter (d. 1614), working in Basel University and describing the cretins in his homeland of Wallis; and the historian Josias Simmler (1574) in Zurich. In addition, the Dutch physician Peter Foreest (d. 1597) observed many cretins in Veltlin. Then almost total silence fell until the second half of the eighteenth century, when the natural scientist H. de Saussure of Geneva studied the problem of cretinism during his travels in the Alps and connected it with sea level and air quality. Surprisingly, cretinism is mentioned only very briefly by Albrecht von Haller who, as director of the Bex saltworks in the lower Rhone Valley (1758–1764), probably had ample opportunity for personal research. He describes cretins as 'only half humans', who are totally unfit for all business of human life, have enormous goitres and often even die because the excrement in the colon has grown to an unbelievable size. Haller is of the opinion that the heat of the sun's rays has perhaps contributed to influencing the brains of cretins to their detriment.

Then from 1780 lively interest was awakened in the scientific investigation of cretinism, with not only travellers reporting its extent and its presumed causes, but attempts being made also on the medical front to penetrate more deeply into its essence. In 1788, for the first time, Malacarne in Turin included a description of

J. Dennison et al., *Endemic Cretinism*,
DOI 10.1007/978-1-4614-0281-7_3, © Springer Science+Business Media, LLC 2011

three cretin skulls in his letters to Peter Frank in Pavia. Two skulls had undergone a detailed examination in Pavia by Ackermann. As a result, that investigator from Mainz sought out the cretins in their homes, and in 1790 set down his impressions in a little book, *Über die Kretinen, eine besondere Menschenabart in den Alpen.* According to the book, cretinism was nothing other than the highest grade of rickets.

Then came a flood of literary preoccupation with cretinism, through the work of Fodéré that appeared for the first time in 1792 in Turin and later in Paris, with a German translation published in Berlin in 1796. It referred especially to the situation in Savoie and in the Aosta Valley. The book is still worth reading today because of its abundance of outstanding observations and opinions. In his anatomical investigations culminating with the assumption of an extraordinary hardness of the brain and spinal cord, Fodéré admittedly travelled down a wrong path. This earned him criticism by Joseph and Carl Wenzel in Vienna, who in 1802 gave a good description of the cranial base, whose alteration gave rise to disorders in brain development. They rejected rickets as the cause of cretinism.

Noted in passing, the cretinous degeneration of the Wallesian population evidently made such a strong impression on Napoleon I, during his military campaigns that took him through Wallis into Italy, that he charged his Prefects with producing an official, topographical-statistical inquiry into cretinism in the Simplon Département (*cit.* Köstl).

In the first half of the nineteenth century we encounter an astonishingly copious literature on cretinism. A detailed monograph by Iphofen (1817) followed the works of Troxler, Demme, Thieme, Stahl, plus the extensive report on cretinism by the *Sardinian Commission*, that had been ordered by King Karl Albert. At the instigation of Troxler and Guggenbühl the Swiss Natural Scientific Society engaged themselves with the question of cretinism firstly in 1830 and then on repeated occasions. In 1834 Autenrieth raised the same question with the Assembly of German Natural Scientists and Physicians. Prime interest was in the geographical extent and the presumed causes of this evil, sought mainly in climatological-atmospheric influences. Associated with this was the question as to the curability of cretinism that was put forward by Guggenbühl and answered by his opening of the first psychiatric hospital for young cretins in 1841 on the Abendberg at Interlaken. His undertaking initially met with approval and gained moral support throughout Europe and America. However it did not achieve the success hoped for, and became a miserable failure after about 20 years. From the Noric Alps and Württemberg, Maffei and Rösch (1844) published studies that belonged among the best written at that time.

The anatomical investigation of cretinism received a massive boost through the outstanding work of B. Nièpce who in 1851 produced detailed reports of several autopsies, and through the important work of Virchow (1856–62) in following up the Lower Franconian endemia from Wurzburg. He devoted his attention particularly to the physical proportions of the cretin skull, and came to the conclusion that the skull deformities often had an autonomous character and, for their part, determined the development of the brain. He was responsible for the doctrine of premature synostosis of cranial bones, to which he ascribed a major role in the origin of cretinism. As the pathogen of goitre and cretinism, Virchow proposed a miasma whose lesser effect presented goitre and the greater effect: cretinism.

At the instigation of the Swiss Natural Scientific Society the epidemiology of cretinism in Switzerland underwent a detailed exposition by Meyer-Ahrens (1854). In France Nièpce (1851), Fabre (1857), Morel (1863), St Lager (1867) and Baillarger (1873) studied not only the geographical extent of goitre and cretinism but also the aetiology in great detail, admittedly without coming to any definite conclusions on the latter. The internal connection between goitre and cretinism throughout the world is accentuated in these works. H. Bircher (1883) and Allara (1892) dealt with endemic cretinism and the *sequelae* of total thyroidectomy in a similar manner, but with the addition of clinical pathology. Bircher traced mainly the Swiss epidemiology, Allara the Italian.

The work of Th. Kocher (1892) brought a completely new point of view of the pathogenesis of cretinism. Starting from the major discovery of *Cachexia thyreopriva*, he drew a parallel between cretinism and the outcome of total thyroidectomy, explaining the former as precocious suppression or severe disturbance of thyroid function. For the first time, a severe, endemically occurring disorder in the development of the entire organism was traced back to an endocrine gland. From this point on, in the eyes of many researchers, endemic cretinism was nothing other than an internal secretory disorder – hypothyroidism.

In his first publication in 1883 Kocher attempted to explain the clinical picture of *Cachexia strumipriva* through anaemia, deducing the latter from an atrophy of the trachea as a result of vascular repression. The first reference to the 'breakdown in physiological function of the thyroid gland' as a cause of cachexia was by Rud. Grundler in 1885. The author came to this conclusion during a study supervised by P. Bruns, when he observed three cases of total extirpation in Brun's clinic, and witnessed the trials by Schiff and Wagner. He writes, 'Analysis of all the symptoms makes it likely that with *Cachexia strumipriva* we are dealing with a disorder of the central nervous system that can happen only when the presumed activity of the thyroid gland, viz. its metabolic involvement, is diminished'. Cretinism was automatically included in the problem and threw the question of the nature of thyroid function into the centre of the debate. The exchange of ideas between Kocher and Horsley, and the research by Hofmeister, Ewald, Leichtenstern and Murray brought progress. Around 1890–1893 the proponents and *Assistents* of Kocher and Langhans considered the basic question as settled – cretinism in its various stages is a deficit in endocrine function.

Subsequently, Kocher's point of view found partial agreement, and was supported in both the anatomical and clinical aspects by new investigations (Langhans, Beyon, Weygandt, Wagner von Jauregg, Cerletti, de Quervain, Wydler and Eggenberger). In some quarters it also came up against quite strong resistance (H. and E. Bircher, Dieterle, Scholz and, in part, Ewald), with changes in the cretin's body being perceived as a direct consequence of noxious goitre. Admittedly, in recent times opposition to Kocher's opinion has steadily quietened down.

Not completely however—in 1923 Finkbeiner attempted to resolve the problem of endemic cretinism from an anthropological point of view by perceiving cretins as the degenerate remnants of a primitive 'race', basing his argument on a few older authors from the beginning of the previous century. Admittedly Finkbeiner accepted the doctrine of hypothyroidism in part as well.

Also, Gamper and Scharfetter (1928) agreed with the hypothyroidism theory only with a certain constraint; relating the inhibition of growth and development of the various organ systems to a single exogenous noxious goitre, with the failure of the particular thyroid gland occurring only in the sense of a strengthening of this inhibition.

Finally, it must be mentioned that our knowledge of the geographical extent of cretinism in European countries and in other parts of the world has been significantly advanced by the ongoing work of Flinker, Marañón, Marimon, Höjer, MacCarrison, van Bommel, Simons, Eerland and others.

Chapter 4
Epidemiology

1 Statistics

Since endemic cretinism has become the focus of special attention for both physicians and lay scientists, we also have information on its frequency and geographical distribution. What was astonishing at the outset was the consistency of its occurrence in highly discrete regions – its connection with certain mountain ranges, valleys and river courses. Here its occurrence can always be traced back over an extended period – at least several generations. For many foci of cretinism, for example that of Valais, we are absolutely certain that they are already centuries old, and that cretinism can therefore be regarded as a textbook case of an endemic disease. We are unaware of any sporadic epidemic outbreaks of cretinism, such as have been described here and there for common goitre.

Of course it should not be suggested that the endemic disease must be maintained at the same strength over a long period of time. It has even been reported from various places that cretinism was in decline, and was even disappearing in certain areas, such as in Switzerland's Aargau canton (E. Bircher). Admittedly Dieterle and Eugster disagree. Recently Rupilius was virtually unable to find any child cretins or youthful cretins in the cretinism pockets of Steiermark, whereas older cretins were still relatively common.

In the poor-houses of Berne canton, the inventory of older cretins is somewhat greater. By comparison, the 'younger generation' has rather declined in the last decade. Whether this is related to the decline of classical goitre achieved over the last 12 years through iodine is not open for debate here. It is possible that some borderline case was made socially acceptable by early-intervention administration of iodine, thereby involving medical care.

Unfortunately, reliable numerical data that can actually be compared are rarely found, for example in Lower Franconia where, in 1930, Willer was able to locate only 15 cretins, compared with the 133 that were declared by Virchow in the years 1840–1841. Admittedly the latter value may not be accurate, since Virchow doubts that all cases were correctly diagnosed or statistically acquired.

Generally speaking, statistics are a black mark in the aetiology of cretinism. For one thing, the acquisition of precise statistics encounters stern resistance in many

J. Dennison et al., *Endemic Cretinism*,
DOI 10.1007/978-1-4614-0281-7_4, © Springer Science+Business Media, LLC 2011

regions because cretins are kept hidden, out of misguided shame. Virchow graphically described how, during a foray into Lower Franconia, he exposed an organised conspiracy, among even the educated. However, the border between cretinism and the norm caused even greater difficulties, for without a detailed yet time-consuming investigation it is barely possible to recognise borderline cases of cretinism. Also, one investigator will include certain mental or physical characteristics in cretinism whereas to another investigator they indicate something else. Thus in larger areas all recording of statistics that cannot be carried out by one single investigator will markedly depend on various subjective factors and deliver dissimilar results.

Consequently we do not have a single, precise set of statistics relating to any larger region. Major statistics, for example those of the Sardinian Commission, are based solely on multiple surveys carried out by the various physicians who had been sent questionnaires. The bureaux where these data were subjected to critical examination frequently complained that on the one hand there was no sharp distinction between cretinism and common idiocy, and on the other hand the numbers of cretins recorded were too few. The same situation applied where lay people such as teachers and clergy were brought in to survey the numbers of cretins.

Likewise, the numbers recorded for Austria (Wagner von Jauregg) and Northern Italy (Allara) amounting to 100–300 cretins per 100,000 head of population in some provinces might be rather too low. The figure of 1,000 cretins for 100,000 population reckoned for Switzerland by Finkbeiner is, as he himself concedes, arbitrary and in any case totally imprecise.

2 Geographical Distribution

In 1883 Hirsch gave an overview of the geographical distribution of cretinism in his manual of historical/geographical pathology which to date is unsurpassed, achieving the highest possible level of precision. Admittedly his copious data may be quite dubious in places, and no longer valid, but the purely geographical determinations might generally apply even now, with a supplementary correction here and there. With regard to recent surveys of cretinism, only the most significant ranges of distribution will be presented here.

2.1 Europe

Predominantly identified is the entire region of the *Alps*, where cretinism is endemic to the northern and southern slopes. Distribution appears to be not quite so regular in the east–west direction, with two maxima standing out clearly – one in the east and one in the west.

The western includes mainly the valleys of Savoie with the river courses of the Isère and the Durance; the northern and western parts of Piemonte, particularly the Aosta Valley and the Rhone Valley in the canton of Valais; and the Swiss midlands in the cantons of Fribourg, Berne, and Aargau (river courses of the Saane and the Aare). Foothills extend from there through the Swiss midlands and the Voralpen as far as Lake Constance and the Rhine, with the headwaters of the Rhine being encountered in Graubünden canton. Virtually corresponding with this, the endemic disease covers a zone: on the southern slopes of the Alps; in the northern valleys of Lombardia, through the Ticino canton as far as Veltlin; and the headwaters of the Brembo, Seria, Oglio, Mella and Chiesa rivers. The Etschtal and the northern part of Veneto are smitten by cretinism to a much lesser degree. The only exception is the headwaters of the Tagliamento on the southern slopes of the Carnic Alps, where the number of cretins rises once more (Pighini).

The eastern centre of cretinism lies in Styria and Carinthia, where the river courses of the Drau and the Mur are heavily afflicted, but cretinism is also widespread in Salzburg and Upper Austria, along the Salzach and the Traun. Outliers run eastward from there to Lower Austria, and southward into the Krain. The connection with the western centre is through the somewhat milder Tyrolean endemic zone in the Inn valley, through into Upper Bavaria, Allgäu, and the Vorarlberg, while at the southern foot of the Alps the Venetian foci already mentioned lead over into the western dispersal zone.

A second great mountain range recognised as a homeland for cretins (see also Marimon) is the Pyrenees where the endemia prevails to a significant extent on the northern and southern flanks, continuing westward as far as the Spanish provinces of Asturia and Galicia. The other portion of the Iberian Peninsula is by no means free of cretinism. We are grateful to Marañon and Goyanes for the information that by far the heaviest focus in the vicinity of the Spanish–Portuguese border north of the Tajo is in Las Hurdes, with smaller foci occurring in the region of Avila and Segovia as well as in the south near Albacete (Murcia) (Figs. 1 and 2).

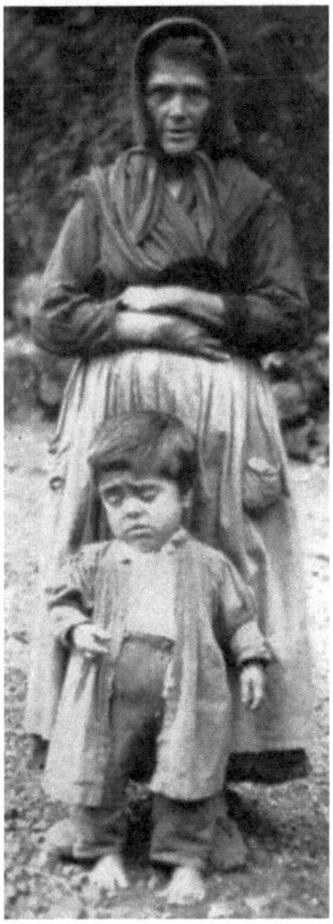

Fig. 1 Hydrocephalic dwarf cretin from Ribota (Asturia). Goitrous mother, prematurely aged (after Marañon)

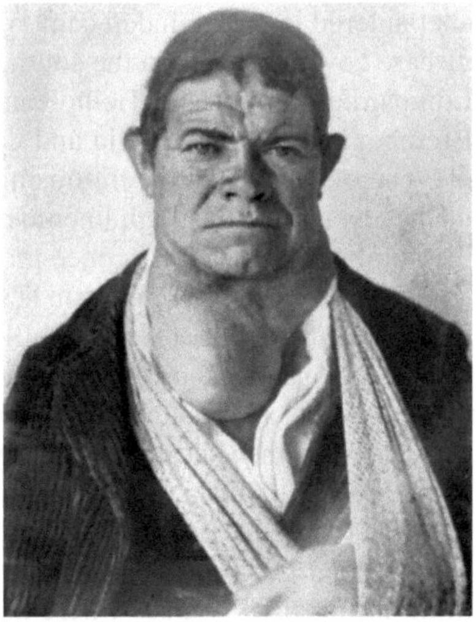

Fig. 2 Goitrous cretin from the Pyrenees (after Marimon)

The endemic disease appears in a significantly lesser degree along the Appeninnes on the Italian peninsula. The northern slopes in Liguria and in the Emilia come into special consideration, with smaller groups said to exist also in Umbria and in Abruzzo. I saw a typical cretin in Amalfi on the Gulf of Salerno, but in central and southern Italy cretinism seems to play only a minor role. In recent times small clusters have been found in Sicily (Coppola) and in Sardinia (Ottonello, Riquier).

A northern connection with the alpine distribution range is brought about by moderate clusters in *Alsace* and *southern Germany*, where cretins are found in the Rhine valley and the Vosges valleys, and also in the side valleys of the Black Forest and the Swabian Mountains, the headwaters of the Neckar and its tributaries Kocher and Jagst, and of the Main (Lower Franconia). However the recent investigations by Willer, mentioned above, demonstrate how cretinism has very much receded here. Similarly, cretins have become very rare in Baden (Aschoff). It is doubtful whether cretinism still occurs in central Germany (the Thuringian Forest) or in the Saxon and Bohemian valleys of the Ore Mountains. According to written accounts by Professor Berblinger, in Jena sporadic cases of cretinism are to be found in Thuringia at least.

In the areas of France distant from the Alps and the Pyrenees, in Belgium, Holland and Denmark, and in the north German lowland plains endemic cretinism is unknown, in spite of mild epidemics of goitre having been reported quite recently in isolated areas of these countries, for example in the area around Utrecht (de Josselin de Jong); Danzig (Feldmann); and East Prussia (Justus). In England too, where endemic goitre is quite widespread in the Midlands (around Derby), cretinism is absent.

For a long time *Scandinavia* was considered free of cretinism, until Dedichen located a minor cluster in Modum on the Tyri Fjord (north of Oslo). Furthermore, Höjer has recently discovered cretinism in its classical form in southern Sweden, on

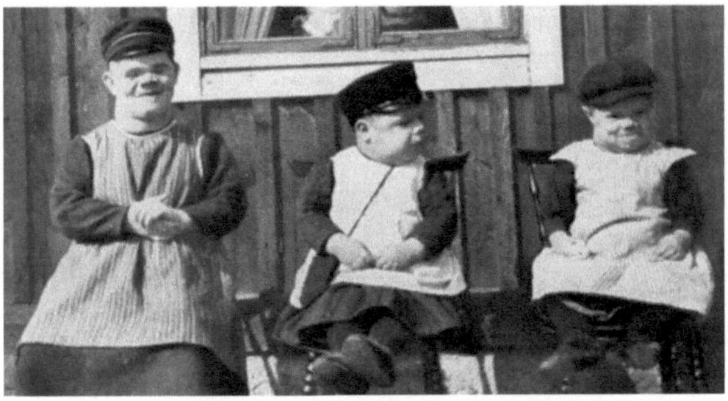

Fig. 3 Cretin siblings from Smårland, 30-, 20-, and 18 years old (after Höjer)

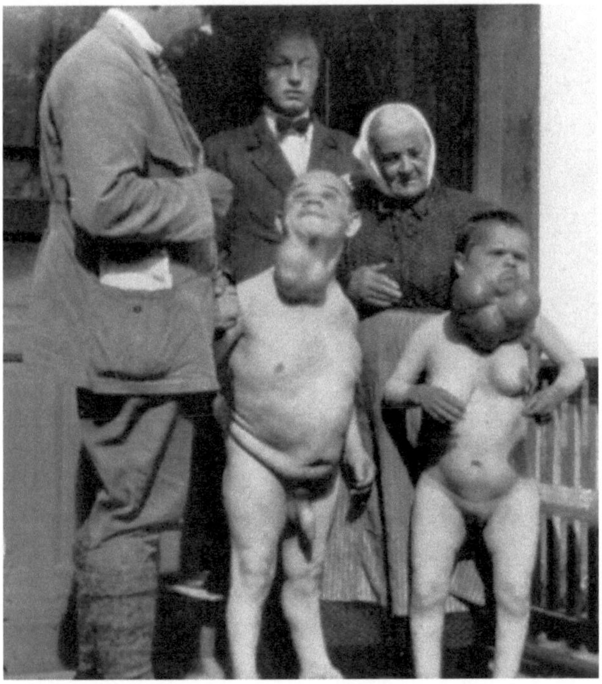

Fig. 4 Cretins from Sweden with a normal-sized (171 cm) mother (after Höjer)

the high plateau of Smårland (Figs. 3 and 4) – indeed it seems fairly widespread there (1‰ full cretins). In *Finland* cretins are so rare that we cannot talk of an endemic disease (Adlerkreutz).

We must not forget the occurrence of cretinism in the *Hungarian Lowlands*, where the Danube island of Schütt harbours a very considerable number of them (Lendvay), and the island in the lower reaches of the Mur boasts a similar pattern (Wagner von Jauregg).

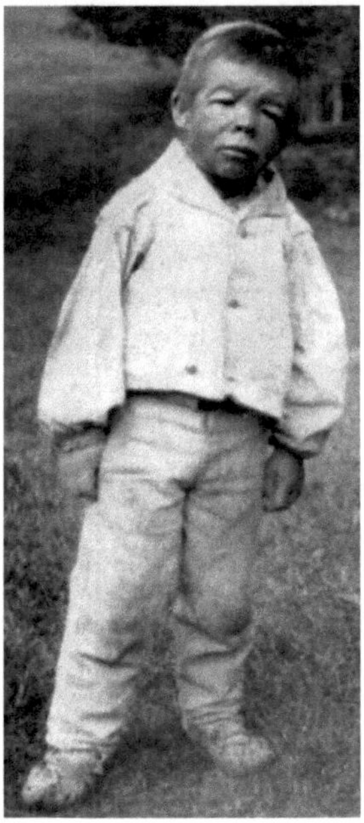

Fig. 5 Cretin without goitre, aged 32, from the Carpathians (after D. Adaroenko)

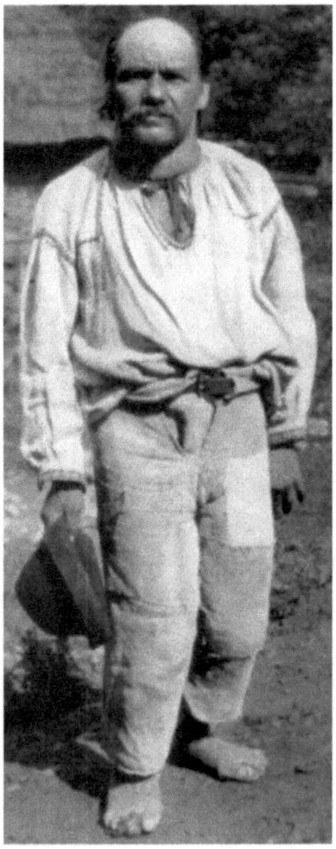

Fig. 6 Cretin with goitre, 50 years old, from the Carpathians (after D. Adaroenko)

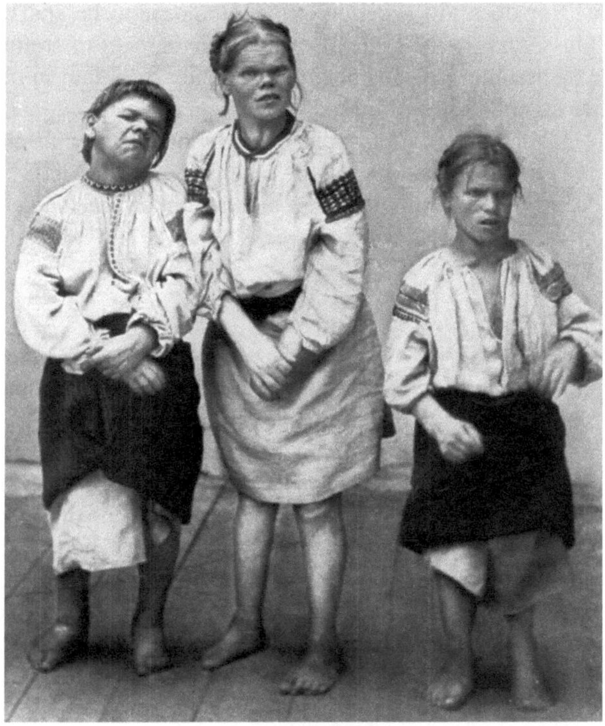

Fig. 7 Ukrainian cretin farm women (from A. Flinker)

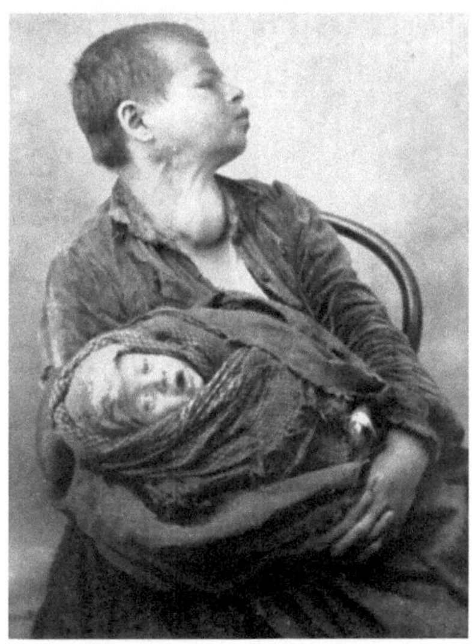

Fig. 8 A 28-year-old Jewish cretin and child, from the Bukovina (from A. Flinker)

Further east the endemia includes the *Carpathians* with cretins throughout (Campeanu, Adaroenko). Their numbers are especially great in Bukovina where there are endemic clusters particularly in the broad, deep river valleys near the plains. The river courses of the Moldava, Suczawa and Czeremosz are particularly affected (Flinker) (Figs. 5–8).

Nor does the *Balkan Peninsula* appear to be spared from cretinism – at least Taussig has found quite a considerable number of cretins in Bosnia, from which we may assume that the endemia is equally prevalent in other Balkan states, although we do not know for sure.

In the *Russian Plain* we know so far of only a single cluster between Lakes Ladoga and Onega (Oldekop). On the other hand, cretinism is widespread in the *Caucasus*, occurring especially in the Svaneti region on the southern slopes (Arndt).

2.2 Asia

As in Europe, cretinism relates mainly to the great mountain ranges, and is therefore most prevalent in the highlands of Central Asia.

We find it in the *Pamir* region (Korownikow, Pereschiwkin) and in *Eastern Siberia*, particularly in Trans–Baikal, but less so in the goitre area of the Lena (Arndt). After that, the *Himalayas* are the focus of a very widespread, severe goitre endemic zone with cretinism present as well. The Indian population of the southern side of the range has been very thoroughly investigated by MacCarrison although cretinism is said to occur also in *Tibet* and in the northern part of China, and likewise in the mountainous parts of *Burma* and *Cochin China*. However, this information is old (see Hirsch) and should be re-examined. Cretinism is unknown in *Japan*, while on the other hand it is endemic in *Ceylon*.

We are very well informed on the occurrence of cretinism on the *Sunda Islands* (Figs. 9 and 10). *Sumatra* is particularly affected – recently van Bommel found an

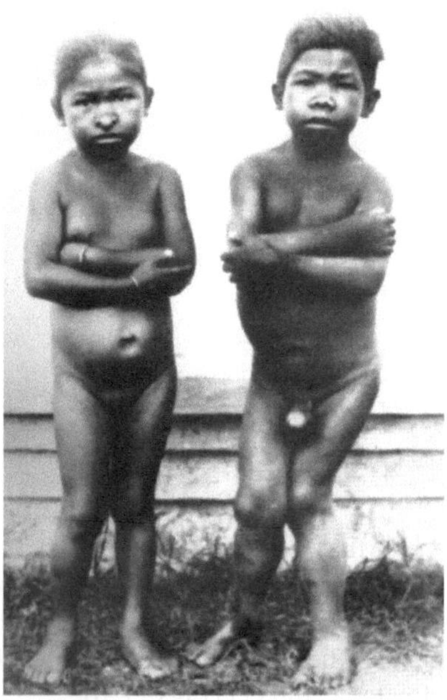

Fig. 9 Fully grown siblings without goitre, from Java (after Eerland)

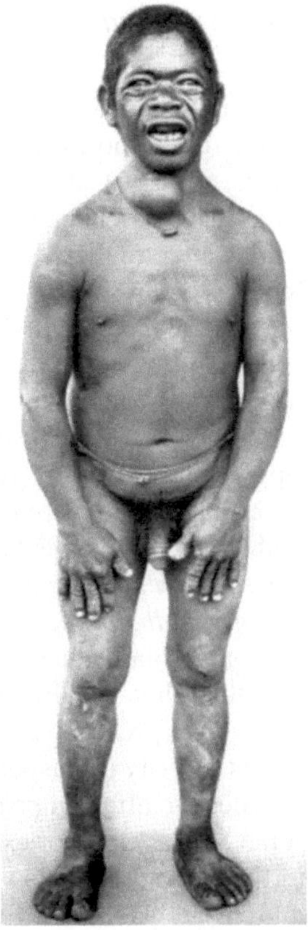

Fig. 10 Goitrous cretin from Sumatra (after von Bommel)

extremely-pronounced focus (0.9% of the total population) in the *Alas lands* (Aceh), and Simons likewise. In addition, cretinism has been detected among the markedly-goitrous Bataks, the mountain-dwellers of Sumatra, in the vicinity of Deli. It is also said to occur on Borneo and Bali, nor is the interior of Java spared (Eerland).

2.3 Australia

Nothing is known of cretinism in Australia and the South Sea islands, although goitre is endemic to New Zealand and Tasmania for example (Hercus et al.).

2.4 Africa

Reports on cretinism in Africa are very unreliable. They all come from long ago, and most likely they are hardly medically certified. Cretinism is said to occur among the Berbers, among the negro tribes of the Kong Mountains in the upper course of the Niger, and in the interior of Madagascar.

2.5 America

In North America we are aware of large areas of goitre in the Great Lakes area, as well as in the north-western United States between the Rockies and the Cascade ranges, as far as California and northwards into Canada, but virtually all recent data agree that this endemic goitre is not encumbered by cretinism, or minimally so. Cretins are rare there. Nevertheless, Jackson estimates their numbers in the United States as being several thousand, and recently reported 512 cases. Cretinism is said to be on the increase in the American goitre regions, especially Wisconsin.

Still further south in the *Cordilleras* (Andes) of Central- and South America in the midst of severe goitre among the population, endemic cretinism is said to occur frequently as well. However, for the most part the only information available was supplied by travelling researchers in the beginning and middle of last century. Nevertheless, the more recent accounts of Kraus and his co-workers leave us in no doubt that cretinism is fairly widespread in northern Argentina and also in Brazil.

Cretinism is, therefore, spread over virtually every part of the world and occurs both in middle latitudes and below the equator. According to our current information, only Polar countries are totally free of the endemic disease.

Although it is evident from what we have said that endemic cretinism mainly follows the great mountain ranges, we still have to free ourselves from the idea that its severity corresponds with sea level. Rather, as with goitre, the intermediate altitudes are affected primarily, in some places the deeply gashed valleys as well. In the Swiss Alps, for example, the Rhone valley is heavily affected; likewise the northern foot of the downs and the foothills of the Alps (400–1,000 m), whereas in high valleys like the Engadin (1,400–1,800 m) cretinism is unknown (note from Dr Ruppanner in Samaden). According to MacCarrison, similar patterns occur in the Himalayas where endemic goitre linked with cretinism increases from above downwards. Further, it is reported by Flinker that in the Carpathians it is just the broad river valleys approaching the plain – not the mountain range itself – that is the extent of cretinism. And finally we remind ourselves of the occurrence of cretinism in the lowland plain (the Danube islands of Schütt, and Carelia).

On the other hand, one most emphatic result from the geographical survey was that cretinism is a *disease of inland people.* It does not occur in the immediate vicinity of the sea nor on the coast itself. When cretins were seen on the Ligurian coast (Lombroso) for example, they were individuals who had come originally from the neighbouring valleys of the Appennines and the coast was within easy reach (Eggenberger). *Nowhere at all has an endemic cluster been found on the sea coast.*

3 Racial Affinity

The geographical spread of endemic cretinism has demonstrated quite clearly that it cannot be confined to one particular 'race' since it occurs among the Caucasoids of Europe, the Hindus of the Himalayas, the Mongoloids of central and east Asia, the

Malay mixed population of the Sunda Islands, the Indians of South America and probably among certain African Negroid tribes. In endemic areas as well it cannot be proven beyond doubt that one race is exclusively or predominantly affected by cretinism.

Although it might appear that in Europe alpine people in particular tend toward cretinism (Figs. 29–31, on pages 39-40), closer examination reveals that this is not so. Probably the great majority of the cretins in the alps do indeed belong to this alpine cluster, but neither are the Nordic nor the Mediterranean groups immune, as evidenced on the one hand by the cluster in southern Scandinavia (Figs. 3 and 4) and on the other hand those in Spain and central Italy. Especially instructive is the situation in the Carpathian valleys of the Bukovina where Flinker found representatives of completely diverse population groups – Romanians, Ukrainians (Fig. 7), Germans, Hungarians, Gypsies and Jews (Fig. 8) – affected by cretinism in exactly the same way. In Bosnia it is the southern Slav-Serbian population that provides cretins.

We find a similar situation in Asia where likewise totally different groups such as Indians, Mongoloids and the Bataks of Sumatra (closely related to the Malays) can show cretinoid degeneration, as can the hybrids of Alas land on Sumatra (Fig. 10).

Finally, it is reported from the province of Salta in northern Argentina that Europeans, Mestizos and Indians living there are frequently affected by cretinism (Mantegazza, cited by Lombroso), while remarkably the Negroids are said to be spared.

Even conceding that the anthropological investigation of many regions is still inadequate, it can still be argued with some certainty from the material available *that cretinism is not a 'racial' attribute*, but afflicts the population of certain geographically circumscribed areas, completely independently of 'race'.

4 Relation to Endemic Goitre

It was noted in the Introduction that the most intimate connections exist between goitre and cretinism; indeed the relationship may briefly be stated: *nowhere does endemic cretinism appear independently – it is always tied to endemic goitre.*

Also, very recent meticulous investigations by Dieterle and Eugster have resulted in a complete synopsis of cretinism and goitre for certain areas of the cantons of Zürich and Aargau in Switzerland. The localised, solid attachments of both phenomena to certain houses have been preserved, totally unchanged over a period of 20 years. According to Eugster, the lower storey of old houses is a focus for goitre and cretinism.

Yet in no part of the world has cretinism been observed without concomitant endemic goitre. Only confusion with common idiocy could lead to contradictory claims. Thus, even in the last century, the perception has permeated through most researchers that cretinism and goitre also have some kind of connection in their manner of development (Fodéré, Iphofen, Rösch, Virchow, B. Nièpce, Morel, Saint-Lager, Baillarger, Allara, Lombroso and others). This came about through the high frequency of goitre among cretins. Only in a few older papers (Ackermann,

Maffei, *the Sardinian Commission*) is the view expressed that goitre and cretinism occur independently of each other, and only by chance in the same locations. This view found support in the accurate observation that often the most severe cases of cretinism have no goitre and even have a reduced thyroid gland. But this is only an illusory contradiction, which has been removed by a more-precise histological investigation of the cretin's thyroid gland and, above all, by examination of the gland's functional performance.

However, quite recently, a new champion for the independence of cretinism has appeared: Finkbeiner maintains that 'goitre and cretinism have nothing directly to do with each other'. Admittedly, therein lies the concession that possibly an indirect connection exists between the two. Finkbeiner based the above statement on the fact that with goitre it was always women who were more often affected than men, whereas with cretinism males predominated. However, this objection has no bearing for, even though in adult goitre statistics the female sex is indeed more frequently affected, the childhood situation, at least during severe endemic goitre, is often directly the opposite, with boys more frequently affected by goitre than girls (Marthe, Woelz) or again both sexes almost equally affected (Dieterle, Hirschfeld and Klinger, Kerzmann). Also, no sexual difference can be determined among newborns affected by goitre (Wegelin). Thus, early childhood is the determining time for the development of cretinism. However, Finkbeiner did not take into account the distribution of goitre during this period.

Finkbeiner's opinion has also been refuted by Pfaundler who determined the syntropy between goitre and cretinism and found an index of 41.6. This means that 'both states would be found combined in an individual 41 times more frequently than would have been expected if they (directly or indirectly) had nothing to do with each other'. Pfaundler determined this high syntropy among patients in the children's clinics at Graz and Munich.

This leads us to a further point. Not every goitre region is also home to endemic cretinism. While listing the zones of distribution of cretinism we mentioned that certain goitre countries were unfamiliar with cretinism. *Only severe endemic goitre is connected with endemic cretinism.* This is true primarily of the endemic goitre that follows the great mountain ranges of Europe, Asia and America, whereas milder goitre endemias, goitre affecting the lowlands and areas near the sea coast are, almost without exception, free of cretinism. I recollect the goitre endemic to Holland, Danzig and East Prussia. In Russia too, in spite of mild endemic goitre, the greater part of the European region is spared from cretinism (Arndt), and the same is true of North America. These are, for the most part, regions where individuals affected by goitre show a tendency toward hyperthyroidism, Basedow/Grave's disease. We will see later that the goitres of such endemias also differ anatomically from those of the other endemias related to cretinism. It cannot be emphasised too highly that the anatomical and functional picture of particular endemic goitres is extremely variable. Cretinism finds the prerequisite of its development only in a rigidly fixed morphological and functional behaviour of the goitrous thyroid gland, and is therefore restricted also to certain goitre regions.

Chapter 5
Course and Clinical Pattern of Cretinism

We can obtain an overview of the course of cretinism and its clinical appearance only if we keep its two main anatomical and clinical forms separate – *cretinism without goitre* and *cretinism with goitre*. Admittedly, as will be seen in the section on pathological anatomy, the borderline is not sharply defined. For instance, in cretins with early atrophy of the thyroid gland we often find anatomically tiny goitrous nodules that do not attract attention clinically, and, at most, can be palpated only during more detailed examination. In addition, it can happen that early atrophy of the gland's parenchyma is connected with the development of even bigger isolated nodules. The case must then be assigned anatomically to cretinism with goitre, in spite of its developmental path being that of a cretin without goitre. Such nodules can be intrathoracic and detectable only by x-ray (the case in Fig. 23). Finally, the not uncommon transitions in the clinical picture demonstrate that no sharp border can be drawn temporally and anatomically between early and late atrophy of the thyroid gland. Clinically then, we lock onto *early atrophy* when, irrespective of the type of intellectual defect, the delay of body growth stands out, and we assume *late atrophy* when physical development shows a fairly normal tempo during the initial years of schooling. You could object that this is an *a priori* assumption, but in actual fact it is confirmed by the histological findings in the gland.

The observation that there are cretins *without* goitre and some *with* goitre had already been made at a time when the connections between cretinism and the thyroid gland were not so clearly exposed as they are today. In this respect, the absence of goitre was a mystery for those researchers for, based on the general observation of the connection with the goitre malady, one had to assume, while not knowing, how one might explain the absence of goitre in the most severe cases of cretinism. The meticulous observer Maffei in particular came up against this. In spite of wanting to separate the two of them, his statements mention goitre and cretinism in one breath. Rösch, who avoided speculative thoughts as much as possible and kept to objective observation, came so close to the correct explanation almost 100 years ago that we will quote his statement. He says

J. Dennison et al., *Endemic Cretinism*,
DOI 10.1007/978-1-4614-0281-7_5,

> Furthermore, even though it is true that not all cretins have a goitre and, as I have observed, that often cretins of the highest level, the very image of cretinism, are not afflicted with goitre as well, it is nevertheless true that most cretins present a more or less substantial goitre, and that with children who subsequently become cretins the goitre is frequently congenital. Therefore we cannot be wrong if we designate endemic goitre (called 'Alpine goitre' by Troxler), to be the first sign of cretinous degeneration not only in general, but even among particularly ravaged individuals as a major evil belonging to cretinism – the first link in the chain of degrees and forms of cretinism...... mothers, midwives, and physicians have recounted many examples of children who have brought sizeable swellings into the world. Such children frequently die early. If they survive, then usually the swelling disappears quickly but the children develop poorly and almost always decline into cretinous degeneration.

Fodéré said the same thing in 1801:

> Most children destined to become cretins are born with a small goitre the size of a nut. Those who do not have goitre nevertheless bear the characteristics that show that they will enter that class.

Conversely, we come across investigators who adhere to the schematic, textbook description of dwarf myxœdematous cretins with the retracted root of the nose – the not uncommonly normal or almost normal adult cases of goitrous cretins, whom you might popularly call goitrous oafs – and those investigators create a unique category for them: thyrogenic simpletons or idiots. We will see later that simplification does not support such a subdividing – it is superfluous.

Cretins with goitre dominated most of the earlier statistics and this is still true today. Statistics from institutions give a relatively practical overview, bringing together a large amount of data on cretins. It reveals that in the Berne canton substantially two thirds of the cretins are afflicted with a clearly identifiable goitre.

Furthermore, in the first half of the last century, cretins were graded according to their *level of degeneration*, and their level of intellectual competence and practical versatility were used as criteria rather than their physical condition. We still use this classification as the most convenient, and present it as follows.

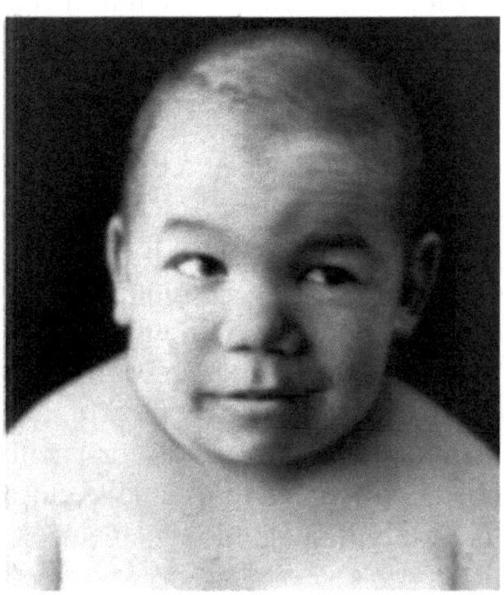

Fig. 11 A 12-year-old cretin without goitre (we note in this and later cases that the ages given in later references relate to the age-year in which the investigation was undertaken. This can give rise to considerable error since some cases have been under observation for 10 years or more); note the roguish glance

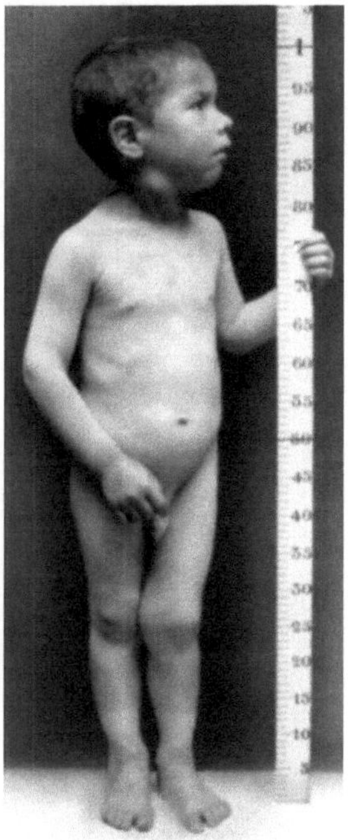

Fig. 12 Goitrous half-cretin, 5½ years old

The most severe *third* grade includes those cretins who are incapable of any task, who can neither speak nor appear to comprehend the spoken word, and whose whole existence is limited to being fed. Their intellectual life is near zero, and they would perish if human society did not keep them alive artificially. They are roughly at the same level as cases of thyroid deficiency, of congenital myxœdema whose compensatory glossal thyroid gland is quite recognizable, placing them somewhat higher than the most severe cases of congenital myxœdema, who normally die before puberty. Also, among those third-grade cretins incapable of performing tasks, closer examination often reveals a spark of intellectual life: a good memory for people and expressions of appreciative recollection of material pleasures.

Ranged in the *second grade* are cases of those who are incapable of independent activity but are able to carry out certain simple tasks in the fields or around the house under close supervision, and have the capacity for achieving an understanding of their surroundings, in a primitive manner.

Cases of the *first grade* are capable of reading and writing; learning lighter manual skills and becoming to some extent independent in life.

Such cretins also marry, be it among themselves or with normal partners, and are capable of producing offspring.

The frequently used designations of full-cretin for the third, half-cretin for the second, and cretinous or cretinoid condition for the first grade seem less advisable since they are more easily subjected to arbitrary amendments than the more schematic classification into grades, particularly where the first grade is concerned.

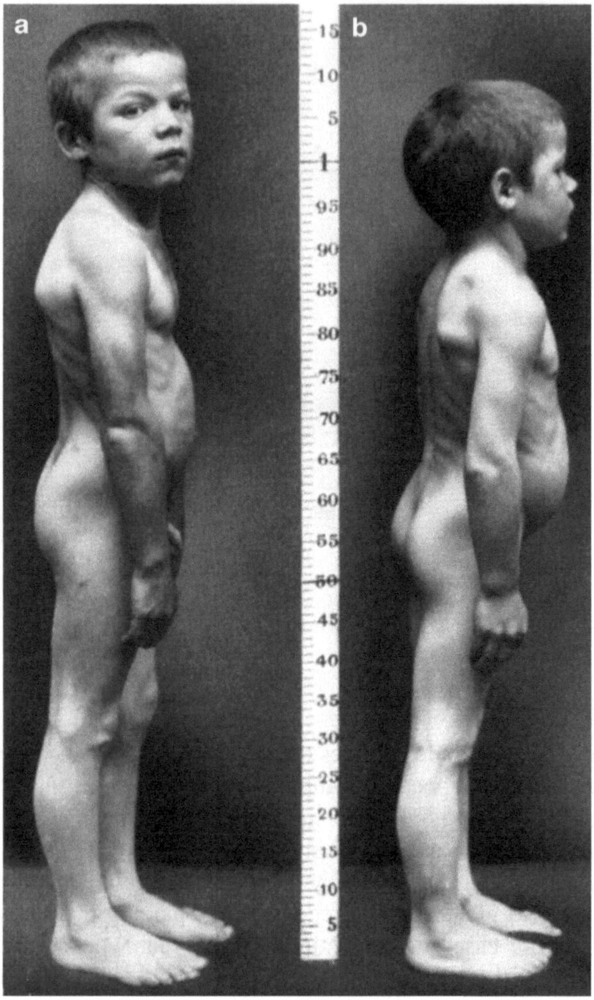

Fig. 13 Two cretins without goitre, 11 and 9 years old

Between these three grades there are fluid transitions according to intellect. The picture becomes even more complex when we take into consideration the presence or absence of goitre and other physical attributes as well.

In actual fact, we find cretins of all three grades in both the goitre-free and the goitrous types. The most we can say is that in the goitre-free type with early atrophy of the thyroid gland the *physical* attributes are more evident, while from the point of view of their *intellectual* capacity we not uncommonly also find first-grade cases among them. Thus in reality there are no 'standard cretins' and we entirely agree with Maffei when he says

> I cannot let it pass without comment that among several physicians there seems to be an opinion that there is a prototype of cretinous body form and, sadly, in so many writings we encounter the popularity of this view. It is the outcome of a lack of practical experience, amidst flourishing fantasy.

If we follow the *development of a cretin from birth*, we generally find that during the first year of life, before the child has teeth and begins to walk and talk, nothing in particular is noticed, such as an occasional neonatal goitre. Cases where a diagnosis can be made in 2- to 3-month-old infants, as Wagner and Diviak assume, might, in their opinion, be rare exceptions. We can accept Fodéré's 'congenital cretinism' only in a pathological sense, not in a clinical sense. From our own observations, where cases can be diagnosed very early we are usually dealing with congenital hypothyroidism, not with endemic cretinism. Often, even during the breastfeeding period, there is a striking loss of interest in their surroundings, compared with the behaviour of a normal child, and sluggishness of movement. During the second year of life, the signs become more pronounced: dental development is delayed and often irregular, and what stands out to the parents is that their child does not learn either to speak or to walk. Of course both of these disorders are still not diagnostic for cretinism, since they also occur in primary cerebral deficiency and mongoloid idiocy. More indicative on the other hand is the frequent occurrence of physical growth retardation and increasing bloat from a type of myxœdema.

In the fourth year of life, in view of the seldom-absent goitrous illness of the mother and the affiliation with a cretin region, the diagnosis cannot be mistaken any longer. In severe cases, their fate is already sealed before school age.

Their gait is arduous, and they have possibly learned to speak several words; however, school education is out of the question. Their neck is not only straight but we can palpate the trachea abnormally easily in spite of the myxœdema – a sign of thyroid atrophy. From all of this, but more particularly from the loss of interest and the muscular lethargy, the child can be distinguished from the restless mongoloid idiot in 'perpetual motion'. Much rather, the child resembles a case of non-cretinous myxœdema, but in this case the myxœdema is usually pronounced; we could say the brutishness is of a higher level were we not doing a disservice to the animal. Pronounced macroglossia indicates non-cretinous thyroaplasia.

Maffei is quite correct about the onset of the first signs:

> I did not find any child that I would dare recognize and declare with any certainty as a cretin before the usual period of dental work; nor did I find any who, having completed the fourth year of life, had only just begun to become a cretin. I feel that I can assume that congenital cretinism certainly does not develop after the fourth year of life.

Somewhat later than in the goitre-free cretins, usually during school age, is the fate of the *goitrous* cretins decided, at least externally. Goitre makes a definite appearance in the early years of their school life. They seem to have a certain level of developmental ability, but often they must be given up after the very first year of schooling as hopeless. In other instances, educational efforts do succeed in getting some of the children to read, write, and even do arithmetic. However, the cretins that do go on usually stay in their classes and are discarded after a few years if no remedial attempt is made in a special class for the weakly endowed. There, possibly,

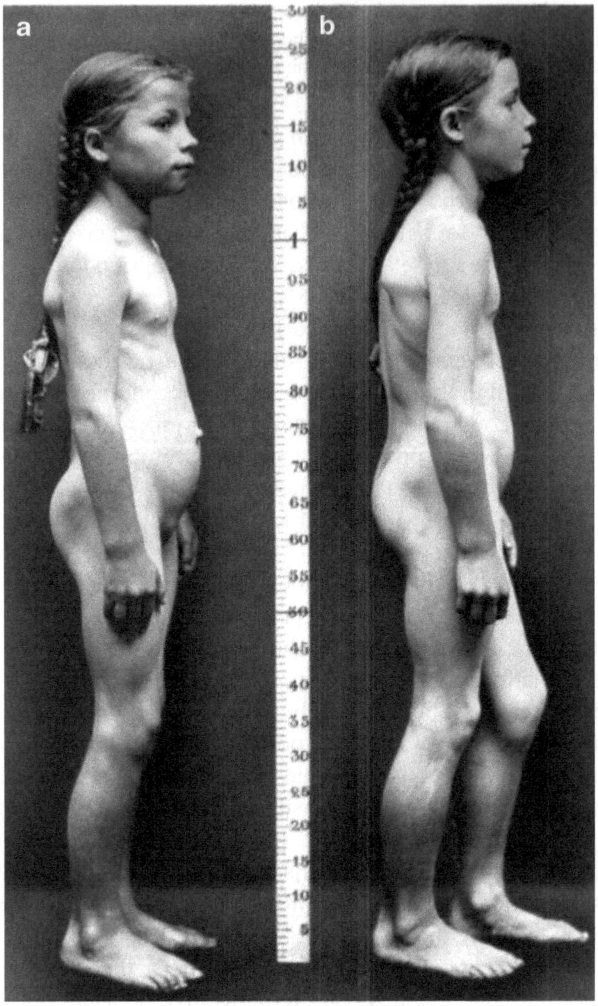

Fig.14 Two half-cretins with goitre, 13 and 12 years old, sisters of the two preceding cases

something can be salvaged from the brain that was probably already deficiently developed while still *in utero*. However, this facility is not normally available until the end of the primary school stage.

In a few severe cases, primary school is finally completed successfully, with 2–3 repeat years; likewise the usual religious instruction, for which the cretin as, even though partially, a spiritual person, shows more interest than for the arithmetic lesson.

Meanwhile the goitre, if appropriate treatment is not carried out, has continued to grow and, not uncommonly, tracheal compression requires surgical intervention, even at this early stage. Rösch says

Fig. 15 Mongoloid, feeble-minded, 9 years old

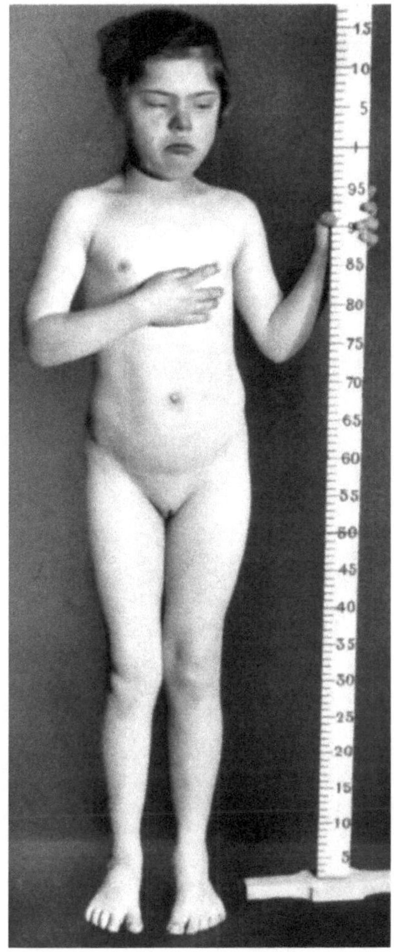

In villages and houses where cretinism was present I often saw children of 10–14 years old with distinct, hard goitres the size of a hen's egg, and these children always had a leucophlegmatic, cachectic appearance; they were physically and mentally sluggish, and close to degeneration or actually already there.

We had left the non-goitrous cretin at the school gate; let's go back to him! He remains a dwarf among his siblings and school mates, and indeed he is, as a rule, a 'cheerful fellow' compared with the taller, goitrous cretins. His mental capabilities are not always level with his growth and, not uncommonly, he is capable of acquiring the simplest elements of school education. Again, at times he demonstrates an originality that is usually lacking in the goitrous cretin. He presents a less 'feeble-minded' impression than his goitrous fellow-sufferer, for whom we acknowledge the accuracy of the later description 'thyrogenic idiot' or 'goitrous imbecile'.

Fig. 16 Chondrodystrophy, 8 years old

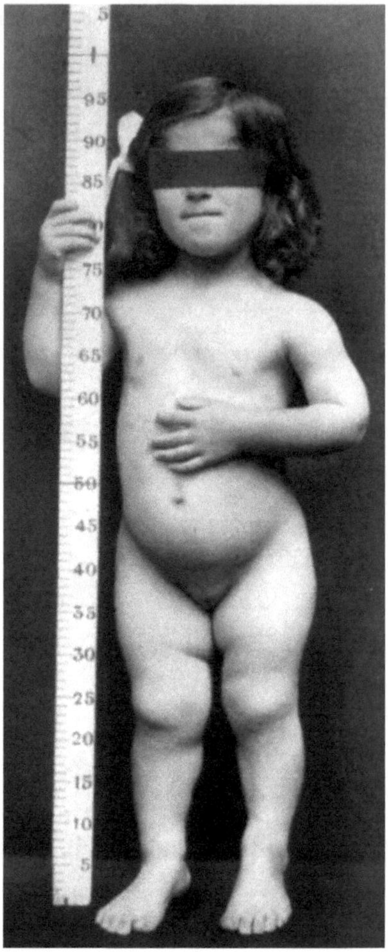

From time to time *deafness* provides a considerable obstacle to school education. This can also be at a high degree with quite a reasonable intelligence. Often, only raising them in a deaf-and-dumb institution is successful in bringing out what has lain dormant inside them, and making them worthwhile.

When the young cretin has left school, he quickly shows whether he can enter employment as a farm labourer with a farmer, or whether he can learn a less physical and more intellectual manual skill, or whether he has to be placed immediately in an institution. Generally, fewer physical demands can be made on the dwarf cretins than on a taller, goitrous cretin. The former settles more on a door-to-door salesman occupation, which he pursues with the greatest possible love but also with his unique local knowledge and even with a pronounced business sense.

The *puberty period* impinges neither on one type nor on another type, and neither on one sex nor the other, nor on their emotional life. Maffei says in this regard, 'That which we call youth, the springtime of life in other men, is virtually non-existent for

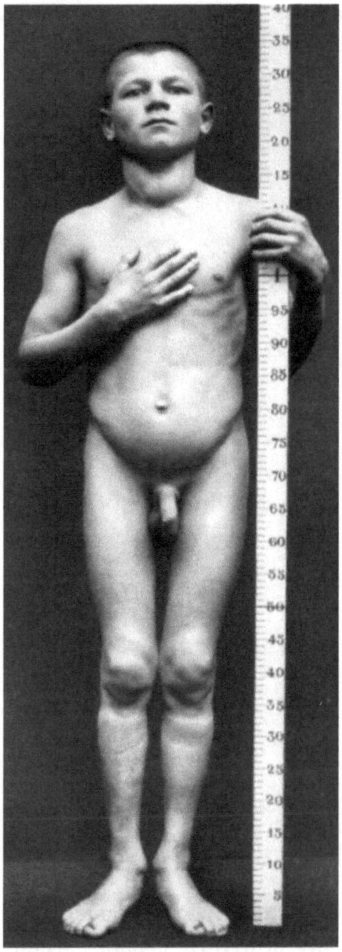

Fig. 17 Goitrous cretin, 16 years old (so-called thyrogenic feeble-minded)

the cretin. From the long-lasting boyhood he passes over directly into manhood. The fully-cretinous girl follows the self-same cycle – never flowers, never withers.'

In dwarf cretins, males especially, the secondary sexual characteristics are more or less strongly retarded and, as we shall see later, he never ever experiences the period of maturity. The same is true of the females, at best with the exception of the occasionally almost-normal development of the breasts. In the case of the goitrous cretin, pubertal development is completed in a normal manner, at least gross-anatomically, but here too without deeper repercussions on the personality. The unfettered development of sexuality, from time to time observed particularly among non-cretinous male *idiots*, is absent among cretins, and masturbation, in contrast to earlier claims (Fodéré), refuted incidentally by Maffei, is extremely rare.

Once the cretin's generally-achievable physical and mental level is attained, albeit more slowly, the rest of his life follows a peaceful pattern of fulfilment. He

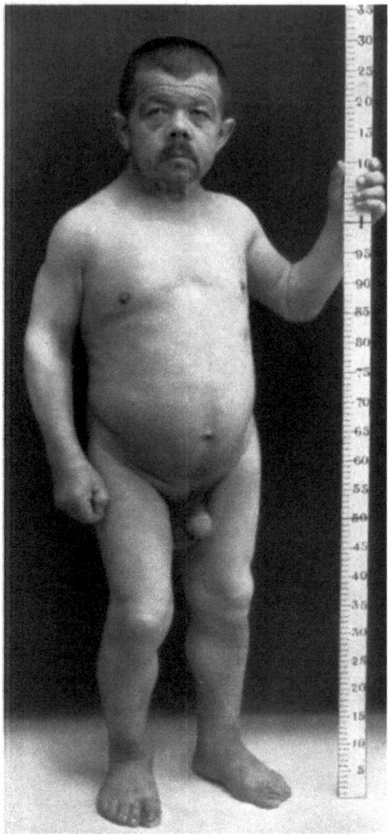

Fig. 18 Cretin without goitre, 53 years old ('House cretin' of the Berne surgical clinic)

stays the same for years and, without having ever looked youthful, he seems to age only slowly. He is happy when he finds himself with a minimum of work (although he can also muddle through life's requirements), or when he (if incapable) finds food, rest, and a modest fulfilment of his smoking needs in an institution.

Sheltered from the vicissitudes of life, he not uncommonly reaches advanced years in such institutions, and he is apparently not stricken with any more severe form of illness than are his fellow inmates who have healthy thyroids. According to a survey among our five biggest institutions, a large proportion of cretins achieve a relatively good age under the favourable conditions within the institution. In the Bärau Institute, for example, the average age of the 12 cretins who died between 1929 and 1933 was 70.6 years.

Ten of them were 68 and over. According to the physicians in the institutions, the main causes of death were decrepitude, failure of the circulatory system, and, in *one* institution, tuberculosis; malignant tumours were the rarest illness.

A distinct *exacerbation of the appearances of cretinism* is generally no longer observable beyond the developmental years. We could even say that the fate of most average cretins is determined much earlier – for some at the time of birth; for others

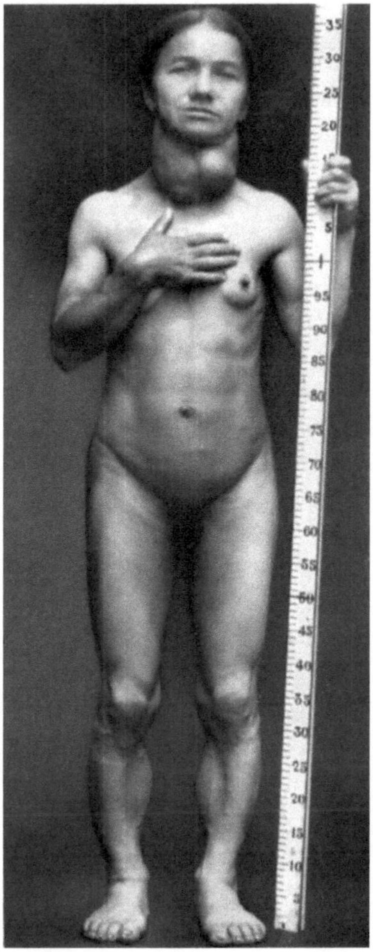

Fig. 19 Goitrous cretin (thyrogenic feeble-minded), 44 years old

during the first years of school. This does not rule out the occasional inflammatory lesion of the thyroid gland leading to rapid deterioration in the thyroideal symptoms.

We observed this in a dwarf cretin *inter alia*, based on the precise details of an elder sister. Like his dwarf-cretin brother he was able to speak to some extent, before beginning school, but then with scarlet fever involvement he lost this ability and became totally incapacitated, while his brother, in spite of his cretinism, worked himself up to the position of an institutional gardener.

We would be sceptical of information on *spontaneous improvement* of cretinous symptoms. This would apply equally to the functioning of a thyroid gland damaged in its earliest conception and to events that, with some degree of probability, we would have to attribute to an extrathyroidal source. At most one could imagine that a change of environment, for instance from the mountains to the sea early in life,

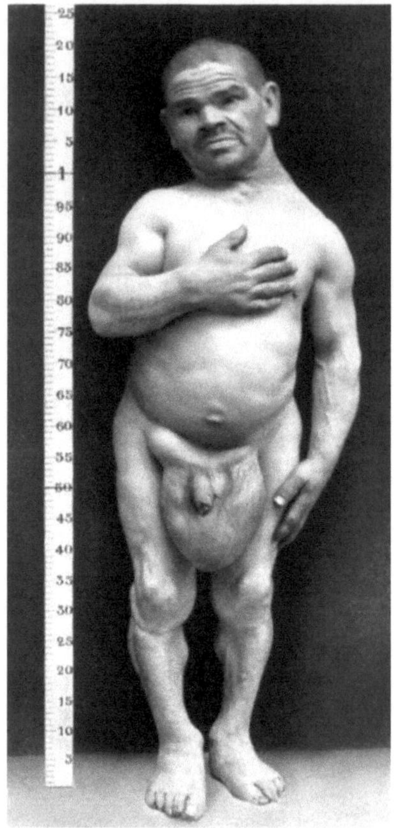

Fig. 20 Cretin with multiple hernias, 52 years old

might salvage something of the thyroid gland and its function. On the other hand, we have to remember that much can be retrieved for an individual through upbringing that cannot be reckoned in a clinical sense as an improvement in his condition. Furthermore, the intellectual development of cretins proceeds so slowly that certain advances that we might tend to include as 'improvement' are actually in line with natural development. By way of exception, a thyroid gland apparently condemned at the start of the school years to atrophy can, subsequently, mature while remaining goitrous, and can influence skeletal growth more favourably than expected. Had Dr Guggenbühl been more familiar with the diagnosis and prognosis of cretinism, he might not have engaged in the unfortunate paedagogical experiment on the Abendberg near Interlaken.

Comparative findings made in 1833 by school medical officers of the Berne canton on 30,000 school children entering the fourth, fifth, and ninth years are significant for the evaluation of the *influence of endemic goitre in children.* This survey was undertaken at the instigation of Dr Lauener, the school physician. The summary of results is subdivided into goitrous regions of the Bernese Oberland, the Central Plateau and the lesser-afflicted Jura (though the latter is not entirely goitre-free). We will come back to the results of these statistics in the individual sections of this chapter. In summary though we can point out that for hearing and speech distur-

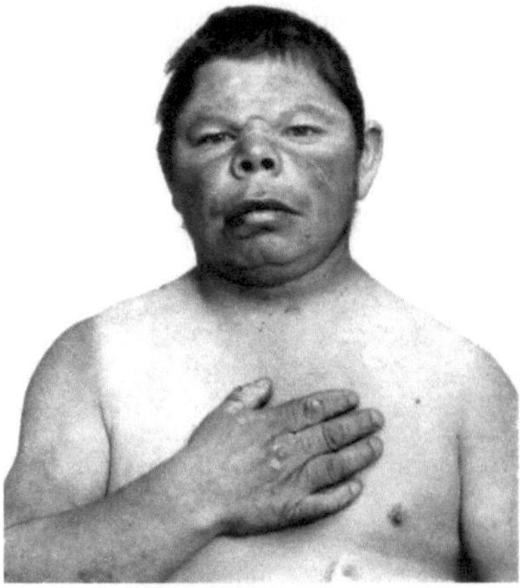

Fig. 21 Cretin without goitre, 32 years old

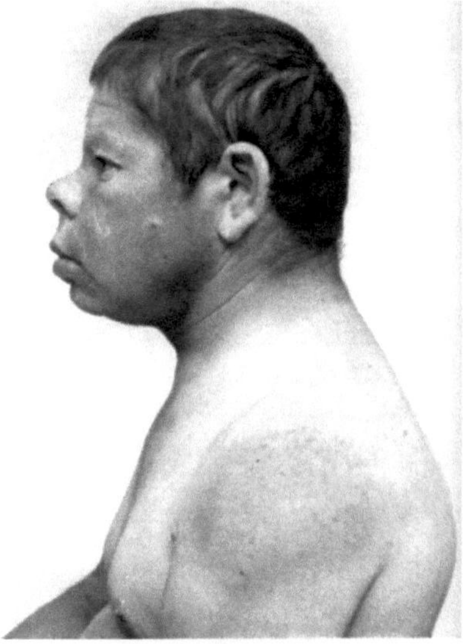

Fig. 22 The same individual

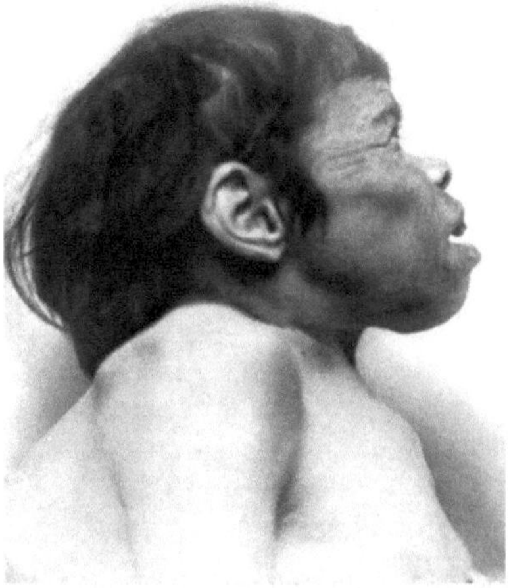

Fig. 23 Dwarf cretin with small intrathoracic goitre in addition to high-grade atrophy of the body of the gland; simian features

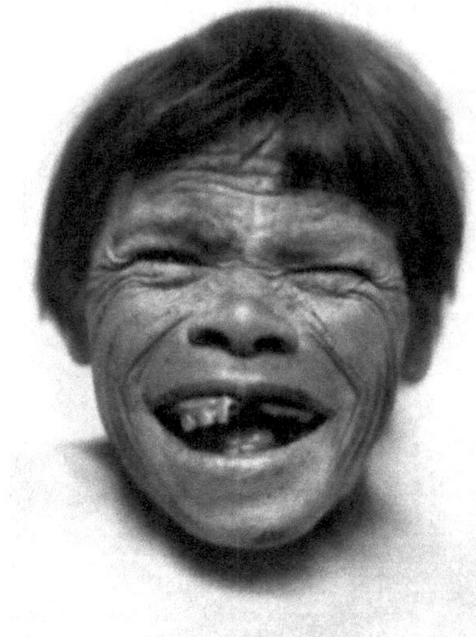

Fig. 24 The same individual

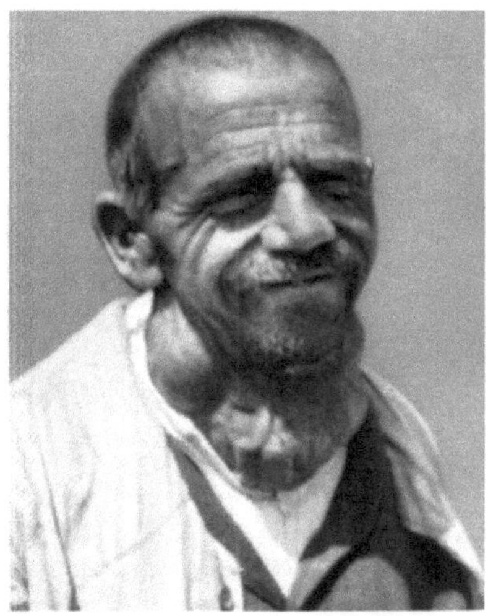

Fig. 25 Goitrous cretin

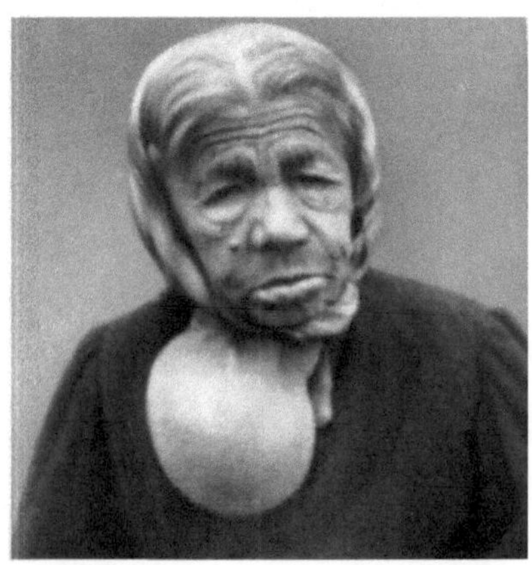

Fig. 26 Cretin with pendulous goitre

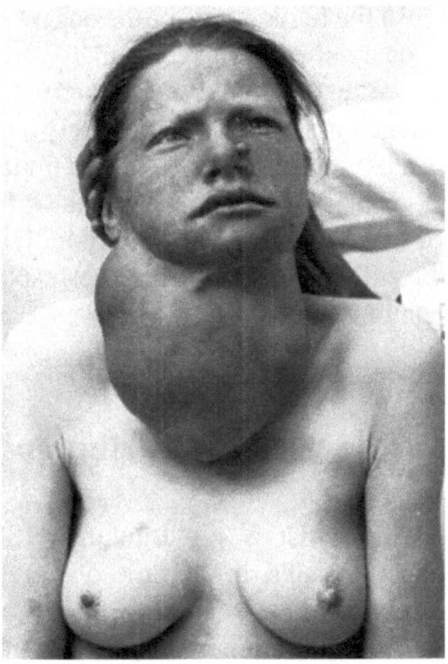

Fig. 27 Grade 3 cretin, 32 years old; *Struma nodosa parenchymatosa et colloides* (from Wydler, Case 53)

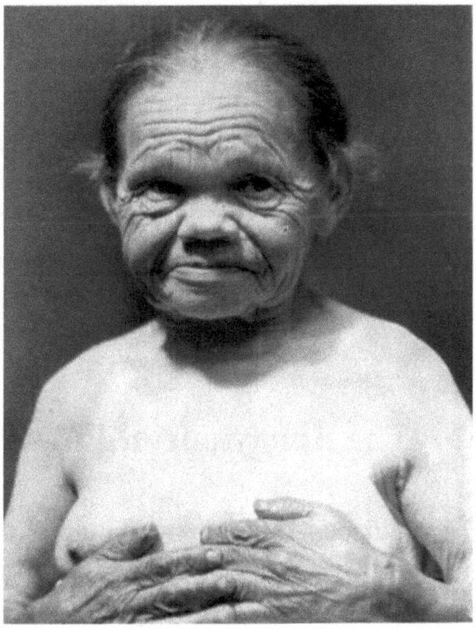

Fig. 28 Dwarf cretin without goitre, 69 years old

bances, adenoid proliferations, cardiac disorders, hernias, and intellectual debility, goitre-free Jura is two to three times more favourable than the goitrous regions of the canton. On the other hand, there is no difference in the comparative values for general bodily weakness, visual disorders, dental caries, general posture, or pulmonary diseases. Thus during school age in the Oberland and the Central Plateau, within the goitrous region, the incidence of pronounced goitre climbs from 16% and 13.6% respectively to 25.3% and 25.6%; and in the Jura from 2.3% to 12.4%. By comparison it is mentioned that barely 1% of cases of induced goitre are observed in the Jura, whereas on average 15% of cases occur in the rest of the cantons.

In the border zone of the endemic region, goitre has a tendency to regress spontaneously after the age of puberty. Berne school statistics provide overwhelming evidence that endemic thyrotoxicity acts also through physical disorders that are not directly attributable to it, namely adenoid growth, heart disease, and hernias. We will discuss the significance of this finding in greater detail in the chapter on pathology.

Following this brief overview of the developmental process in cretins, we will go on to discuss the behaviour of individual organs and organ systems. For many details we will also refer to the corresponding sections in the chapter on pathological anatomy.

1 The Sexual Distribution of Cretinism

Earlier statistics (e.g. Baillarger 1873; Austrian Statistics 1906) show a preponderance of males, in the ratio of roughly 10:7, in both France and Austria. However, idiots were included also, in France at least. Were only the goitrous cretins taken into consideration in France, then the sex ratio would be approximately 1:1. Statistics from a single, meticulous investigator would be more reliable if they did not suffer from the error of small sample sizes. In 123 cases Flinker found a sex ratio of 4:3; Scholz (106 cases) a ratio of about 2:3; Wydler (in our sample of 118 cases) likewise 2:3. A census that we undertook recently in three cretin institutions (107 cases) produced a ratio of almost 1:2.

If you consider that in the middle of a severely endemic region the goitre ratio is 1:1 from school age on, then a similar ratio might be expected for cretinism as well and, in fact, this is the case. The desire to draw any kind of conclusions from variations is unjustified so long as the numerical size does not match 'chance occurrences' in the data summary, but does allow a uniform evaluation of cases.

2 The Behaviour of Physical Development

In the discussion of growth behaviour the necessity of keeping both outlined groups, the *goitrous* and *non-goitrous* cretins, separate has already arisen.

From observations on pure athyroid patients, we know that the more complete the breakdown of thyroid gland function, the greater is the retardation in growth. Should cretinous damage of the thyroid gland proceed as far as total abolition of function, then, irrespective of other pathogenic components in the cretin, we would have the image of the athyroid individual with his adult stature of around 90–100 cm, and severe retardation in the formation of his centres of ossification. The thyroprival nature of this retardation becomes evident from the influence of thyroxin treatment.

In one case of hypothyroidism that we published, after just 4 months of thyroxin administration, development of the hand skeleton went from the level of a 4-year-old to that of a 7-year-old.

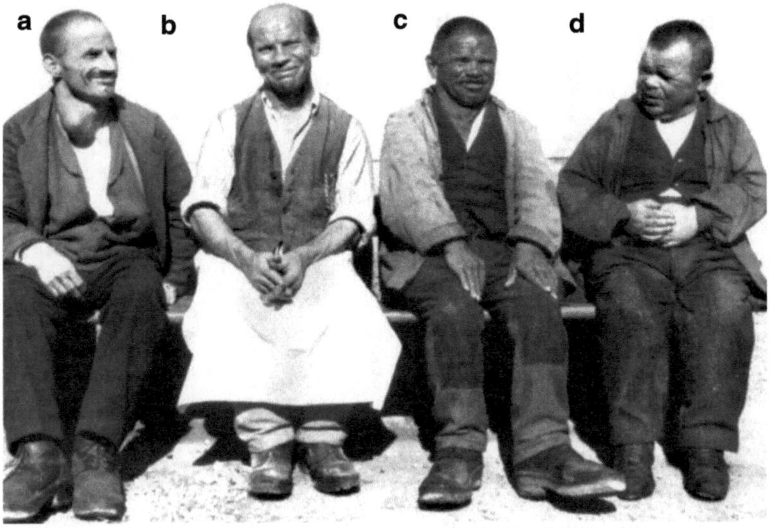

Fig. 29 Group of cretins: (**a–c**) goitrous; (**d**) without goitre (Riggisberg Institution)

The greater the availability of functioning thyroid tissue to the cretin up until the end of his growing years, the more his skeletal development and body proportions will approach those of a normal human. What has not been satisfactorily considered in skeletal investigations of cretins thus far is that there is no typical cretin skeleton, but well-nigh all levels occur – from the athyroid skeletal type right up to the normal skeletal type. We say 'well-nigh' because the small, omnipresent remnant of the gland must cause certain variations among cretins. The material in anatomical collections comes mainly from the skeletons of dwarf cretins – cases where we find precocious anatomical atrophy of the thyroid gland. Until now, bigger cretins, being of less interest, were not incorporated in collections. Anatomical examinations of the material are thus inevitably biased.

This is true particularly of the intrinsically meticulous measurements by Finkbeiner, whose Bernese material comprised exclusively dwarf cretins. He describes them as 'thoroughbred cretins', a term for which he certainly cannot set any clinical bounds. He ascribes open epiphyses to atrophy of the thyroid gland; whatever in his opinion does not conform with the bony structure of athyroid patients, he regards as primitive features that might connect these people on the one hand with certain polar people and on the other hand with Neolithic pygmies and indirectly with the fossil Neandertal group. In spite of a lack of evidence, if we assume also that Finkbeiner's athyroid comparative skeleton from Graz is actually that of an athyroid (as seems likely), then the differences between the cretin skeleton and this athyroid skeleton are also understandable, without having to fall back on pygmies and the temporally-distant Neandertals.

After all, the cretin is not a pure athyroid. His thyroid gland still performs to some extent in the most important period of life for the skeleton, and his bone

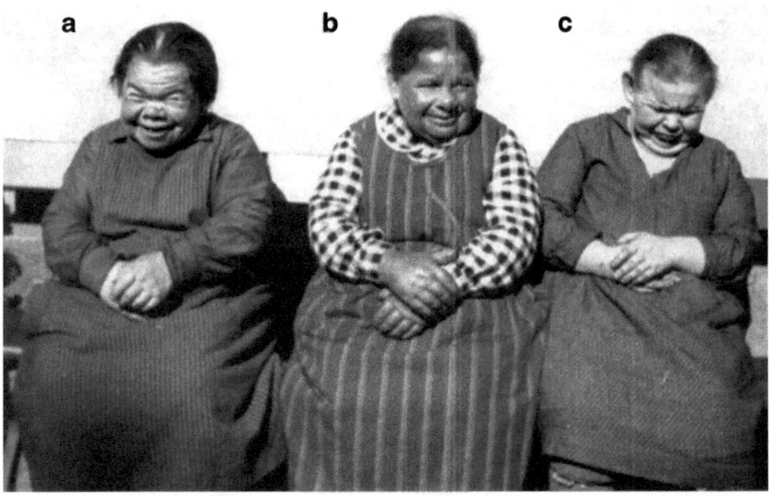

Fig. 30 Group of cretins without goitre (Riggisberg Institution)

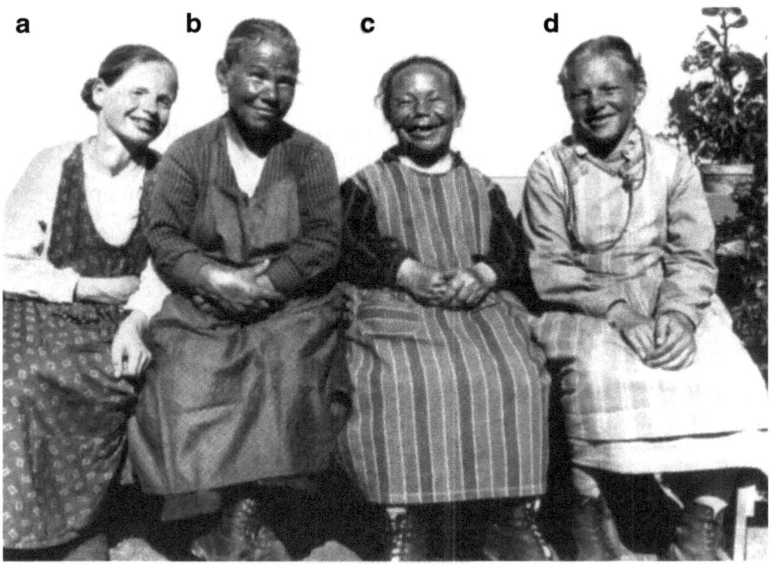

Fig. 31 Group of goitrous cretins (Riggisberg Institution)

formation will therefore not present the pronounced early childhood or neonatal characteristics of the athyroid skeleton. That Neolithic pygmies and the 10,000-years-older Neandertals can be mentioned by Finkbeiner in the same breath might, on the other hand, raise a few murmurs among the prehistorians.

What is said for the bone forms examined in isolation by Finkbeiner must also be said of skeletal proportions in general. To some extent this allows the proposal of a

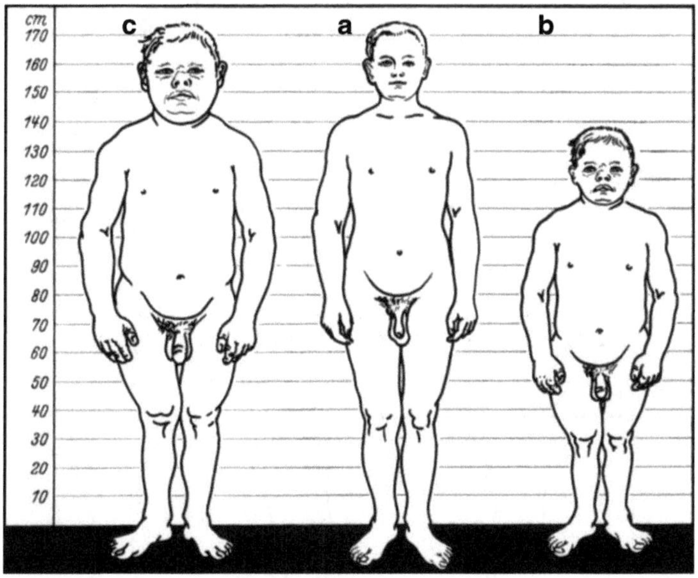

Fig. 32 Bodily proportions of a cretin without goitre: (**a**) normal 32-year-old male; (**b**) cretin of the same age; (**c**) the same individual scaled to the size of the normal male – head abnormally large, trunk abnormally long, lower limbs abnormally short

'dwarf cretin type' but not, in short, a cretinism 'type'. Figures 32 and 33 demonstrate well enough what we mean.

Among the factors determining body growth are not only the age of the individual and the effectiveness of the thyroid gland, but also the rate at which the skeleton develops, independently of the thyroid gland. We might theoretically expect that this is the same in all people of the same sex and the same 'race'. A glance at the differing body sizes of people with healthy thyroids under the same external conditions demonstrates, however, that this is not the case, and that the growth type in individuals is still dependent on factors that have nothing to do with thyroid glands and cretinism.

Putting aside these unknown factors, we note that cretins without goitre but with major growth disorders are found generally in the centre of the endemic region, while the taller, goitrous cretins are more frequently encountered towards the periphery – an observation that does not rule out numerous exceptions.

Wydler's compilation from our clinic (Table 1) demonstrates that about a quarter of our cretins are normal, average size, while the remaining three quarters show growth retardation, and about 7% are genuinely dwarfs.

In actual fact, this material gives exaggerated stature values, since the majority of these cretins came to the clinic for goitre surgery, so that their statures were above the real average for cretin size. All non-goitrous cretins presented dwarf stature. The *macrogoitrous* cretins exhibited generally greater body length than the *microgoitrous*. (Table 2) from Wydler shows this clearly.

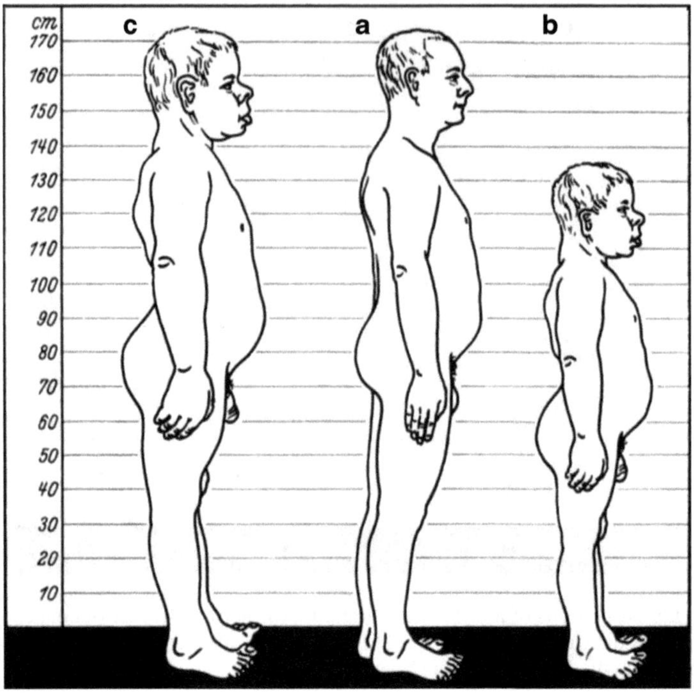

Fig. 33 The same, in profile

Table 1

	Body length (cm)						
Age (years)	110–120	121–130	131–140	141–150	151–160	161–170	171–180
1–5	–	–	–	–	–	–	–
6–15	3	1	2	3	–	–	–
16–30	–	–	3	9	8	3	–
31–40	–	1	–	8	6	5	1
41–50	–	–	1	7	6	9	1
51–60	–	–	1	4	4	–	1
61–70	–	–	–	2	2	1	–
71–80	–	–	–	2	1	–	–

Of 18 cretins with relatively minor goitre (40–150 g), 16 are abnormally small and only two attain average or normal size. In contrast, we find two dwarf cretins with large goitres of 200–300 g and 400–600 g; 23 cases abnormally small, large goitres notwithstanding; and 42 cases attaining average and, occasionally, normal body height. Dwarf cretins with large goitres are encountered only rarely, and macrogoitrous cretins generally attain greater body length than microgoitrous cretins. Thus there is a well-known inverse causal relationship between body length and goitre mass.

Table 2

Body length (cm)	Gram weight of the gland, estimated after removal, and remnant tissue						
	40–100	101–150	151–200	201–300	301–400	401–500	501–600
121–130	–	–	–	1	–	–	–
131–140	5	–	–	–	–	1	–
141–150	5	6	10	6	5	1	1
151–160	–	1	11	7	7	3	–
161–170	–	1	3	9	3	1	2
171–180	–	–	–	1	–	1	–

From Hirschfelder's examination of our material comes a numerical presentation of skeletal development – the *development quotient*: the age corresponding with the skeletal development divided by the chronological age. Athyroids show a developmental limit of 80–90%, i.e., a quotient of 0.8–0.9 evaluated from wrist and knee joints.

In juvenile non-goitrous cretins (dwarf cretins), the quotient comes to about 0.5; and in juvenile cretins with goitre, about 0.25. In other words, dwarf cretins are underdeveloped by about half their age; goitrous cretins by about a quarter of their age.

As E. Bircher and von Wyss have already observed, development of the epiphyseal ossification centres is not inhibited equally throughout the skeleton. For example, inhibition in the hand region increases from the forearm peripherally. In contrast, we find the hip joint quite markedly inhibited. This unequal influence of the various skeletal parts leads to disproportionate growth in dwarfs, whereas the growth disruptions among athyroids are said to be proportionate. Admittedly, this latter assertion applies only with certain limitations.

As a general observation it must be added that delay in the formation of centres of ossification and in the ends of cartilaginous joints is still not synonymous *a priori* with delay in longitudinal growth and, conversely, normal appearance of the centres and normal closure of cartilaginous joints do not guarantee normal lengthwise growth. That last statement is substantiated by those forms of non-endocrine dwarfism or small stature where even premature closure of cartilaginous joints can occur alongside (hereditary) small stature.

2.1 *The Individual Parts of the Skeleton*

2.1.1 Skull Behaviour

While the majority of the cretins closely examined so far are generally recognized to be *brachycephalic*, this is due in part to their coming from alpine lands, where the brachycephalic type is, by far, predominant. Therefore, cretinoid disturbances in growth themselves tend towards brachycephaly. It is well known that brachycephaly is not based on premature ossification of the cranial base, as Virchow wrongly assumed; this has been demonstrated both by Langhans and by Wegelin

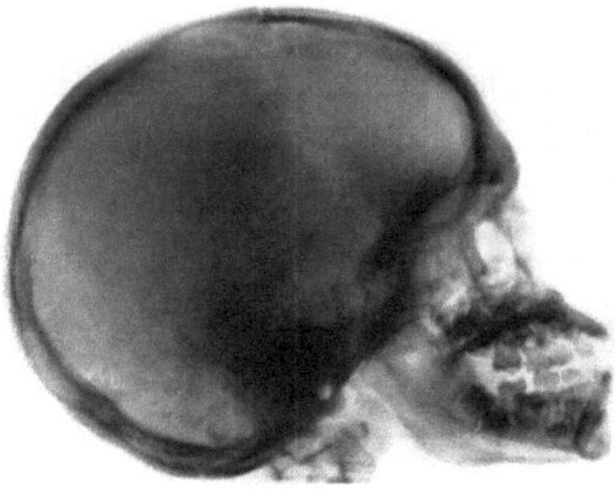

Fig. 34 Thyroaplasia, 17 years old. Case from Fig. 118

(Stoccada). Corresponding with the other skeletal anomalies, however, there is a *delay* in ossification of the cranial base, with reduced activity of the remaining, abnormally lingering cartilaginous zones. This growth delay exceeds that of the cranial vault so that despite the relatively small brain, there develops a relative shortening of the cranial base with associated contraction of the root of the nose. The *calculated cranial capacity* is, on average, somewhat below normal, as all measurements so far show (Scholz; Finkbeiner), admittedly with a range including above-average values.

Finkbeiner found a male cretin mean of 1340 cc (1142–1647 cc); and a female mean of 1211 cc (1030–1440 cc). The reduction in cranial capacity diminishes in significance when, as Finkbeiner correctly suggests, we place it in proportion to the body size of the individual in question.

Another feature to be considered when estimating the cranial capacity of both cretins and athyroid people is the frequent occurrence of *Hydrocephalus internus*. Irrespective of the range, brain mass corresponds, generally within normal limits, with the calculated cranial capacity (Wegelin, see later).

There is no question of relating it to *microcephaly* or anything similar. Whoever sees a microcephalic individual alongside a cretin would hardly want to make such a connection.

It is obvious from what has been said so far that the most pronounced cranial changes – the most distinctive cretin type – occur among dwarf cretins, i.e., cretins with premature atrophy of the thyroid gland without goitre formation, and that here, therefore, the inherited characteristics of the individual are most greatly repressed by cretinism. The longer time the thyroid gland has had to influence skeletal growth, the stronger the familial and racial type manifests itself while the cretin type is blurred. Thus, even among goitrous third-grade cretins, while they present an otherwise virtually normal body growth, we also find a cranial form corresponding with the racial and family type of the person in question.

In the *facial skeleton* the prognathism among dwarf cretins is astonishing, helping to impart the 'monkey face', while in this aspect the fully grown cretin retains his familial appearance. We refer those who want to delve deeper into the cranial dimensions recorded so far to the studies by Scholz and by Finkbeiner.

From Mayrhofer's meticulous investigations, *tooth formation* reveals numerous structural anomalies, indicating early germ damage, and leading as a rule to major

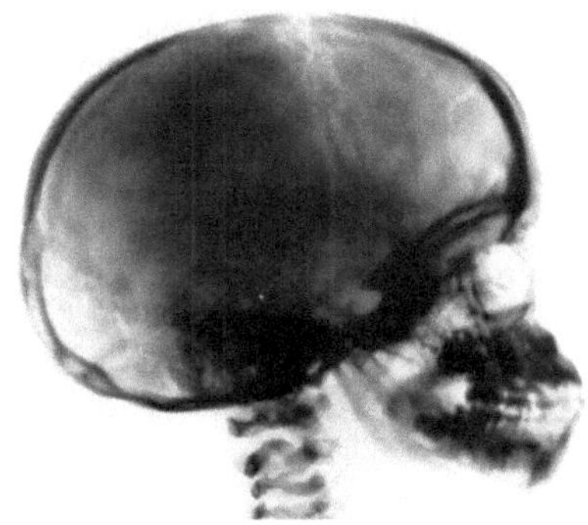

Fig. 35 A 12-year-old cretin without goitre. Case from Fig. 11

neglect of the dentition. On the other hand, the cretin does not appear to be more greatly affected by dental caries than his compatriots. At least there is no evidence to the contrary. Mayrhofer even talks of an often astonishing degree of caries immunity. Investigations in the Berne canton reveal that schools in low-goitre Jura show just as much dental caries as those in the goitrous region of the canton (Lauener). Parhon and Goldstein emphasize dentition delays; Scholz the relative frequency of positional anomalies. For further detail on dental relationships, see Eggenberger among others.

As for the *rest of the skeleton*, from the thicker appearance of the limbs earlier researchers were easily tempted to assume a robust bone structure as well. This is not always true, and radiology has demonstrated that a greater proportion of cretin skeletons belong to the gracile type, females especially. Using radiographs of hand and knee joints from our material, Hirschfelder found the following proportional values:

Skeleton of the hand		Skeleton of the knee	
1. Dwarf cretins without goitre (15 cases)			
Very stocky to moderate	46%	Very stocky to moderate	33%
Stocky to normal	20%	Stocky to normal	27%
Normal	7%	Normal	20%
Gracile	27%	Gracile	20%
2. Dwarf cretins with goitre (22 cases)			
Very stocky to moderate	4.5%	Very stocky to moderate	27%
Stocky to normal	50%	Stocky to normal	27%
Normal	36%	Normal	31.5%
Gracile	9%	Gracile	13.5%

Here females, as normal, reveal a tendency towards the gracile form. Thus, there is no strict parallel between hand and knee joints.

We refer readers to Finkbeiner's measurements for details on the limb bone dimensions, again emphasizing that these are significantly related to the dwarf type, and simply cannot be described as characteristic of cretinism.

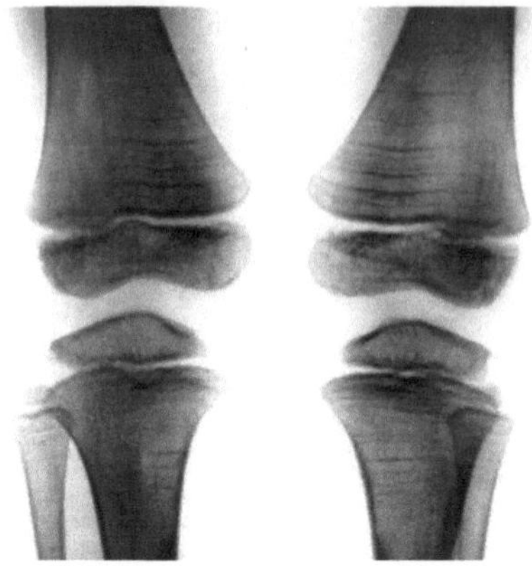

Fig. 36 Skeletal knee of a 9-year-old cretin without goitre, with well-defined trabeculation

The *delay in the appearance of the bony centres of ossification among dwarf cretins* is particularly striking in the limbs. The succession of their appearance is, however, normal (von Wyss, personal observation).

We often also find a certain delay in ossification among goitrous cretins too. However, the latter do approach the norm, to a certain extent, as is the case with stature.

From what is said, and Wieland emphasizes, comparison of the skeleton of the hand, particularly the wrist, with that of a normal individual of similar age, belongs among the essential diagnostic tests, though experience is needed in interpreting the result. Delay in the development of bony centres of ossification is indicative of thyroid insufficiency, but not yet with any certainty for endemic cretinism. On the other hand, by their appearance in goitrous cretins, normal centres of ossification are no proof of thyroid function being normal over the whole range.

Pronounced trabeculae in the structure of the metaphyses occur especially in the distal end of the femur and the proximal end of the tibia. We cannot consider them specific to hypothyroid conditions since, for example, they are found also in marble bone disease – certainly not an endocrine condition – and, conversely, in the majority of cretin skeletons they do not exceed the normal range, or else they are absent.

Of the *joints*, the hip is most commonly altered, and the most severely, even though in many cases, particularly in women, it may remain normal right into old age. Together with the carpus it shows the greatest delay in development of the centres of ossification. The femoral head centre of ossification is normally well developed even in the third year of life; in some instances among cretins we find only traces even in the 12th year.

In thyroaplasia the femoral proximal epiphysis shows a similar elective retardation. Sometimes, at a later stage of development, changes occurring in the proximal epiphysis are more reminiscent of *Osteochondritis dissecans*, and at other times, Perthes' *Osteochondritis deformans juvenilis*. The head retracts more and more in breadth, becomes flattened, and is often dented by a central groove; not uncommonly it also deviates posteriorly. The neck remains short. In later years, frequently into the fifth decade, the femoral head increasingly assumes the mushroom or sad-

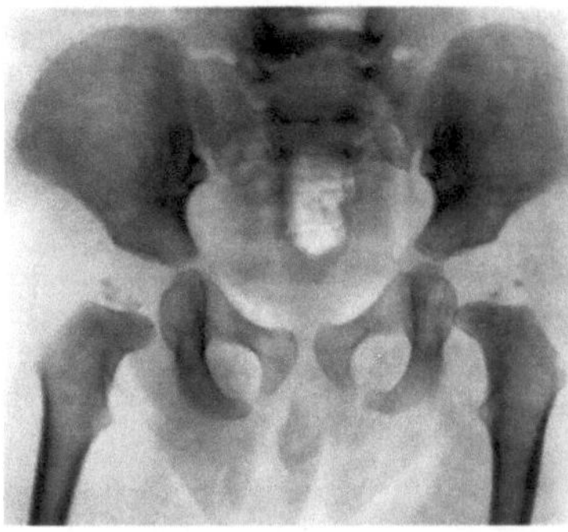

Fig. 37 Pelvis presenting thyroaplasia; 12-year-old boy. Case from Fig. 57b

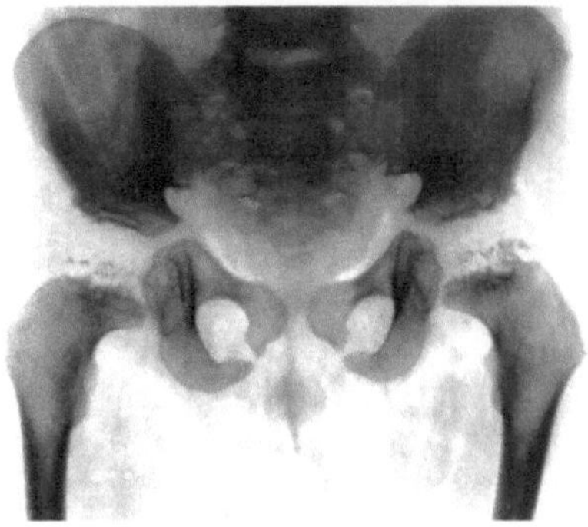

Fig. 38 Pelvis of a 12-year-old cretin without goitre. Case from Fig. 57a

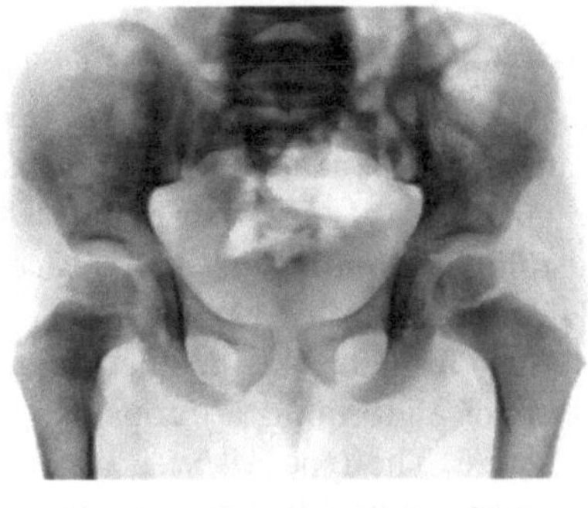

Fig. 39 Normal bony pelvis; 3 years old

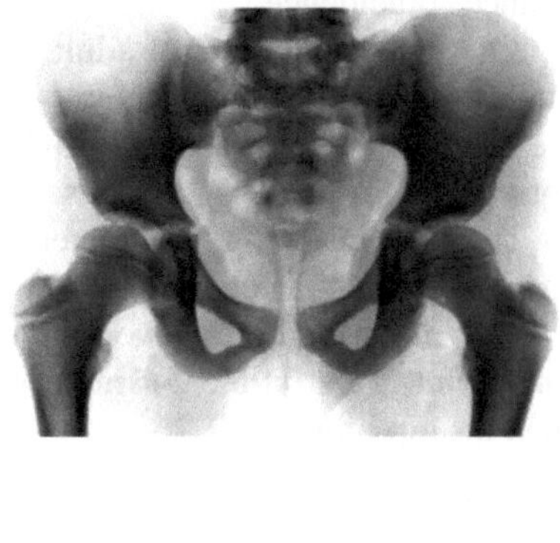

Fig. 40 Pelvis of a goitrous 13-year-old half-cretin. Case from Fig. 14a

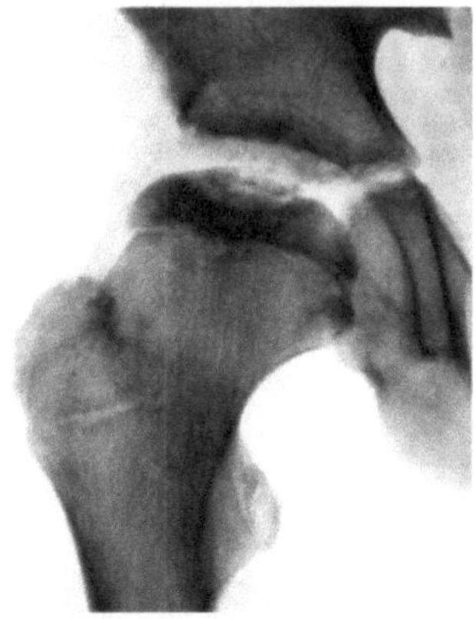

Fig. 41 Cretin hip resembling *Osteochondritis deformans juvenilis*; 16-year-old female cretin with mild goitre

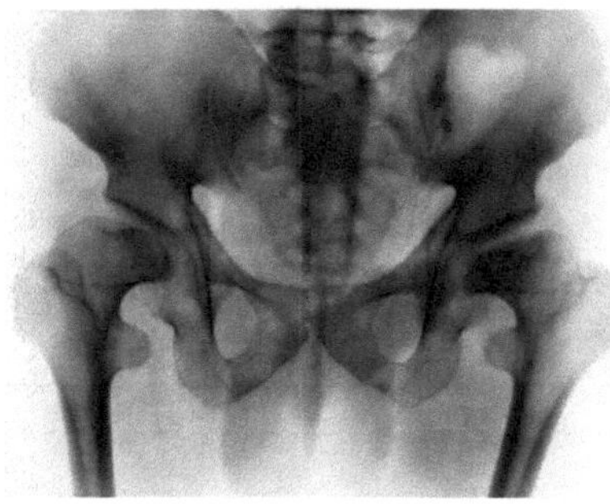

Fig. 42 Pelvis of a 38-year-old cretin without goitre

dle shape of deforming arthritis. The regions of the lesser and greater trochanters also show changes in shape, while in the acetabulum we find delay in ossification, flattening, and adaptation to the shape of the femoral head. The 'cretin hip' is distinguished, as Looser has emphasized, first by its progression but then through the histological finding of both *Osteochondritis deformans juvenilis* and the usual, deforming arthritis.

Seen from the outside, the later stages of cretinous arthropathy resemble those of common deforming arthropathy, with marked rim excrescences and joint body structure. The type *Arthritis sicca* with premature cartilage atrophy and moderate deformation may be observed exceptionally in radiographs, but rather seems to be a chance coincidence.

Among 34 hip joints of adult cretins (21 with goitre, 13 non-goitrous; 13 male and 21 female), in our sample, Fristmann found normal hip joints only twice (females, with goitre). If we grade these changes, from slight alterations in head form right through to the most severe deformities, the results are as follows:

These values imply a greater tendency of non-goitrous (dwarf) male cretins toward the most severe changes.

Scabell verified a relatively high frequency of *Osteochondritis dissecans* in the knee joint of our clinical sample. Nevertheless, the knee is far more often normal than the hip joint.

Table 3

	Total	With goitre	Without goitre	Male	Female
I. Grade	15	13	2	2	13
II. Grade	8	4	4	2	6
III. Grade	6	2	4	6	–
IV. Grade	3	–	3	3	–

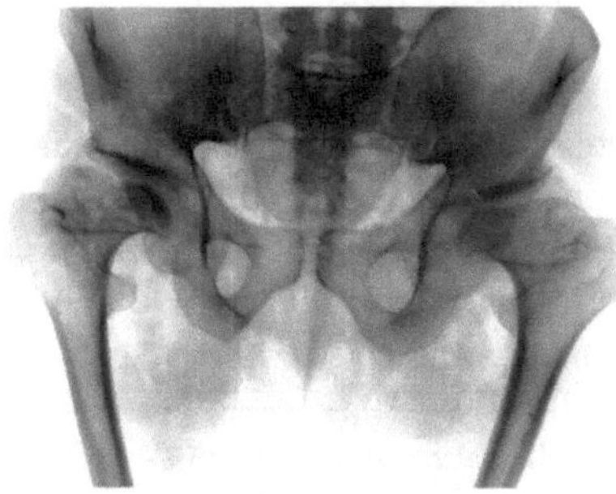

Fig. 43 Pelvis of a 43-year-old cretin with goitre

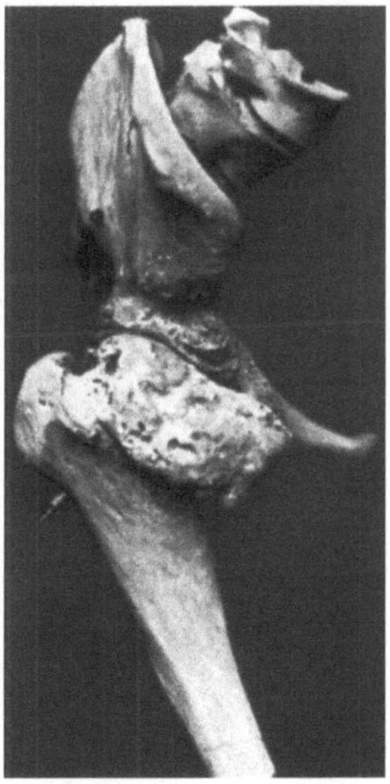

Fig. 44 Hip of a 39-year-old male cretin

E. Bircher has described cretins' *Humerus varus*. Deformational changes there are far more rare than in the hips.

Alterations of the *pelvis* have attained particular importance because of the birth disruptions they cause. The cretin's generally narrowed pelvis was first described in detail by P. Müller in Berne in 1880. B. Müller made the same discovery 50 years later, also from material in the Berne Obstetric Clinic, while Eggenberger confirmed it in the Appenzell canton – in over 10% of births he hypothesized a pathological sequence of events caused in part by endemic goitre.

2.2 The Skin and Its Appendages

Besides the skeletal structure, the behaviour of the *skin* is usually an indicator of cretinism. Where it occurs, myxœdema distinguishes it from other forms of mental deficiency but not from congenital thyroid-deficient myxœdema. It is recognizable from the dense, usually pallid, wax-like puffiness of the skin, which cannot be banished by finger pressure, as with genuine œdema. We will leave the histological evaluation to the pathologists. This myxœdema, which normally attacks the entire body but is most strikingly expressed on the face and hands, is usually a temporary condition. It is most easily influenced by compensatory mechanisms with all the appearances of hypothyroidism, and hence it is least pronounced in older cretins. After the age of puberty the myxœdema usually regresses over time, and in most cases only the gross, remarkably wrinkled skin of the forehead remains. We still find pronounced levels of myxœdema in older cretins, especially those without goitre (Fig. 59).

The *skin shade* among cretins is generally a yellow-grey tone with a dash of brown, more or less – you could argue that the cretin exhibits a brownish skin tone ('maroons'). In assessing the brown pigmentation it should not be forgotten that most cretins come from the country and, whether from working in the fields or pleasantly doing nothing, they spend a lot of their time in the sun.

That the yellow sallowness is not based on anaemia can be confirmed by case-by-case blood analysis. Even though haemoglobin and erythrocyte count tend to be reduced in cretins, haemoglobin depletion as a rule is not one of those features that could explain the skin pallor by itself.

Remarkable also is the *dryness* of the skin and its tendency to fine desquamation. This sign too is found to a pronounced degree only among dwarf cretins and

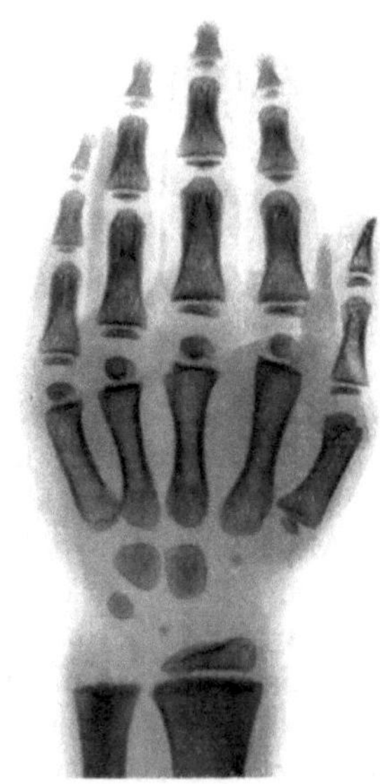

Fig. 45 Hand skeleton of an 11-year-old cretin without goitre. Case from Fig. 13a

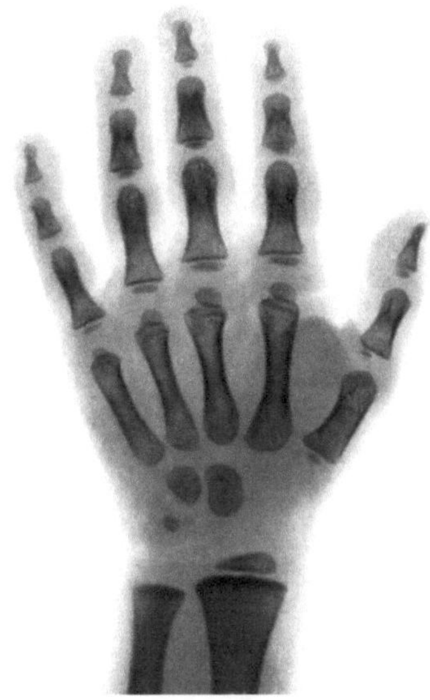

Fig. 46 For comparison: normal hand skeleton; 5 years old

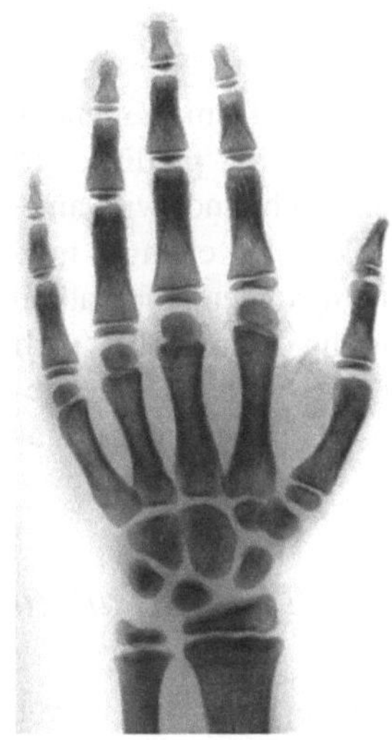

Fig. 47 Hand skeleton of a 13-year-old half-cretin. Case from Fig. 14a

regresses to a great extent when body growth and hair covering become normal. Observations in well-run institutions and clinics show that this is not a lack of cleanliness, as Finkbeiner alleges.

Hair growth among cretins without goitre is generally sparse over the entire body, with the scalp hairs fuzzy and bristly, but not showing the level of degeneration found among athyroids. Among taller cretins with goitre, hair growth generally matches the local norm. From time to time you come across *Cutis verticis gyrata*.

Fig. 48 For comparison: normal hand skeleton; 12½ years old

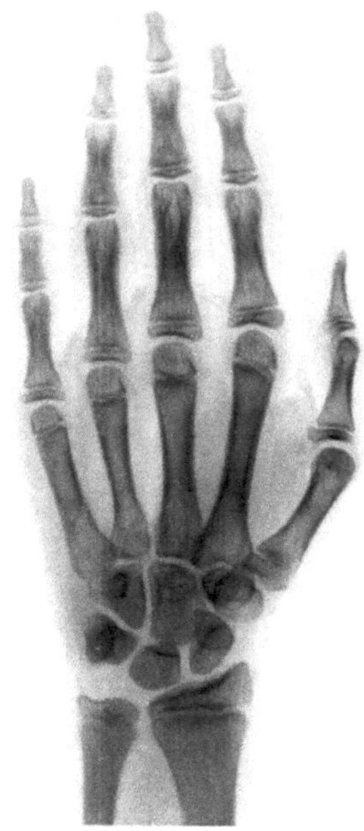

Apart from the tendency to dryness, desquamation, and crust formation on the scalp hair, a predisposition to eczema is ascribed to cretinism. We have observed eczema but not with any surprising frequency.

The skin changes mentioned are particularly more pronounced among congenital, myxœdematous, athyroids than among cretins; among the latter, more pronounced among dwarf cretins with thyroid atrophy than among cretins with goitre. The same is true of changes to the nails. On the other hand, cretins are spared skin diseases based on increased sweat secretion.

2.3 *The Musculature*

Deficiency of the entire body structure is apparent in muscle development as well. Among myxœdematous, adolescent cretins without goitre, the underdevelopment of the musculature is partially concealed by the myxœdema. Among juvenile, goitrous cretins on the other hand, the gangling constitution appears early. Occasionally during his teenage years but sometimes only after those developmental years, the goitrous cretin is distinguished both by his somewhat stooping posture and by his unaided stumbling, shuffling gait. For all that, the cretin is in a position to strengthen his muscles by exercise, at least if his intellectual development makes this possible. Innumerable first- and second-grade cretins, particularly those with goitre, work as farm labourers and farm girls and, as such, accomplish a substantial amount of physical labour. The cretin without goitre prefers to apply himself more quietly,

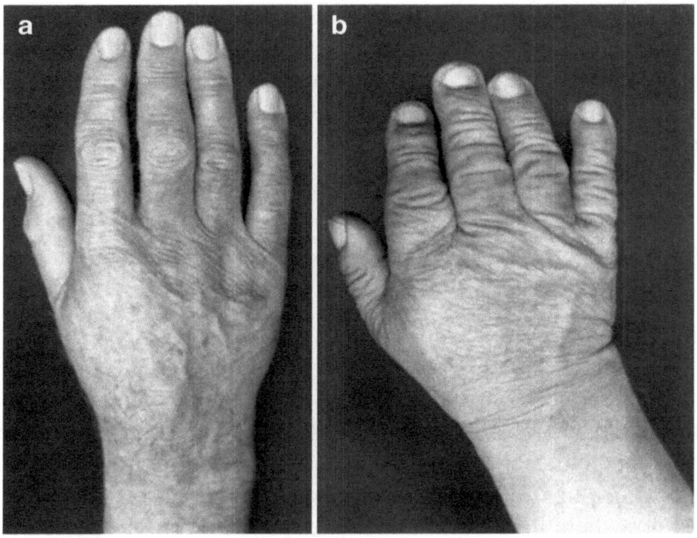

Fig. 49 Hand of a normal 63-year-old man (**a**); and of a dwarf cretin of the same age with atrophied thyroid gland (**b**). Case from Fig. 18

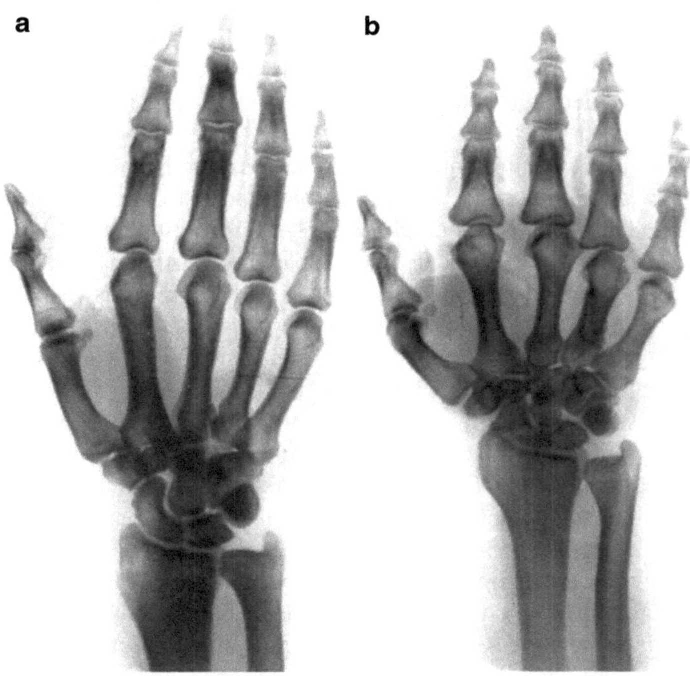

Fig. 49a The corresponding radiographs

since he is made wretched not only by his muscular weakness but also by his skeletal structure. Related to this muscular weakness is the cretin's well-known tendency to abdominal herniation. Among school children, hernias were observed about three times more frequently in the goitre region of the Berne canton than in the low-goitre Jura (Lauener).

2.4 *The Behaviour of the Endocrine Glands*

2.4.1 The Thyroid Gland

The very definition of cretinism establishes that we are dealing first and foremost with the thyroid gland. We will expand on its functional behaviour in cretinism in the section on pathological physiology; here we shall restrict ourselves to presenting the clinical findings. Histology is relegated to a special section.

Up until now there have been no definite findings from the *period of infancy*, for who could predict that the tiny baby would turn into a cretin. Reports of anamnestic reactions point to diffuse neonatal goitre, as mentioned by Rösch, but we do not know how often such a finding might actually arise. At most, we can be sure, based on statistics and pathological–anatomical studies (Wegelin), that in the endemic zone by far the majority of children come into the world with an enlarged thyroid gland. Yet although thyroid atrophy would occur during the first year of life and could be determined by palpation, we have no definite information. From findings during the first years of schooling, we can only conclude that it *is* possible. No neonatal autopsy so far has detected an atrophy of the thyroid gland.

Also, we have little information on the macroscopic behaviour of the thyroid gland up until starting school, since children suspected of cretinism are usually presented to the physician at about school age. At this juncture the finding is usually clear-cut – either the thyroid gland is not palpable or it is barely palpable. We can feel the trachea lying under the skin, so to speak, and accordingly we diagnose early atrophy of the gland. In other cases, we find a diffuse, goitrous enlargement that occasionally behaves as such right up to puberty. Histologically it presents the type of parenchymatous enlargement with colloid deficiency and images reminiscent of the Graves–Basedow type (adolescent goitre of Gold and Orator), but always connected with symptoms of degenerative change. These sorts of observations were described in our clinic by Doubler in 1922. Despite physical and mental symptoms of incipient cretinism, symptoms of cardiovascular erethism are observed in such (girl) children as an exception at puberty.

These symptoms are reminiscent of a transient hyperthyroid condition (Doubler). In early cretins, a diffuse goitre can even exhibit a vascular character in exceptional cases. Since the systematic administration of iodine in schools, the histological type of adolescent goitre has become rare, in our experience, and has been replaced by diffuse colloid goitre.

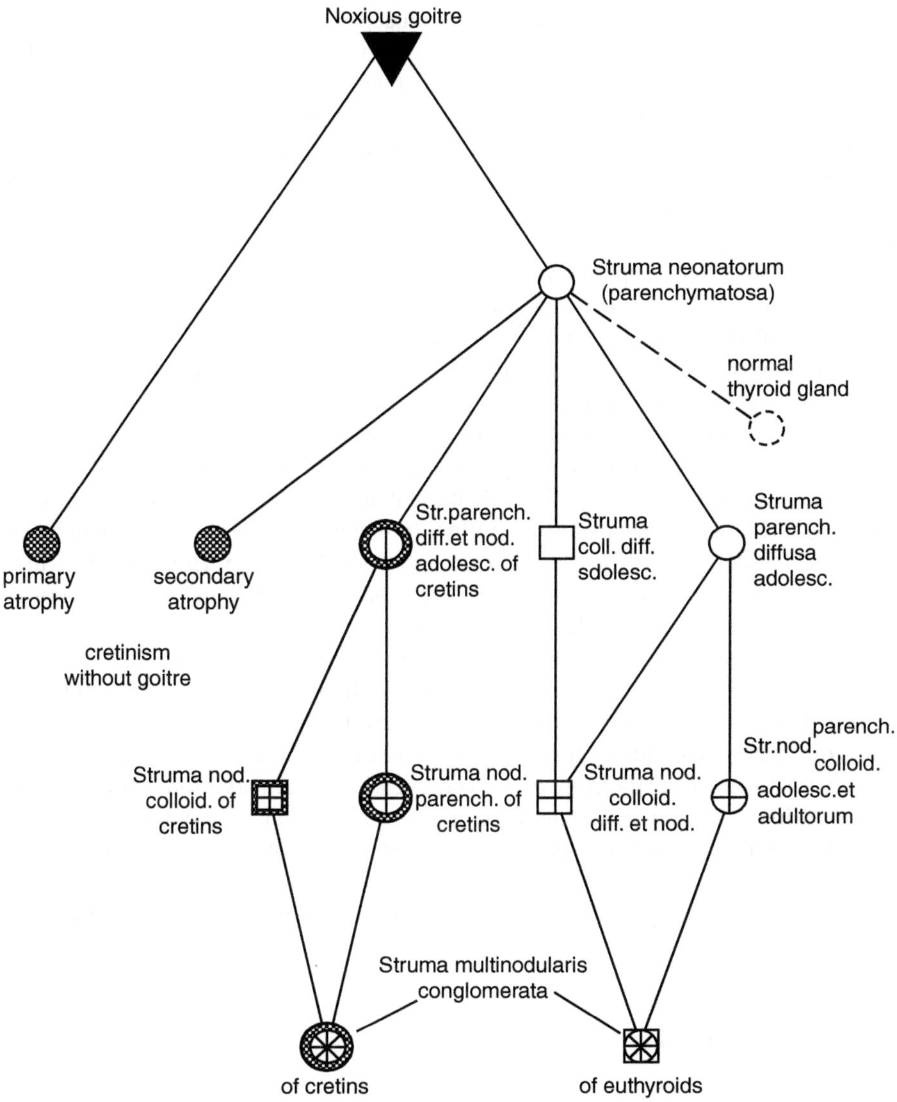

Fig. 50 Endemic goitre tree

In other cases we have found rudiments of nodulation in the first years of school – in 6% of Bernese school children before the adoption of iodine treatment. In a region of severe endemic goitre, early, extensive nodule formation always arouses the suspicion of incipient goitrous cretinism – a suspicion approaching certainty when, coincidentally, there is a retardation of intellectual development.

During the post-pubertal period, both types of dwarf cretinism steadily develop – thyroid atrophy on the one hand, and normally growing cretins with nodular goitre on the other. The nodular goitre shows the same macroscopic forms that we see among non-cretinous goitre sufferers, and evolves sometimes towards the coarse, nodular form, and in other cases more towards the small, multinodular form. In the latter especially, the thyroid gland appears frequently embedded in a loose, soft tissue whose physical characteristics are more clearly visible from palpation than from eventual surgery. For all that, the surgeon is pleasantly surprised by the ease with which he can strip the goitre from its wrapping, in cretins. In this respect, cretinous goitre stands in stark contrast with Grave's goitre.

At the beginning we mentioned, as an intermediate form between goitre and absence of goitre, those cases where individual goitrous nodules were embedded in the atrophic thyroid glands and even early atrophic glands.

In later years cretin goitre undergoes all the changes that we are familiar with in the goitre of euthyroids – fibrous degeneration, cyst formation, calcification, inflammation, and, finally, it can become malignant as well.

All of this confirms every observer's finding that clinically and macroscopically there is no typical cretin goitre. The only thing that we can say is that a pure, diffuse, colloid goitre has not been seen in cretins. In exceptional cases, combinations of diffuse and nodular colloid goitre do occur, as we shall see later. However, the *usual cretin goitre* most frequently observed in the centre of an endemic region is *parenchymatous, nodular goitre*, which occurs also among non-cretins.

After what has been said so far, there remains a gap to fill – the macroscopic and, as we shall see later, the histological study of the thyroid gland of cretins between birth and school age. Such a study requires careful, periodic examination of the necks of the child candidates for cretinism up until the moment when the diagnosis is confirmed – i.e., over the course of several years – and, in addition, better use and centralisation of the autopsy material, which is currently far too limited. Put simply, once this problem is acknowledged, ways and means of solving it will also be found.

The *in utero* developmental history of the cretin thyroid gland will be discussed elsewhere.

2.4.2 The Parathyroid Glands

Among ordinary cretins, clinical signs by the parathyroid glands are non-existent. Only rarely is Chvostek's sign clearly positive. The value of 17% that we ourselves proposed earlier has, after more extensive tests, revealed itself to be too high. We should not be deceived by the lip twitch that appears among cretins and non-cretins alike when palpating outside the zone of a facial nerve root and even during palpation of the neck. Our earlier co-workers have probably occasionally gone astray; the same applies to Mathez's data, since our own tests on part of the same sample produced much lower values. Also, Mathez's theoretical reduction of the blood calcium level does not exist in practice. Furthermore, extremely rarely have we found values lower than 9.0 mg% among cretins. Streit's data from 31 cretins in our clinic, of both types and in all stages, rather more frequently (45%), reveal a drop below 10.0 mg% compared with data from normal people (25%), but never below 9.0 mg%. This demonstrates that the environmental factor or the nourishment factor does play a certain role among cretins and non-cretins. In 27 cases from among our *clinical* material Saegesser never found values below 10 mg%. Streit's cases were for the most part examined in institutions, where a few control cases also gave values below 10 mg%.

The fact that Wegelin (see later) found the parathyroid glands unchanged in cretins corresponds with the normal blood calcium level.

We will go into detail about the significance of these findings when we discuss so-called 'nervous cretinism'. The only comment here is that the opposing behaviour of thyroid glands and parathyroid glands is of theoretical interest. The noxious agent of goitre evidently acts very selectively on the endocrine system, and we see from this that it simply does not involve making a multi-glandular disorder out of cretinism. It would be easiest to imagine that the parathyroid glands might be *mechanically* damaged by goitre. Theoretically, such a possibility cannot be rejected out of hand and can occasionally be true of one or other case. But then in the same way, this must also be the case for non-cretinous goitre patients, among thousands of whom we have so far never seen a clinically recognizable hypoparathyroid individual. MacCarrison's case of sclerosis of the parathyroid glands has, anatomically speaking, so far remained isolated. In endocrinology, we must stick to the bare facts, and not let the endocrine glands spring into action like chess pieces, in support of some theory or other.

2.4.3 The Sexual Glands and the Sexual Organs

Clinically there is also a difference between the two groups of cretins in the behaviour of the genitalia. In non-goitrous *male cretins* the external genitalia remain more or less infantile for a long time, and in severe cases they never achieve normal development. The testicles remain small, and show the histological changes that Wegelin will discuss later. Hairiness retains a hypogenital character.

The penis develops slowly, often remaining somewhat retarded in its development, while in other cases it attains dimensions that offhand would ensure normal functioning. In older texts the scrotum is often described as flaccidly enlarged, even though the sex glands remain small. Such flaccidness does occur, but this is not a general rule. Also, the most pronounced underdevelopment of the external genitalia among cretins is nowhere near comparable with those that we see among the *adiposo-genitalis* hypophyseal type (see Fig. 51) and among primary eunuchoid conditions.

Among cretins of average normal height with goitre, genital development, broadly speaking, is anatomically normal.

In *females* we find less-clear differences between non-goitrous dwarf cretins and normal-sized goitrous cretins. Among the former, axillary and pubic hair remain in a relatively infantile condition, while their development among normal-height goitrous cretins can be normal. Obviously, further intermediate stages lie between the two extremes. Breast development falls outside the line, whereas among non-goitrous

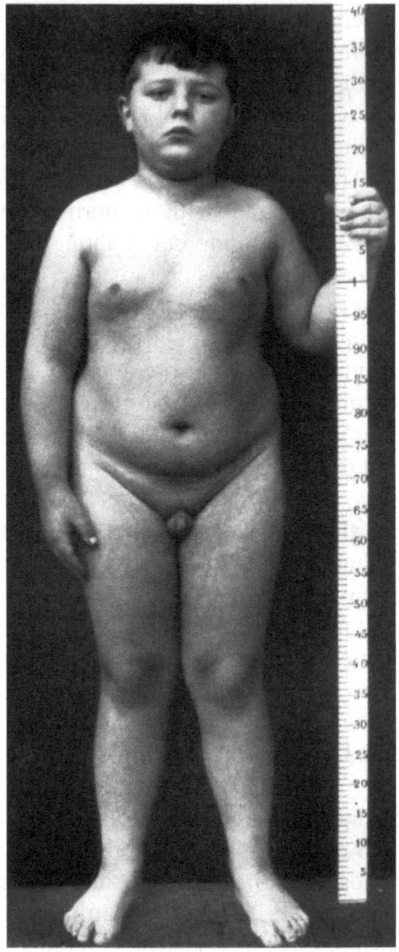

Fig. 51 *Dystrophia adiposogenitalis*; 9 years old

dwarf cretins without special fat deposits we occasionally find them quite well formed. Guggisberg observed that the internal organs often showed an infantile character.

As for *functional behaviour*, the sex drive in full cretins of both sexes is equally non-existent, and the previously alleged lechery is, as we have seen, a fable that has possibly arisen from confusion with certain non-cretinous mentally-deficient forms.

Likewise, among dwarf cretins with reasonable development of the intellectual faculty and of the genital apparatus, the tendency, and probably also the capacity, for sexual activity is, as a rule, completely lacking. Therefore, inmates in this category cause few problems for staff in institutions. Among goitrous cretins the possibility of sexual activity depends on the extent of genital development, and cretins at this level not infrequently marry, as mentioned earlier, and raise offspring.

However, even in the best instances, one has the impression that their achievements in this regard are below average.

In females, menstruation is sometimes totally absent or late in onset, and is scant and irregular. However, according to observations from our cretin institutions, it is often, alternatively, abnormally strong. Functional behaviour of the sexual apparatus approximates the norm to the same degree as body growth. Among female cretins of the second grade, with more or less pronounced dwarfism, activity not infrequently leads to pregnancy, with a normal outcome. Accurate statistical data on their children's condition can be compiled only with difficulty. These infants leave the maternity facilities before potential cretinism can be recognized. From occasional observations we can assume that children of half-cretins are capable of normal development. On the other hand, the half-cretin in Fig. 56 was the son of half-cretin siblings. As yet there is no statistical evidence that under similar environmental conditions half-cretin mothers raise cretins more frequently than do goitrous non-cretin mothers. Maffei's information on this point is slanted too pessimistically when he writes:

> All the children that I saw coming into the world from half-cretins suffered hydrocephaly or atrophy, were stillborn or soon died. However I have no wish at all of denying that female half-cretins of the highest level are capable of conceiving a child and even in due time bringing him, live, into the world.

According to records from the obstetrical clinic in Berne we find that generally births among cretins occur after the full gestation period. Birth complications due to anomalies in placental development are no more common than among women with healthy thyroid glands. On the other hand, as previously mentioned, according to reports from the same clinic (B. Müller), the observation made 50 years earlier by Peter Müller still applies – the generally narrowed pelvis is particularly common in the goitrous region of the Berne canton. Today the geographical distribution of this pelvic anomaly fully coincides with distribution of the most severe goitre, and of endemic cretinism.

Careful study of the goitre of neonates led Guggisberg to discover that the physique of goitre-afflicted newborns – whether or not they later become cretinous – is already inferior at birth by comparison with children with healthy thyroids. This finding is consistent with Eggenberger's information that, since the systematic distribution of iodised cooking salt in the Appenzell canton, cases of congenital debility have dropped from 3.6‰ to 0.6‰. Wieland on the other hand regards the assumption of a thyrogenic 'congenital debility' as not yet satisfactorily substantiated.

2.4.4 The Hypophysis

There has been a lot of dispute over whether the *hypophysis* too participates in the clinical picture of cretinism. Individual histological findings might make us think so (cf. Wegelin). One such assertion theoretically closed the gap somewhat, in that today we recognize the close connections between the two glands. In actual fact, there is nothing so far in the picture of cretinism likely to be attributable to functional damage to the hypophysis.

On the other hand, it is clear that, also among cretins, the hypophysis plays the role of a hormonal link and regulatory apparatus between brain and thyroid gland. It is also conceivable that its activity is somehow influenced by the thyroid gland's underperformance. Such an influence is corroborated by the almost invariable enlargement of the anterior lobe. Since the same finding applies to cases of congenital thyroaplasia, we have to assume that it is a secondary response to the failure or deficit in thyroid gland function. The hypophysis therefore does not participate *primarily*, in the sense of a multiglandular disorder, in the cretinism picture – it suffers the consequences of thyroid gland damage *secondarily*, possibly attempting to readjust the system by hyperplasia of its own glandular portion.

We will not go into details of the *other endocrine glands* because, so far, no case for a primary participation in the clinical picture of cretinism has been made for any of them. On the other hand, what has just been said about the hypophysis probably applies to several of these as well. The hormonal connections between thyroid gland, liver, and pancreas allow us to assume that these organs too are affected, at least functionally, by the poor performance of the thyroid. Poor testicular performance is considered secondary in both cretinism and thyroaplasia.

2.5 *The Intestinal Tract and Its Glands*

Among cretins the intestinal tract shows no gross anatomical changes and no characteristic functional defects. Rather, when the intestinal tract and its function is compared with the irritable bowel activity of Grave–Basedow patients, this is not a cretin characteristic – the inertia of intestinal function is simply a growth disorder, and a sign of degeneration. Furthermore, nothing relating to liver or pancreatic defects has been observed among cretins.

Apart from the tendency to constipation, the question of whether the cretin is especially predisposed to gastrointestinal tract disorders does not lend itself to a definitive answer. We have very rarely seen benign stomach ulcers among cretins, in spite of their frequent occurrence among the male portion of our rural population. We have occasionally encountered carcinomas among cretins and half-cretins, gastric cancer in particular, but not often enough to assume a special predisposition. Given the impossibility of drawing a sharp line between euthyroid and hypothyroid forms of endemic thyropathy, a much broader problem presents itself, emphasized initially by Bayard, and later by Stiner, Eggenberger, and others: does endemic goitre or, more accurately, endemic thyropathy require a predisposition to malignancies? Both Bayard and Stiner support this supposition with statistical calculations from Switzerland, and Eggenberger assumes that among hypothyroids the anatomical basis is a hypoplasia or dystrophy of both the gastric and intestinal mucosa. We will discuss this question critically later.

2.6 The Blood Vascular System

The recognition that connections exist between the development of the vascular system and cretinism arose from the following observation.

Years ago, when we wanted to screen blood from the arm veins of a large number of cretins, it struck Dr F. Starlinger, our registrar at the time, that the collection procedure was much easier from goitrous cretins than from non-goitrous cretins. He drew a major conclusion: as a consequence of the breakdown in thyroid function the vascular system remains in a hypoplastic state when the breakdown comes into effect during the first years of life. If it impacts on development only later, and perhaps somewhat less rapidly, then venous system hypoplasia no longer occurs and, at least at first glance, we find the normal pattern, even to strongly developed cutaneous veins. Wegelin's discovery that cardiac dimensions are small among dwarf cretins corresponds with this. Of course autopsy findings give no measure of the picture in the living, especially when viewed by radiography. Even a small, flaccid heart can enlarge passively to considerable size, because muscular weakness allows the enlargement. In actual fact, the cretin heart seems rather large on x-ray, even if it does not reach the size that we regularly find in athyroid hearts.

Of significance in this regard are the findings of Feer and Guggisberg in goitrous neonates. According to them, normal heart diameter increases from 5.1 to 5.7 cm in markedly goitrous neonates. Feer traces this back to involvement of the thymus. Guggisberg, on the other hand, noted that cardiac enlargement often occurred without the thymus being enlarged. He therefore assumed that the damaged goitrous heart had not grown to meet the increased demands of the first stages of life, by comparison with the healthy heart, and had accordingly enlarged. Therefore, when faced with neonatal goitre, we should not immediately conclude cretinism – alongside the endocrine element in functional defects in the gland, we should also consider the mechanical element of vascular obstruction and respiratory difficulties. The fact emerging from Lauener's school investigations, that heart defects among school children in the relatively goitre-free Jura are only half as common as in the part of the Berne canton heavily beset by endemic goitre, is remarkable. ECG, radiological and kymographic investigations undertaken on several of our cases of cretinism and thyroaplasia in conjunction with the medical clinic (Prof. Frey) and Dr Weber are briefly summarised: the heart–lung quotient lay within normal limits, as it did also in our numerous goitrous cretin patients, while not taking into account secondary diseases of the vascular system. Nor did the ECG reveal anything spectacular. In athyroidism and cretinism the kymogram revealed Stumpf's Type 2 movement, recognized by reduction, or total loss, of movement in the performance arena – a sign of inferior constitution and rapid fatigue during loading tests. This finding, which admittedly we regard as merely a trial run for the more extensive investigations planned, falls at least within the range of our ideas so far. We expect further information, in particular from our parallel studies of the vascular system in goitrous and in non-goitrous cretins.

The microscopic investigations of the *capillary pattern* systematically undertaken by Otfried Müller on healthy and sick men prompted Jaensch, Wittneben, Gundermann, and Hoepfner to use capillary microscopy for the detection of constitutional and endocrine anomalies in childhood, and to use them principally in the diagnosis of cretinoid conditions. Investigations undertaken by Miss Gehri under our direction have demonstrated that anomalies in the capillary pattern certainly do indicate defects in development, but also that those defects are not pathognomonic for cretinoid conditions. Admittedly, around 80% of cretins show moderate to major changes in the capillary pattern. However, we find similar proportions for idiocy as well – an outcome of primary diseases of the nervous system. At the same time, a minimal number of cases in every group of developmental defects show a normal or barely changed capillary pattern. The ratio of major changes among cretins increases in proportion with the intensity of the cretinism.

The following summary of the subjects in Berne shelters studied by Miss Gehri amplifies what has been said:

	Disruption of capillary structure				
Grade of cretinism		Normal (%)	Mild (%)	Moderate (%)	Severe (%)
1. Disruption of the capillary structure in cretinism: 155 cases					
(a) Mild	16 cases	6.25	25	42.5	25
(b) Moderate	46 cases	8.7	19.5	32.6	39.1
(c) Full cretin	93 cases	3.2	9.6	39.7	47.5
Percentage total		7.1	13.0	29.0	51.0
2. Disruption of the capillary structure in primary, neurological, non-cretinous idiots: 51 cases					
		6	19.5	41	33.5

These observations are confirmed in the most recent publications of Jaensch, Gundermann, Wittneben, O. Müller, and K. Bock. The limited capillary development is stripped of its specific characteristics, and becomes a general sign with limited development that can arise genotypically or be acquired. Jaensch and Gundermann even discovered that, as they had assumed, on the goitre-free North Friesian islands, capillary defects were common among school children as a result of inbreeding. In spite of this, they lay the main emphasis on thyroid gland insufficiency as the cause of capillary defects, even today. This is based partially on their discovery that among their samples from the relatively goitre-free High Jura, they found significantly greater percentages of capillary defects than in the goitre-free areas of Germany.

They blame this occurrence of thyroid gland pathology on the loading which, in its terminal branches, would be expressed only through more capillary stigmatisation.

We will discuss the grounds of validity *for* and *against* those authors' positions in another section.

The question at issue, whether we should be restricted to investigating nail cuticle capillaries or whether, like O. Müller, we should extend to other areas of the skin, can be answered as follows: from the standpoint of scientific research Müller is undoubtedly correct. For clinical and endemiological studies, particularly involving school children, the nail cuticle is the site where case-by-case comparable results are most easily obtained.

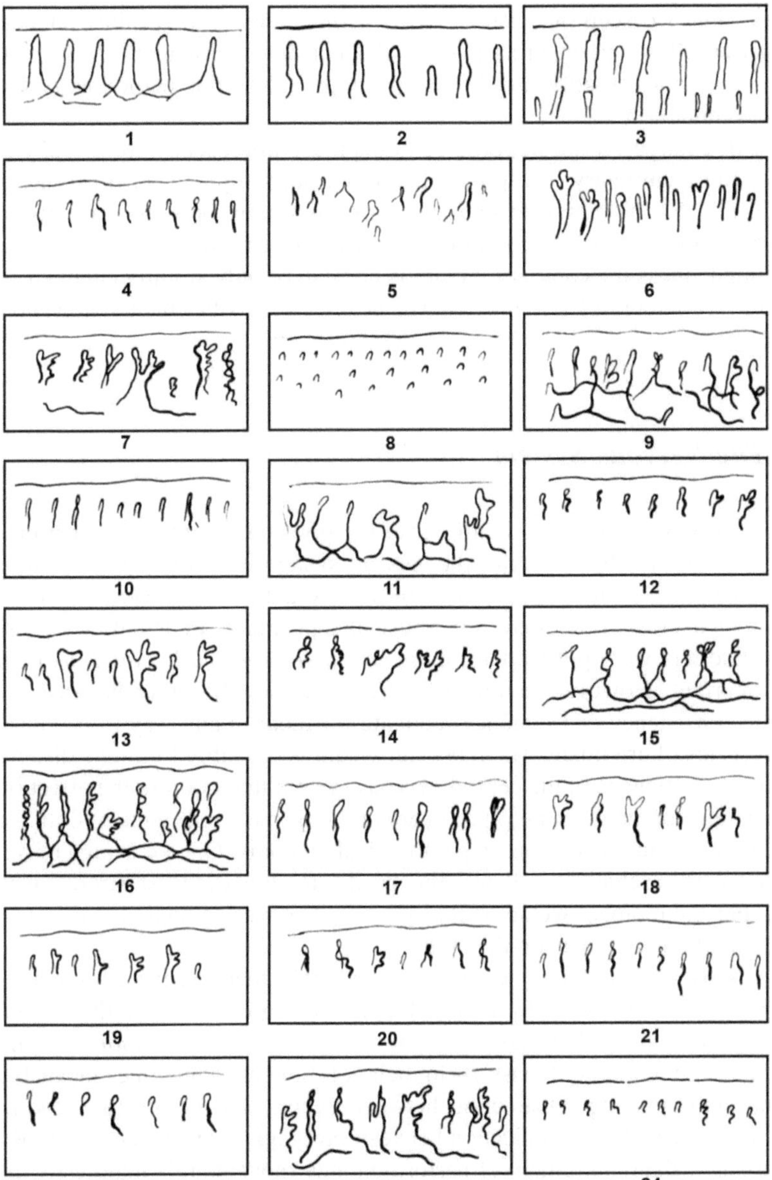

Fig. 52 Capillary forms: (**a**) Normal forms. *1*, Normal child 6 years, *2*, normal adult 31 years; *3*, normal adult 82 years. (**b**) Non-thyroidal disruptions. *4*, chondrodystrophy (Fig. 16); *5*, *Dystrophia adiposogenitalis* (Fig. 51); *6*, mongoloid feeble-minded (Fig. 15). (**c**) Athyroid. *7*, 14-year-old (Fig. 57b); *8*, 18-year-old (Fig. 118); *9*, incomplete athyroid (probably lingual thyroid) now 20 years (Fig. 119); *10*, normal sister, now 14 years (Fig. 119). (**d**) Non-goitrous cretinism with thyroid gland atrophy and dwarfism. *11*, 14 years (Fig. 11); *12*, 52 years (Fig. 120), non-cretin goitrous mother of the same; *13*, 17 years (Fig. 13a); *14*, 32 years (Fig. 21); *15*, 61 years (Fig. 30a); *16*, 63 years (Fig. 30b); *17*, 63 years (Fig. 18). (**e**) Goitrous cretins and half-cretins. *18*, 14 years (Fig. 12); *19*, 18 years (Fig. 14a); *20*, 23 years (Fig. 17); *21*, 35 years (Fig. 29a); *22*, 53 years (Fig. 55); *23*, 53 years (Fig. 31c); *24*, 60 years (Fig. 31b)

Even while we keep our distance from taking sides in the evaluation, capillary examination allows us insights that we did not have prior to O. Müller and his school. Even more broadly, and free from any prejudice, the methodology deserves further examination.

We will enlarge on the importance of capillary microscopy for therapy further on. We offer a summary of capillary pictures from sample cases illustrated in our book, in Fig. 52. No athyroid individual, or any cretin, presents a totally normal capillary picture, whereas in chondrodystrophy, Frölich's syndrome, and mongoloid feeble-mindedness the capillary picture is normal, or only slightly changed.

For the behaviour of *blood* in cretinism we refer you to the chapter on pathological physiology.

2.7 The Nervous System

From the very beginning of scientific investigations on cretinism, authors occupied themselves with the behaviour of the nervous system in cretins (Ackermann). This is fairly obvious, because appearances of intellectual failure attracted just as much attention on average as anomalies in physical appearance. In actual fact, gross anatomical findings were put forward more often, *Hydrocephalus internus* being the most important. However, neither hydrocephalus nor the other isolated findings show the consistency or frequency requisite for them in any way to be considered characteristics of cretinism. The most significant is probably Lotmar's discovery of fine structural changes in the central nervous system that point to the effect of limitations in development taking place in about the fifth to sixth foetal month. Further details are given in the section on pathological anatomy. Once this area of research is expanded, these changes will probably be able to clarify at least part of the clinical picture. For the moment we are still relying on discovering anatomical facts on the one hand and clinical facts on the other.

If we start with *mobility*, we must immediately mention the extremely severe cases where walking is totally impossible, and all movement is reduced to a bare minimum. These individuals lie like an immoveable mass – *rudis indigestaque molis* (Ovid: 'a rough, unordered mass') – in their cots, and are sometimes incapable even of sitting and standing. Distinction between central and peripheral dyskinesia is impossible, since all communication between investigator and subject is impossible, and, similarly, the requirement of performing any movement is manifestly unavailable. In any endeavour to make such an individual sit up or stand up, he collapses like an empty sack. The entire neuromuscular apparatus from cerebral cortex to periphery has remained inadequate, or become so, after an initial phase of less severe breakdown. These individuals are most easily compared with cases of complete thyroaplasia. We find these conditions both in cretins without goitre and in those with goitre. Pathological findings in their thyroid glands and their brains only rarely come to light, because, unfortunately, these extremely severe sufferers of cretinism do not as a rule die in hospital. They have become rare over recent decades.

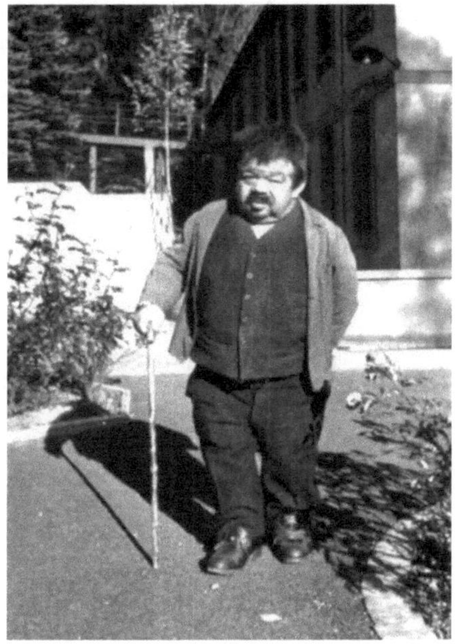

Fig. 53 Cretinism without goitre – anteriorly degenerated cretin hips; heavy tottering gait

In the great majority of cases the cretin is able to move around and generally use his limbs freely. However, he does this with a characteristic slowness and a lack of any degree of emotion. Here again we come across differences between goitre-free and goitrous cretins. Slowness of movement is common to both. We find the very characteristic *wobbling gait* mainly in dwarf cretins without goitre and again in those goitrous cretins near to them in stature. The more normal the body build, the more normal is the gait. However, it is still not totally normal in fully grown, goitrous cretins, who always shows a certain *awkward helplessness*, which distinguishes cretinous disorder from most other forms of nervous system breakdown. Goitre-free dwarf cretins usually have an erect posture; the somewhat bigger goitrous cretins, at least once growth is complete, are flaccidly bent forward. While the gait of goitre-free cretins is very characteristic, that of normally grown, goitrous cretins is, however, indistinguishable from that of non-thyrogenic idiots.

As Scholz and Finkbeiner among others quite rightly point out, skeletal behaviour plays not a small role in the wobbling gait. Stuntedness in an individual of approximately normal girth must necessarily lead to a wobbling gait, without the joints taking a particular part in gait dysfunction.

Of great importance too is the often *pathological construction of the hip joint* and, to a certain extent, the knee joint as well. These have already been discussed. It is obvious that the various levels of skeletal anomaly influence the gait to various degrees. We come across the most severe disturbances of gait from the fifth decade onwards, that is, during those years when, in non-cretins too, rheumatoid arthritis begins to make itself felt. Next we will discuss one final point, the neuromuscular.

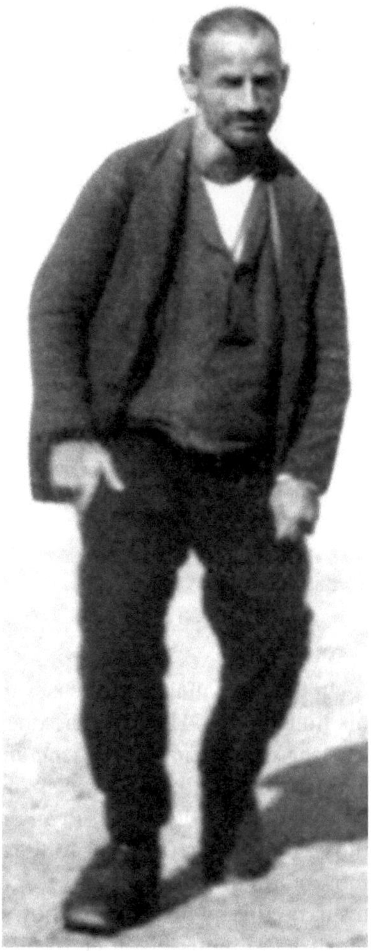

Fig. 54 A 35-year-old deaf–mute cretin with nodular colloidal goitre and atrophy of the thyroid gland (histological diagnosis). Unsteady gait; overlay of cretinism due to massive striatal damage (Lotmar); (birth trauma?)

Disruptions on the part of the *neuromuscular apparatus* are of a complex nature. On the one hand, we have an undoubted slowdown of all mental reactions and all fine gradations, which must necessarily impart a certain ungainliness to the gait, of which the state of the bones and the joints are also a part. However, on the other hand, among roughly half the cretins we see an increase in tendon reflexes – a curious contradiction to the slowdown of mental reflexes. This is expressed in the patellar reflex especially, observed in about half the cases (Scholz, personal observations), right through to patellar clonus. In 47% of our last series of 184 cases it was increased. The periosteal reflex was raised in about a quarter of the cases; the Babinski reflex was clearly positive in 17%, and just as often weak or absent; the Achilles tendon reflex rose in 21% of cases, and was almost equally often weak or absent. In contrast to the tendon reflexes, skin reflexes are in most cases weak or normal, and raised in only a small number of cases.

On palpation, muscle tone was normal in around 60% of cases; in the remaining cases it was nearly equally increased or reduced. During passive movement, muscle tone often seems to be increased on the first attempt, because the cretin does not grasp what is required of him. With careful, repeated study we found it increased far less often – the percentage values just given could represent an upper limit.

Recently an attempt was made (Mathez) to trace the reflex increases among cretins to a co-partnership with the parathyroid glands, and to assimilate a latent tetany. However, such an approach is contradicted by the fact that, as already mentioned, the Chvöstek phenomenon is clearly pronounced only in exceptional cases among cretins, and that there is a total absence of other appearances of tetany among cretins. We have already mentioned that, according to the investigations of our students Streit and Saegesser, the cretin's blood calcium level also contradicts such an interpretation. We cannot even talk of a special 'predisposition to tetany' among cretins. Indeed, following bilateral goitre surgery in cretins, we have so far never observed tetany.

How then are we to interpret these tendon reflex disturbances, especially the increase in the patellar reflex observed surprisingly regularly? Until now we could only say that this appearance certainly does not necessarily belong in the cretin picture, but can be traced back to an injury or developmental defect in the nervous system that depends on cretinism in order for it to appear. We have already alluded to hydrocephalus as a possible cause of reflex anomalies. We now know that it is not infrequently found in severe cretinism – in about half the cases, according to Wegelin. Further investigation of the nervous system, histology in particular, must be handed over to the clinics in order to clarify this major phenomenon. In any case, besides the skeletal features, the neuromuscular disorders just described play a special role in the development of the cretin's gait. We are forced into this conclusion from the fact that the wobbling gait is also observed in cretins with normal hip joints, and that the intensity exceeds what the skeletal proportions might lead us to expect. The awkward, shuffling gait of the goitrous cretins with a normal skeletal structure can be traced back entirely to disruption in the neuromuscular system.

One thing distinguishing cretinism from many cases of primary cerebral feeblemindedness is the absence of actual focal symptoms such as isolated functional damping or stimulation phenomena in the motor and sensory area. We have observed epilepsy in one single, goitrous cretin.

Here also we must argue the case of so-called *nervous cretinism*, as described by MacCarrison and Crookshank. According to MacCarrison, solely by whom we are given a detailed description and illustrations from India, nervous cretinism should have a combination of typical myxœdematous, cerebral palsy and tetany symptoms. Based on an isolated, histological finding, MacCarrison assumes the cause to be damage not only of the thyroid gland but the parathyroids as well, tracing both back to toxic origins. For years we have searched among our patients and our cretin material for just such a disease scenario; we have found nothing that by any criteria could resemble tetany. On the other hand, we encountered over half a dozen cases where, in addition to a pronounced cretinous habitus and behaviour, there were distinct signs of cerebral palsy in the form of spastic hemiplegia or tetraplegia with club feet.

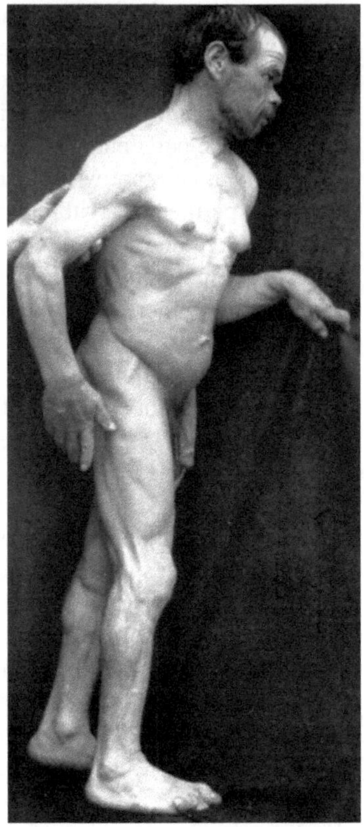

Fig. 55 Cretin with a small goitre and signs of cerebral palsy; 47 years old

According to von Kutschera we could, without any hesitation, simply lump together such clinical pictures with cretinism and various other damage under the term 'endemic dystrophy'. However, such a course of action is not possible because, for example, the cases of cerebral palsy and of mongoloid idiocy which are associated with cretinism, constitute only a minimal number, and because the majority of those conditions occur just as often outside the realm of endemic cretinism as within it. In theory, it might be plausible that cretinism could engender a predisposition for diseases of the nervous system and create degenerative conditions within it. However, as Gamper has correctly noted, there is not a scrap of evidence for this, and so there is nothing else for it but to investigate more of these kinds of incidents in detail, and withhold judgement until we have sufficient material for observation and comparison.

Less tight than the congenital disturbances of the nervous system is of course the association of cretinism with *acquired encephalitic processes*. Here we must simply assume random overlay of a pre-existing cretinism by any kind of secondary, localized or diffuse encephalitis.

The behaviour of the *sense organs* in cretins has aroused special interest. Detailed investigations of the organ of vision are lacking. These are also difficult to perform, because of the defective intelligence of a great number of cretins. The only striking feature from our material, noted also by Scholz and Eggenberger, is the relative frequency of *strabismus.*

The frequent occurrence of *hyperopia*, as Kurz has found, would be interesting, had he not included all the other forms of feeble-mindedness in his investigations.

We have not observed any peculiarities in the *senses of smell and taste* among cretins. Female cretins are very partial to sweets, but this is a universal male and particularly female characteristic. Men smoke whatever comes to hand, but in this they are no different than the average man.

Hearing disorders among cretins have triggered by far the most discussions. In spite of their unavoidable sources of error, not only do the interesting deaf–mute statistics demonstrate that hearing and speech defects are closely related in cretinism, but this can be confirmed by anyone who has the opportunity of observing a large amount of cretin material. From the school investigations in the Berne canton (Lauener), it emerges that hearing and speech disorders are twice as common in the endemic region of the canton than in the relatively goitre-free Jura. Hunziker's statistics rejecting a connection between goitre (not cretinism!) and hearing difficulty are unsubstantiated. These were based on recruiting examinations, which had eliminated pronounced cretins right at the outset. Also, they covered only males, over an age range unsuited to resolving this issue. In Wydler's statistics (111 controlled cases), the cases of deaf–mute (in the normal sense) make up 42%; hard-of-hearing cases with more or less unintelligible speech, 32%; and cases of laboured speech with satisfactory hearing, 25%. Not one single case presented normal hearing combined with normal speech. Our subsequent investigations confirm these findings.

It is evident that we are dealing with a complex process in hearing and speech disorders among cretins, On the one hand, we see cases where hearing disturbances stand alongside reasonable intelligence. These individuals with sufficient intelligence can be taught to speak, like other deaf–mutes. They learn to read lips, like one of our patients with goitrous cretinism – the product of a pregnancy of a half-cretin by her half-cretin brother. In other cases, sound perception over the speech range is only slightly reduced, associated with a reasonable degree of intelligence and only a moderate degree of hearing difficulty. In spite of this, speech is very characteristically clumsy, ponderous, and monotonous, at times only comprehensible to the initiated. No teaching measures can help the individual. Finally, in the most severe cases, hearing capacity, intelligence, and speaking ability all amount to nothing. It is a case of using different vocabulary in order to assemble a complex of a wide variety of disorders, all converging on the abolition of function, but, individually, not approaching this end point along the same curve – in individual cases the disorders come together by different routes.

Thus, the perception defect is limited, partially peripherally and partially centrally. Among low-grade cretins we are dealing first and foremost with a peripheral defect in perception, because they understand the content of what is said, provided that is enunciated sufficiently loudly. Siebenmann, Nager, Oppikoper, and Alexander found changes, particularly in the middle ear and in the capsule of the labyrinth, but not with certainty in the labyrinth itself. Among higher-grade cretins these peripheral defects may also be present, but they are swamped by a defect in central perception based probably not only on an inferiority of the corresponding cortical region (psychic deafness), but on the inferiority of the entire brain that arose *in utero*, especially the intelligence deficit.

A chance coincidence with any kind of ordinary inflammatory hearing disorder can occur, obviously, but it does not carry the weight in the frequency of hearing difficulty that Finkbeiner theoretically ascribes to such a combination. Such gross anatomical defects are missing in most cretins with hearing difficulties.

As with hearing difficulties, so too is the behaviour of *speech defects*. Like the entire motor system, the peripheral vocal organs also work lethargically, under restriction, and lack the fine gradation of environmental influences. Hence speech is monotonous and clumsy, fading into incomprehension. Leading up to this is the central defect: the limitation of intellectual and emotional life and the impoverishment of vocabulary, limited in the end to a few words or syllables, even to incomprehensible grunts. Awkwardness of speech does not parallel the level of hearing defect. Occasionally we find the speech defect very pronounced even with quite reasonable perception of sound, which as such should make well-articulated speech quite possible.

As H. Bircher and E. Bircher have rightly emphasized, in some cases hearing and speech defects are virtually the sole indication of a cretinoid condition to a lay person. From our observations, the clumsiness of speech is more pronounced than would correspond with the level of hearing defect, and from his manner of speech we usually can immediately recognize the fledgling, almost mono-symptomatic cretin.

Comparison with the *behaviour of non-cretinous* or, more accurately, *athyroid individuals* is interesting. Indeed, pronounced myxœdema can exist through even a tiny, partial error in the thyroid gland and also the sluggishness of the neuromuscular system unique to thyroid gland defect. However, hearing remains good while speech is indeed slow, although well articulated. Also, with total athyroids, elementary hearing perception can still be present – reaction to sudden, loud noises, even attentiveness to music. However, as in most severe cretinism, any comprehension of speech and any possibility of expressing themselves in any other way than through inarticulate grunts and bellows is missing. As with third-grade cretins, the dysfunction is so deep-seated, based on primordial development of the particular central brain function, that it cannot be reversed by subsequent substitution therapy. In this regard, it goes much deeper than myxœdema for example, or a defect in hair formation and delay in bone growth.

As far as we know, thorough investigations into the *behaviour of the autonomic nervous system* do not yet exist. Nevertheless, skin dryness and the rarity of blushing among cretins lead us to conclude that, in contrast to what we know of Grave's disease, sympathetic responsiveness among cretins is degraded. It has been believed that, in theory, we could assume that in hypothyroid individuals the pulse rate is slowed by pressure on the brainstem, while the opposite occurs among Grave's sufferers (the 'oculocardiac reflex'). Our investigations carried out in collaboration with Smith have demonstrated that no rules apply for cretins. At most we can assume that play and counter-play between sympathetic and parasympathetic systems are executed more slowly, and they possibly also possess a higher stimulus threshold than a normal or even hyperthyroid individual.

3 The Intellectual Behaviour of Cretins

According to surveys in schools in the Berne canton, *mental debility* is detected almost three times more often in the goitrous and cretinous areas than in the low-goitre Jura (Lauener). A portion of these cases can be directly attributed to cretinism, which, as we have seen, also includes 'thyrogenic dementia' of the goitrous cretins and half-cretins. Other instances during school years remain doubtful – their dependence on endemic thyropathy is expressed only during later development. Whether, as Hoeffner and Jaensch believe, capillary stigmatism causes the rash in the thyroid gland remains unproven. One last group that encompasses the mental deficiency of Down's syndrome right through to inflammatory infections within the skull, and also profound mental retardation, has nothing to do with the thyroid gland, but is found in goitrous regions also.

Pronounced cretinism can empirically be ruled out of the *border zone* of an endemic region. How far milder cases of imbecility fall below endemic thyropathy still cannot be determined with any certainty from the material available. The investigating physicians estimate defective thyroid gland function to be 0.5% of cases studied in the Jura. The boundary between thyrogenic and non-thyrogenic developmental disorders still requires extensive clarification. We shall move on from these to the *unequivocal forms of cretinism.*

The manner in which the cretin's physical behaviour is so far rooted in his immediate family that a sharp borderline cannot be defined applies also to his intellectual behaviour. Many things that in him are expressed as illness are found to be indicated in his surroundings as well – customary characteristics of the place, so to speak. This fact had already attracted the attention of the earliest observers, with every possible variation of the theme expressed in the literature on cretinism. It is conceivable that this irrefutable, underlying evidence of the cretin's deep roots in his family stock has, from the earliest investigations of cretinism (Ramond de Carbonnières) right up until recently (Finkbeiner), given rise to an attempt at an *anthropological explanation* of cretinism. We shall revisit this attempt later. It is merely mentioned here that, despite the intertwining in the soil and ancestral lineage, the cretins of the various 'races' appear so similar that a common pathological element in their condition immediately springs to mind. In 1844 Maffei said, 'The cretin is a sick mammal', and again:

> "We are wrong if we think that cretins are an unique kind of human that propagate themselves. The cretin is a sick person, and cretinism is an illness and not a special human species capable of reproduction by the individuals of that species." His good powers of observation have allowed him to be seen without pathological anatomy. Based on our

current knowledge we can characterize cretins as a pathological brotherhood spanning all races over the entire earth.

There is, in this respect, a close parallel between the mental and physical behaviour of cretins, since limitation of development is characteristic of them both. However, it is not simply a matter of their remaining at an earlier stage – infantilism, neoteny – but right from the start the limitation has certain peculiarities, both physically and mentally – certain adjuncts that distinguish it from other forms of limitation. Here, both between the individual physical manifestations, and also between these and the mental defects, we find a *dissociation*, that, for the alert investigator, despite the common traits, develops the picture of cretinism into a varied one. Even in the area of intellectual development we find dissociative processes that allow clearly different types to peel off.

Even the connections of cretinism to stimulating and boring surroundings, to the problems of the human and neighbourhood story, to the political and social behaviour of the entire local population have assured this special form of feeble-mindedness of a much greater interest than has been bestowed on any other form of dementia. This interest is tangible among all the authors involved with cretinism, not only from a theoretical or laboratory point of view of a pathogenetic, pathological and endocrine problem, but also among authors who have had, and have used, the opportunity of observing cretins over the years within the framework of their home population and have come, so to speak, into closer intellectual contact.

The foundation of the cretin psyche is (as Wagner von Jauregg and, most recently, Gamper and Scharfetter have explained and illustrated by the parallel of athyroids and myxœdematous patients), the slowdown of all mental processes – an 'increasing lack of preparedness for action and reaction, from the simple to the most complex mental performances'. This torpor is expressed both in the areas of intellect and of spiritual life. Incorporated in this, as the psychiatrist Klaesi proposed in a clinical discussion of cretinism, is the 'need for certainty'. The cretin is no friend of risky undertakings. Given two paths he will always chose the safer, even when it is the longer.

Intellectual development shows all the stages in its end result – from respectable, bourgeois mediocrity right down to the most extreme apathy. Where an intellectual life can be spoken of, it ranges from the retention of small things painstakingly learned – a vocabulary limited to a few words and the capacity to carry out the simplest activities in the house and the garden – through to performing a simple, manual task requiring no deep thought. One of our cretins was capable of cleaning a motorcycle; it would be unthinkable for him to correct any type of even the simplest mechanical fault on it. One major exception is the young deaf–mute cretin already mentioned, the son of a cretin and her half-cretin brother, who had sufficient understanding to master his *Meccano* superbly. In school the highest achievements are in reading, writing and religion, whereas mathematics generally is no area for cretins. At most where it is a matter of achieving, he displays a certain interest in numerical values. I gave a few postcards to our 60-year-old clinic cretin, who earlier had earned a meagre living as a peddler from house to house, to sell to his fellow patients. In response to his question I suggested 20 Rappen [0.20 sFr, 1936] per card as the selling price.

Fig. 56 Deaf–mute half-cretin busy with his *Meccano*

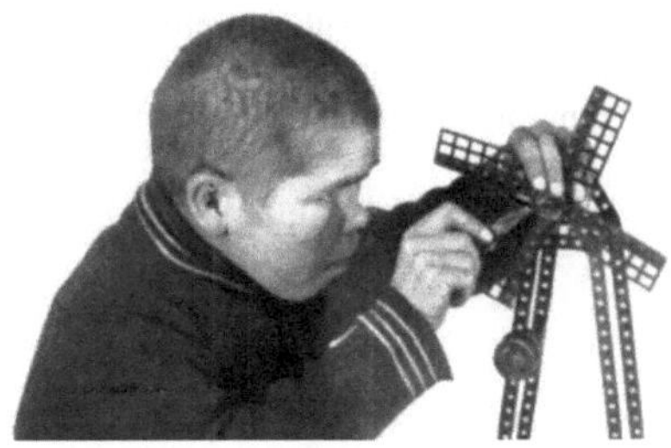

His laconic reply was, "And if someone were to give me 25 Rappen?" The inability to invent something new, even to enjoy novelties, makes him a pronounced conservative and, as far as he can be considered political, a supporter of the so-called 'Conservatives'. In other words he is a classic 'subject'. Regions where cretinism, so to speak, forms the substrate are therefore unsuitable for revolutionary experiments.

The grasp of barely taught concepts is supported by a retentive memory. Even high-grade cretins months later recognize a person who has been pleasant to them e.g. by giving them sweets, even though they saw them only once. Also, as Rösch and Maffei have emphasized, their memory of location is superb, as a rule – the cretin, with his customary observation, never once forgets the route that he took.

> The cretin who has left his hut has nobody whom he can ask, and yet he finds his way back by retracing his route. Seldom does a cretin get lost. People are so certain of this memory of location in the mountain valleys that they never escort a cretin home.
>
> He also finds his way on complicated journeys. When the 'house cretin' of our clinic goes on a visit into the mountains, he takes himself off to the railway station without bothering about a travel plan, presents his ticket and then calmly waits until a train departs. Time and itineraries play no role for this fortunate type of person. Anyhow, after the expiry of his return ticket the man promptly presents himself again and begins the preliminaries for his next furlough immediately, with the comment that his brother had invited him again for next year.

In the same way as with elementary school knowledge, certain concepts of understanding can be taught to cretins without their being capable of picking up the deeper meaning.

A deaf–mute, dwarf cretin woman, incapable of any work, was given cherries by the institution physician, with a friendly, cheery stroke of the cheek. She cast an inimitable comic–serious side-glance at the director of the institution, who was some distance away, because she had been taught that close-confiding was not tolerated – and then gave herself over to gobbling the cherries with relish.

In the next bed to an older cretin was a senile-demented patient who occasionally unnecessarily bared his backside. The cretin, without saying a word, took a needle and stuck it into the exposed body part as a moral lesson.

Related to the conservative tendencies of cretins is their *hoarding instinct.* A proffered cigar is regarded as due, but may not be lit but stored in his pocket to be smoked at a suitable time. The cretin woman offered a bit of chocolate proceeds according to the same principles. It is totally inconceivable what might be discovered in containers among cretins.

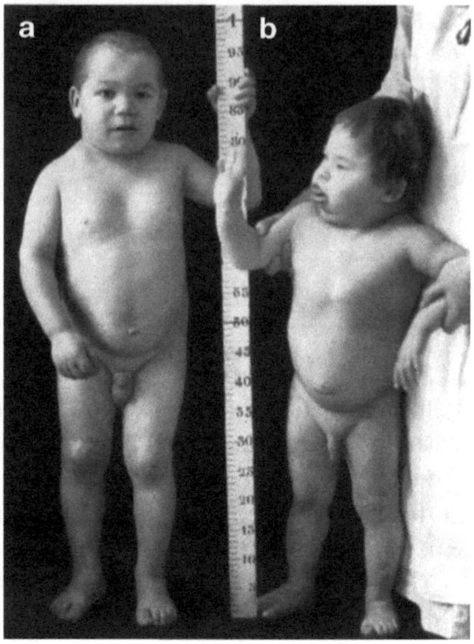

Fig. 57 (**a**) Cretin without goitre, 12 years old, histological thyroid gland atrophy; (**b**) 12-year-old athyroid (surgically managed)

A deaf–mute cretin, incapable of any kind of work, shows me his 'collection' with pride. It consists of a number of pictures of limousines, which he kept in his briefcase. He inspects my car with an appreciative expression and, by signs, he expresses the wish of being able to go for a ride.

The *drive to imitate* of many cretins is remarkable as well.

Our clinic's 'house cretin' had noticed that sick people with a fever were left in bed and that one of his fellow patients was able to make the thermometer rise artificially by rubbing. To give himself a day of rest, he made the same attempt and got it to 41°. That aroused suspicion, even though he would hardly be trusted to do such a thing. When I asked him the reason for his fever, he tried to divert the conversation, and, when this was unsuccessful, he said in a placatory manner, 'It happened only once'.

In contrast to the slow mental reaction of cretins you occasionally encounter a ready wit, reminiscent, in its originality, of what the Swiss call the 'Appenzeller punch line'.

On his Christmas table our house cretin received a packet of chocolate from the institution in whose care he had previously been. He explained to the hospital sister that he would not eat this chocolate. The institution in question should pay more attention to its cooking rather than dishing out chocolate. I asked him later what he would do with the chocolate. He answered without a moment's hesitation, 'I won't eat it, it gives me constipation'. He regarded it as imprudent to let me know the real motive behind his protest. No matter what question I throw at him, with his varied vocabulary and his barely intelligible speech he always has an answer that doesn't compromise himself. He should have been a diplomat.

Self-awareness is not totally foreign to cretins either. A 12-year-old dwarf cretin gazes down with pride at an athyroid of the same age in the same room. In his subconsciousness he is experiencing the distance separating him from the other person. The non-goitrous cretin feels, if he is capable of such thought processes, superior to the goitrous cretin, and expresses this with obvious pride. The goitrous cretin who has undergone surgery is pleased not only about the freed-up breathing but also, at least among the women, about the improved line of the neck. The cretin, too, manifestly experiences the outwardly projecting goitre as something foreign.

Tucked into this mentality is a big chunk of the popular spirit of the mountain farmers with their self-awareness, their ready wit, but also their foresight. This portion of the popular psyche has not been destroyed by cretinism but it has received a particular colouring through the unbroken optimism that good fate has bestowed on the cretin. He follows the Biblical exhortation that Man should not worry about tomorrow, because he doesn't even worry about today. The unpleasant things of life he accepts without or with only a slight grumble, and his entire day's work consists moreover of calmly enjoying the pleasant things and avoiding all the unpleasant aspects, including work, as much as possible. In this sense he interprets and relives Horace's *carpe diem*. It does not depress him that he cannot look after his own support and he would, if he thought about it at all, take it for granted that others should do this for him. When, from time to time, visitors to our charity institutions bemoan the sad fate of these most wretched of all men, we can only respond that, among the demented, the cretin is the privileged one, for nobody enjoys his life more consciously than he does. Admittedly, he does not express his satisfaction with joyous exhilaration but in calm enjoyment of sunshine and peace – a daily pattern whose sole interruption, also pleasurable, is mealtime. As for the latter, the cretin demands, first and foremost, quantity, though he does not value quality as highly.

Regarding work, the cretin comes to terms with it. However, we only noticed some enthusiasm when he observed himself, or saw himself in front of the objective lens of the movie camera. There at least several of them developed a certain, short-lived ambition. This calm enjoyment of life transforms, unnoticed, in the most severe cases into what Maffei so graphically described as *Affektlossigkeit* – periodic or long-term 'brooding'.

Given that the term 'cretin' has been derived from the word *chrétien* with the rationale 'a true Christian because he is incapable of evil', this certainly applies insofar to the middle- and high-grade cretins, who lack the intelligence necessary for a deliberate misdeed, and because for them the concepts of 'good' and 'evil' are, at most, learned. On the other hand, we occasionally see upwellings of rage, even directly dangerous to the surroundings; but usually only episodic, and rarely long-term viciousness.

Maffei says very aptly:

> Without exception, all cretins are subject to rage. With few exceptions the cretin of every type and stage does not recognize mute rage: it is always connected with grumbling, clamouring, or howling roars. Should the cretin happen to be in a full–blown rage, he is to be regarded absolutely as an uncomprehending, totally–wild animal. Without any regard, the instinct to totally destroy the thing that offended and enraged him is fully expressed and, with no choice of means, any item is welcome. Therefore people discourage angering a cretin: don't start anything with the lunatic, you don't know what will happen. With cretins

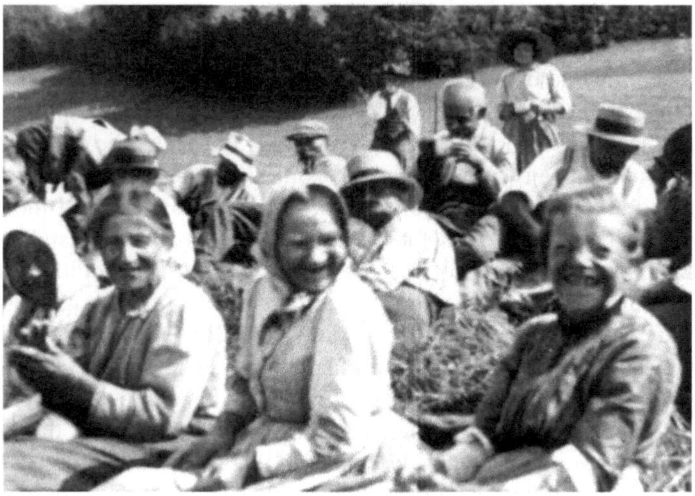

Fig. 58 Cretins in the fields, during the afternoon break

> you are never, ever, in a position to determine when, and on what occasion, and after which encounter, the rage will break out.

These observations are universally confirmed by the superintendents of our cretin institutions. Yet, the rage of the cretin does not last long. As Maffei says, the cretin cannot love anybody, nor can he hate anybody. Our clinic cretin flew into a rage over a fellow cretin who, in his opinion, had behaved in an unseemly manner. He fell upon him and beat him until he himself was out of breath. Then he calmly went to bed to recover, and the rage subsided.

As for *good-fellowship*, the cretin does not have much. He lacks the ability to communicate, and what would he have to impart? He is not equipped for chats over coffee or pub sessions. On the other hand, we see him absorbed for an hour and a day in pursuits that interest him, for instance construction work. Upon questioning, somewhat laconically he make the statement that 'the foreman bellows too much at the workers', or that 'too many people are giving orders'. He therefore has a refined sense of righteousness and sees no special rights for the foreman, 'even when he arrives in a car'.

There are exceptions to the optimism recounted above. During a visit to one of the institutions I came across an older, myxœdematous, dwarf cretin (Fig. 59) whom I knew, in the sickbay.

When I asked him what was the matter, he replied sullenly, 'People are always thinking that you're a dog and want to hang yourself.' In actual fact he had been caught attempting suicide – he was not the first. Also we have repeatedly seen delirious conditions, which necessitated spending time in a mental institution. However, neither depression nor delirium and hallucination belong in the picture of cretinism. These can occur just as often as in other individuals, and the non-cretinous inheritance of behavioural and intellectual tendencies is then added to the

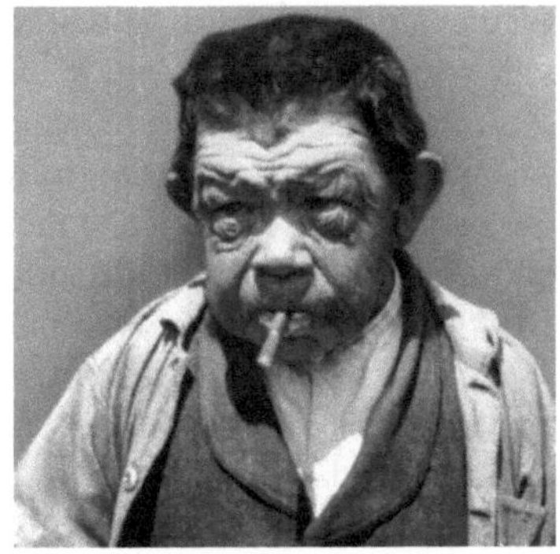

Fig. 59 Non-goitrous cretin with myxoedema

picture of cretinous degeneration where one or other of the two factors dominates the entire picture.

What has just been said relates mainly to non-goitrous, dwarf cretins, principally males. Among female dwarf cretins we found originality and personal opinion less pronounced. They *seem* not only not to think but, as a rule, they think quite little. The goitrous cretin of both sexes more closely approximates the common average. Adjoining rooms of the institutions and 4 p.m. coffee allow them to become familiar with customary conversations over coffee.

Differing from the cretin in regard to mindset is the adult with thyroid aplasia, for example from surgery. This individual retains the memory of what he once was. He is aware of what is missing and we can thus explain his depressed attitude – even to the point of suicide. Follow-up of cases of *Cachexia thyreopriva* from before 1883 during our time as registrars under Kocher dramatically revealed this difference between the inherited and the acquired form of thyroid gland insufficiency.

In the *affective side* of cretin life *gratitude* stands out most especially. Admittedly the cretin momentarily takes amiss the doctor who has requested a blood test. But the good that has been done for him goes much deeper, even when it was mixed with temporary feelings of repugnance. I count no more grateful patients than those cretins whom we had freed from respiratory difficulties by removing their goitres. Whenever I visit the institutions they express their joy with every means available, dragging along cretins still in possession of their goitre and giving me to understand by signs, if they are incapable of speech, that I should operate on them as well. When Maffei stresses that the gratitude is limited only to the memory of the perceived good and the trust emanating from it, this is true in general. In reality, the cretin is hardly in a position to evaluate goodness. Yet occasionally he tries to do just that. Our house cretin was given a good cigar. Although he is a heavy smoker, he holds it up carefully and experiences a palpable joy in handing it over to me.

In the *area of sexuality*, the cretin's affectivity is, as we have already indicated, extremely small; we could even say that in most of them it is totally lacking. This is true of males in particular. The severely afflicted and most of the moderately afflicted male cretins are generally regarded as incapable of procreation, and they also lack any affective attraction to females. Lower-grade cretins may marry, and even bring umpteen progeny into the world. The title of 'Don Juan', even 'Don Juan of the village' is, on the other hand, incompatible with the cretinous predisposition.

Among the females pregnancy is not really rare, even among middle-grade cretins, and provocation, as various observers have stressed, is more common than on the part of male cretins. She then meets with success rather among non-cretin men, and in some cases it is difficult to ascertain who actually was the perpetrator and who was the victim. I saw a half-cretin farm maid who swapped farmyards nearly every year and almost just as often came back to her community with a new child until, after the ninth child, the authorities were prompted to take the necessary steps to put an end to this fecundity through institutional care. That the level of illegitimacy is very high in the cretin region of Steiermark, as Scholz reports, does not contradict the general view of the passivity of cretins in this region. In all cretin regions there are still sufficient individuals whose sexual activity is not dampened, and for the low grade of cretinism it might be well conducted as Maffei said:

> It is the law of nature that speaks out of him and compels him to listen, unconditionally. That feeling which we call attachment, affection, or love, is foreign to all cretins. At a certain stage of life the better half-cretin rather appears to feign an approximation to this. However, on closer investigation this is nothing but sexual instinct temporarily expressed in this manner. The half-cretin woman can probably become a wife, but a wedded wife in the human sense of the word she will never be. The shamefacedness of this child of sociability appears among half-cretins, often in bizarre forms, as an acquired gesture.

Admittedly, a certain sentimentality is not uncommonly observed, even when the feelings corresponding with the cretin psyche remain superficial. When one of our second-grade cretins gave a medical registrar a brass curtain ring as a sign of her affection, a certain symbolism might be interpreted, not just by Freud.

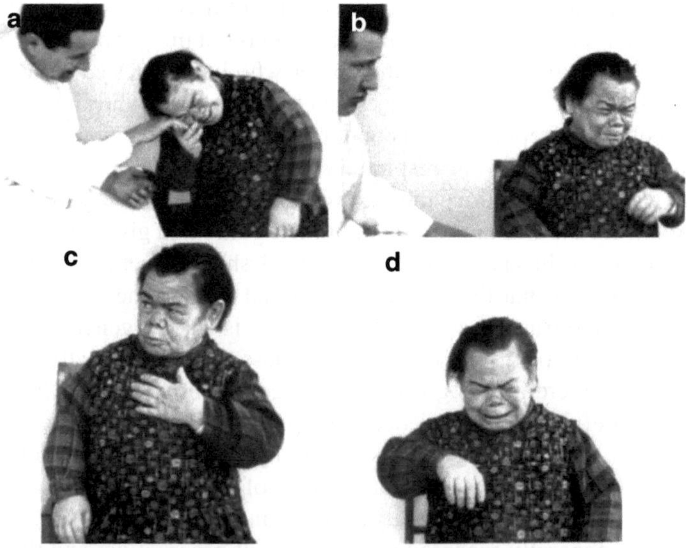

Fig. 60 Mood swings in a 60-year-old deaf–mute cretin; Grade 3

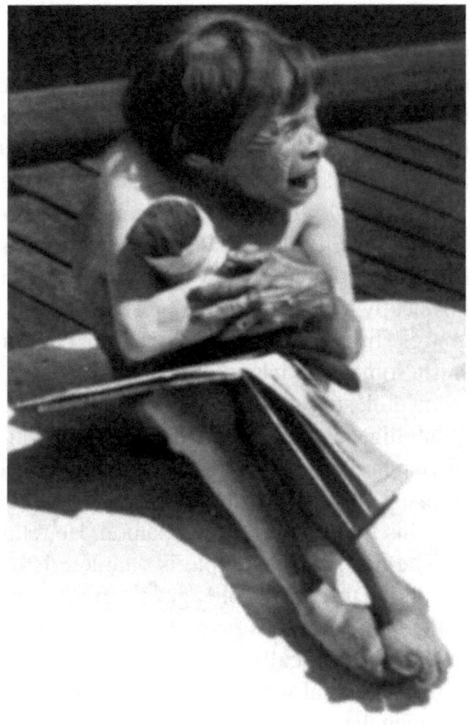

Fig. 61 The cretin woman presses the doll to her, well-nigh with passion, after the picture book has left her cold

The four pictures above were taken of a 60-year-old deaf–mute cretin incapable of any productivity, as demonstrated by her impetuous mood swings. A friendly glance from a registrar induces her to seek caresses. A stern look causes her to pause and, within seconds, brings her to tears. Then in a very short time the smiles reappear. A film star could learn from her mimicry. What might such a temperament have become without cretinism?

In other cases female half-cretins, as highlighted by Maffei, unmistakeably express their desire for sexual freedom but, here too, 'on the far side of good and evil'. Surveillance of female cretins in institutions therefore presents a greater problem than surveillance of males.

We can also observe maternal play with dolls among third-grade female cretins, for whom any sexual impulse has gone, and who generally do not exhibit any other expressions of feelings. This demonstrates how deeply rooted and how primitive is the 'maternal instinct'. For that reason, in any cultural period its regression indicates a major economic or moral decay.

When we then ask ourselves what influence the cretin's *physical type* exerts on his *mental behaviour*, we come to discoveries that are important from the scientific standpoint also.

The usually taller (i.e., skeletal build), goitrous cretin, less damaged in his dermal appendages and his sexual organs, presents a regular reduction of his intellectual abilities in general – a relatively pure form of imbecility ranging from slight awkwardness through to suspension of any intellect: in short, thyrogenic mental deficiency – thyrogenic idiocy in a pure form. In the moderate to severe cases he is simply a cretin. In the mildly to moderately severe cases on the other hand, he is endowed with a different grade of sexuality and with a procreative capacity, and likewise, those female cretins capable of impregnation are, as a rule, burdened with goitre.

In contrast with this, in the non-goitrous dwarf cretins we find a purer form of the cretin mentality described above, with a dash of originality, making the cretin more humanly empathetic towards us than is the usual mentally deficient individual. Physically and mentally, he presents a more sharply defined type than the cretin with goitre. These differences appear from childhood onward, and already the future dwarf cretin sometimes has an impish, joyful facial expression which stands in stark contrast to the dull, stupid expression of the incipient goitrous cretin. The still present vestiges of intelligence are expressed neither in good school marks nor in any ambition to gain such; nor even in a capacity for intense concentration, but in an original grasp of situations. Thus, the non-goitrous cretin exposes less of a progressive stultification than does his future goitrous companion. He retains his 'type' throughout his life.

The following example is characteristic of the psyche of the dwarf cretin from childhood through to old age: a cretin goes past the open door of the registrar's room in the clinic and sees several registrars busy with their pens. 'Communal writing' he says dryly ironically, and goes on his way. In his earlier years he often had to deal with communal writing for his peddler's licence application.

Once the cretin has learned a task, he occasionally sets himself a goal of personal satisfaction by performing to his superiors. When our clinical house cretin helpfully assisted the hospital sister in folding gauze compresses (Fig. 62a), he later proudly reported to me how many hundreds of them he had folded.

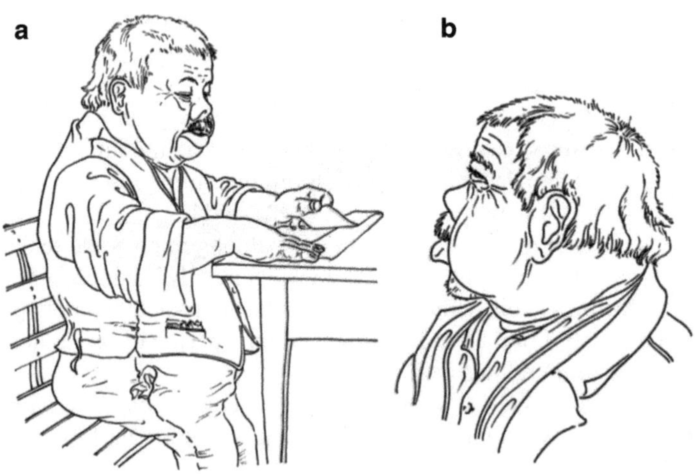

Fig. 62 (**a, b**) The clinic's house cretin folding gas compresses (sketched by one of his fellow patients)

That these two aspects of the disease belong together in spite of their differences is seen not only from the imperceptible transitions between them but also by both types often occurring in their pure form, side by side in the same family (cf. Figs. 13 and 14).

Maffei summarises the cretin's abilities as follows, regardless of the particular type:

> The cretin is given several pictures; he observes objects and forms of the outside world and memorizes them, he gathers a lot of pictures, studies several, even to recognizing many items and storing them in his memory; he is even in a position to summarize several items and their consequences in a picture – even capable of drawing a simple conclusion; – but he doesn't take it any further, he doesn't accomplish anything more, and under no circumstances does he initiate, form, or create an opinion.

This summary is accurate apart from the fact that many cretins who can be regarded as full-cretins intellectually do have a certain degree of discrimination at their disposal. We have already given sufficient examples of this.

One thing more to be noted: Never have we seen in cretins that one-sided, almost phenomenal development of intellectual capacity for numeracy that we have observed in several congenitally mentally-deficient people. Only in geographical memory are certain cretins superior to many healthy people.

We will discuss later the theoretical significance of the disparity in intellectual structure among cretins.

Chapter 6
Pathological Anatomy and Histology

In stressing the regularly-present changes in the thyroid gland in our definition of endemic cretinism, we meant not just morphological variation but also a functional deviation from the norm. The latter implies that the organs downstream from the thyroid gland will be drawn into the circle of disruptions as well, and indeed this is expressed not only in a similarly-disturbed function, but also in the form and structural changes in these organs. Not to mention that the thyroid gland to a great extent dominates growth and differentiation of the animal body – through its effect on metabolism it is in a position to influence the morphological side of cells and tissues as well. Whether all these effects can be ascribed to one and the same hormone is still unknown. The thyroxin isolated from the thyroid gland (its chemical formula made known by Harrington's investigations) might primarily control metabolism and tissue differentiation; however, at a certain dosage, it possesses characteristics for growth. Yet it is quite unlikely that the blood-borne secretion from the active thyroid gland is pure thyroxin, but rather that the thyroxin is present both in the thyroid gland and in its venous drainage, presumably in a bound form (I. Abelin). It will be our task to compare the organ changes occurring in cretinism with the subsequent conditions of definite disturbance in the thyroid gland.

We accordingly present the pathological anatomy of the thyroid gland lying at the centre of early-onset, abnormal, metabolic processes in endemic cretinism, supplemented with discussion of the other endocrine glands, and other organs and organ systems influenced by the thyroid gland.

1 Thyroid Gland

It has already been suggested that the thyroid gland in endemic cretinism displays apparently conflicting behaviour – sometimes a diminution with atrophy of the parenchyma of the gland, and at other times a very considerable goitrous enlargement. The study of the histological changes provides the key to understanding this surprising phenomenon. These histological changes are most strongly pronounced in the reduced thyroid gland. Moreover, since the most severe cases of endemic

J. Dennison et al., *Endemic Cretinism*,
DOI 10.1007/978-1-4614-0281-7_6, © Springer Science+Business Media, LLC 2011

cretinism, dwarf cretins in particular, usually present an atrophic thyroid gland, we might also expect to encounter the purest form of alterations there.

Whereas the earlier literature on cretins (Iphofen, B. Niépce, Rösch, Stahl, Langhans, Bayon) described only the usual goitrous findings, e.g. cyst formation and calcification, it was to Hanau that the honour fell of being the first to report the atrophy of the glandular epithelium and sclerosis of the stroma. His findings were soon confirmed and enlarged upon by de Coulon and Getzova, who examined a greater number of shrunken, cretinous thyroid glands. Several more cases were added later, by E. Bircher, MacCarrison, Hotz, Wydler and Muggia.

I have been able to assemble our own sample of 20 atrophic cretin thyroid glands, the greater portion from autopsy. Atrophy of such glands is often so great that the entire organ is barely larger than the normal thyroid gland of a young child or even a neonate, attaining a mass of 5–15 g (Fig. 63), whereas the normal mass in goitre-free regions is 20–25 g. It is usually grey or greyish-yellow in cross-section and the little, compact lobules are barely recognizable. Usually, with the naked eye, several greyish-red or yellowish nodules a few millimetres in diameter are visible (Fig. 64).

The active, secretory part of the gland is altered both quantitatively and qualitatively. The lobules are clearly smaller than normal, indeed often barely recognizable. Their basic units, the follicles, are similarly more or less markedly atrophied and usually have a diameter of 25–70 μ. However, there are cases where the follicles are to a great extent replaced by a solid, epithelial mass. The size of the individual epithelial cells is extraordinarily variable and, moreover, they are differentiated

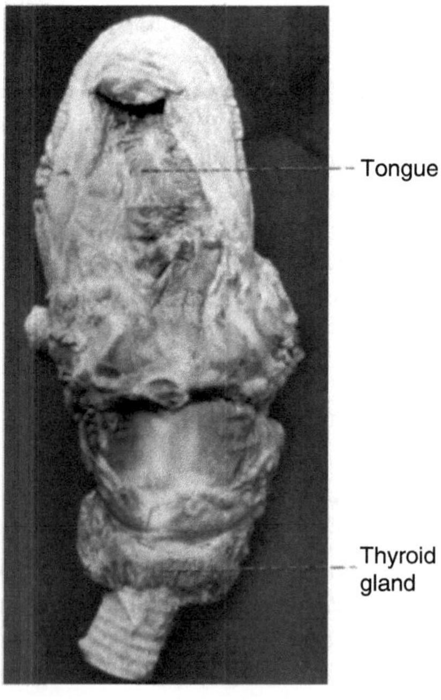

Fig. 63 Atrophic thyroid gland of a 20-year-old cretin

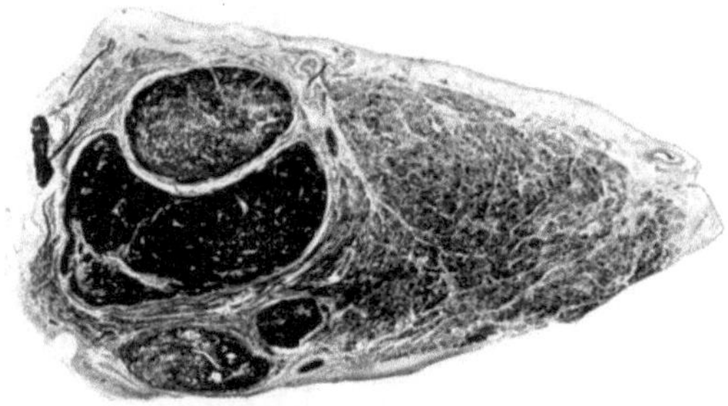

Fig. 64 Longitudinal section through a lobe of the thyroid gland of a 22-year-old cretin. Several adenomatous nodules. Gland weight 16 g×3 magnification

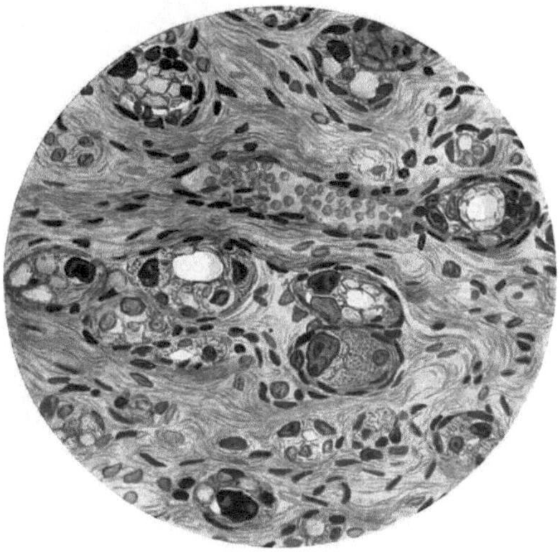

Fig. 65 Thyroid gland of a 41-year-old dwarf cretin. Atrophy of the epithelium with nuclear degeneration. Marked sclerosis

from one another only with difficulty, often being melded into a syncytium. Sometimes they are small and flattened, at other times very big, as though macerated or swollen. A few resemble signet ring cells.

The most striking feature is the condition of the nucleus, to which de Coulon and Getzova in particular have drawn our attention. Size, shape and chromatin content are extremely variable – alongside small, pyknotic and often disintegrated nuclei you may encounter real monstrosities (Fig. 65).

A few swollen nuclei reach a diameter of 30–35 μ and usually then present 'wall hyperchromatosis' with sparsely distributed chromatin granules. Other large nuclei resemble a single, regularly-stained lump of chromatin, but normal-sized nuclei very often contain agglutinated chromatin as well. The form of the nucleus is equally variable, since besides round and oval nuclei, very nearly as often you may find jagged, indented, bell-shaped, hollowed-out, flattened, mulberry-shaped, and thorn apple–shaped nuclei. Added to this is their irregular positioning. In some places, they lie tightly compacted and can form multinucleated giant cells (Fig. 66), while other sites on the follicle wall are virtually divested of nuclei.

The protoplasm of epithelial cells is thickened here and there and darkly stained, although usually pale, swollen and interspersed with numerous, frequently large fat

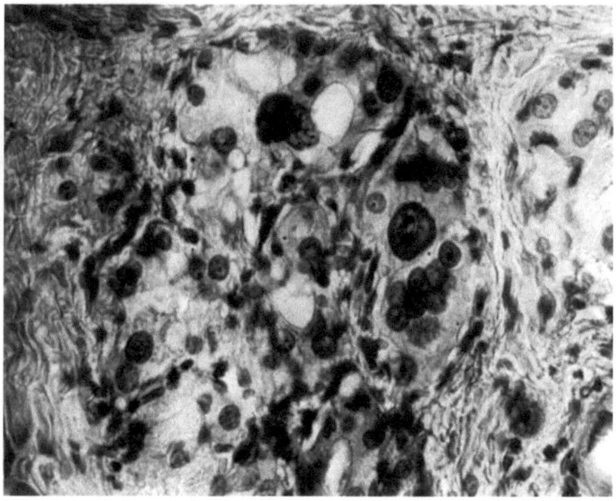

Fig. 66 Thyroid gland of a 16-year-old dwarf cretin. Multinucleated epithelial cells. Giant nuclei

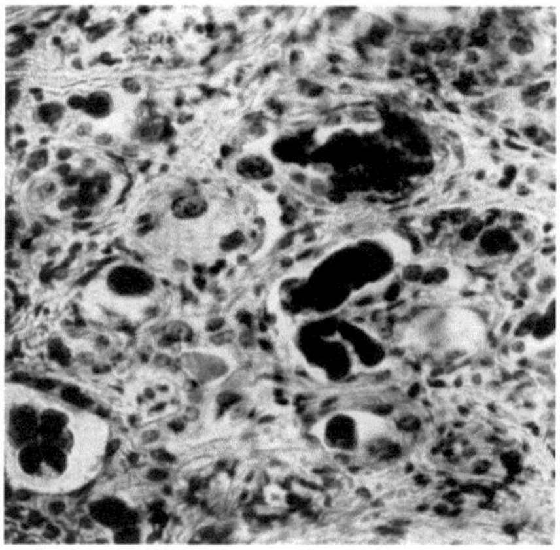

Fig. 67 Atrophic thyroid gland of a 9-year-old cretin. Clumps of thick basophilic colloid. Irregularly sized nuclei

vacuoles. I have not been able to find birefringence in these fat inclusions; from the staining characteristics, we are undoubtedly dealing with composites of neutral fats and lipids, probably phosphatides.

The fatty degeneration of the epithelium represents nothing more than a pathological increase in the normal fat deposition that increases with age. It can reach a high level even in young cretins. Besides this, congestive degeneration also occurs with fat-free vacuoles. On the other hand, I have never encountered glycogen storage.

In addition to fat, the cytoplasm often also contains a yellowish to brownish granular pigment that becomes clearly visible after the dissolution of fat, and represents nothing other than lipofuscin. This material is usually present in much greater quantities than normal for the age of the individual.

The mostly rounded or oval follicles – cylinders are rare – contain (when they are not shrunken and empty) a colloid that is quite predominantly thick, sharply defined and shines markedly (Fig. 67). Often several lumps lie alongside one another in the same follicle. According to the staining, the colloid is usually basophilic, but its border can also be eosinophilic. Vacuoles are absent, and fat droplets are found extremely rarely as inclusions in the colloid, which forms a compact mass. In the fresh state within the stain, there is a yellowish-brown or greenish tone here and there which can be based on an admixture of 'wear and tear' pigment. This colloid is certainly very old, since degeneration of the epithelium usually does not enable any fresh secretion. Since it can be resorbed only with difficulty, or not at all, during epithelial breakdown it often becomes trapped in the middle of connective tissue. Admittedly, in lower grades of atrophy you can also come across thin, eosinophilic colloid in individual vesicles. However, most colloid originates from a 'vanished secretory period' (Getzowa, 1905).

Stronger atrophy of the parenchyma never happens without simultaneous proliferation of the connective tissue. Therefore, it occurs during *sclerosis*. Again the interlobular septa are often very significantly thickened, with the periarterial connective tissue in particular proliferated, but there is also proliferation of the intralobular stroma consisting mostly of cell-deficient, coarse-fibred, connective tissue. Regeneration of elastic fibres does not take place, or only in a very small area. Here and there the stroma includes free, fat droplets, arising probably from disintegrated epithelium. Furthermore, a substitution of the broken-down glandular tissue by fat tissue is possible – the latter's big, round cells lying between the remains of the atrophic follicle – yet to a greater extent this occurs almost only in older cretins over 50 years of age (Fig. 68). However, fatty tissue proliferation can already be clearly pronounced even in the fourth decade.

I have seen lymphocyte infiltration in only a small number of cases (Fig. 69). Usually it is a case of only sparsely-distributed lymphocytes, not great clumps. The breakdown of the epithelium therefore takes place so gradually that, as a rule, it does not evoke an inflammatory reaction.

In the study of the *vascular system*, it is most surprising that in the cretin's atrophic thyroid gland, the arteries relatively rarely present sclerotic changes, whereas, according to the investigations of Isenschmid, Sanderson, Schaer and Clerc, sclerotic

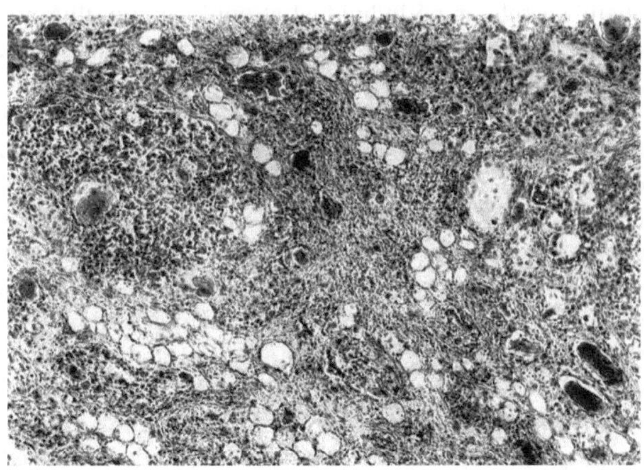

Fig. 68 Atrophic thyroid gland of a 57-year-old cretin. Fatty tissue replacing glandular tissue

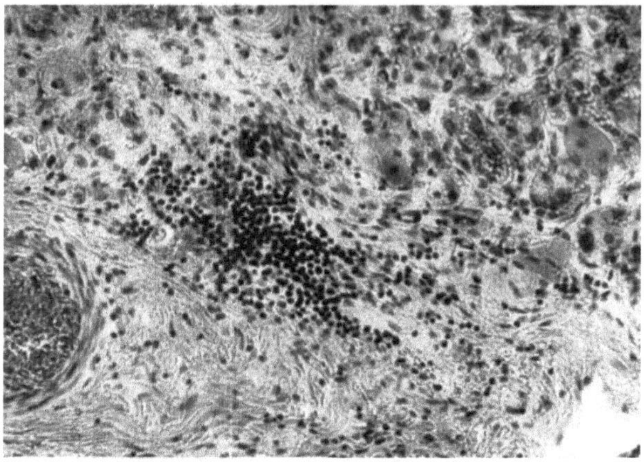

Fig. 69 Thyroid gland of a 75-year-old cretin. Infiltration of lymphocytes into interlobular tissue

changes are very common in the goitrous glands of non-cretinous individuals, with onset even during childhood. This demonstrates that the atrophy cannot be the outcome of vascular alterations. Only among older cretins do we encounter here and there thickening of the *intima* by hyaline transformation and fatty degeneration, as well as splitting up of the *Elastica interna*. However, I have never seen the calcification of the internal elastic membrane very common elsewhere. In the small arteries, the buds that project from the intima into the lumen, as discovered by M.B. Schmidt in the normal gland and extensively described by Getzowa, are very beautiful to see. Recently, however, these have been explained by Gilpin as simple indentations by portions of the vascular wall, while Kux, quite rightly in my opinion, regards them as muscular sphincters. The veins as a rule are wide, and filled with blood or coagulated serum. The capillaries, too, are often quite well developed; they lie on the inner surface of the thickened, intralobular septa and cause the epithelium to arch a little inwards. On the whole, you get the impression that the blood supply of the vesicles is no worse than in the normal situation. Where the epithelium has decayed or forms only little lumps, you can even find entire balls of capillaries. Finally, as for the lymphatic vessels, in no individual atrophic, cretin, thyroid gland have I seen any lymphatic vessels filled with homogenous, colloid-like content, which belongs with the characteristic picture of the normal thyroid gland.

The uniformity of atrophy and sclerosis is interrupted at this point by *regenerative epithelial proliferations*, hardly ever absent from any gland. Very often they resemble the extremely small adenoma dispositions described by Hitzig, Michaud, Krämer and others. Very small, indistinctly delineated groups of vesicles are raised up from their surroundings through a well-maintained epithelium with small, regular cells, and dark, round nuclei. The protoplasm of this epithelium is mostly fat-free, more basophilic and markedly bordered against the lumen, or there is a branching duct with a cylindrical or cuboid epithelium, similar to the so-called central canal of the normal glandular lobules (Aschoff), from which small vesicles pinch off or rebuild by budding. Such vesicles often contain thin, eosinophilic colloid with vacuoles – secretion is therefore in full spate, and since

Fig. 70 Horseshoe-shaped, large-nodular goitre of a 31-year-old cretin, 161 cm tall (From Wydler (1926))

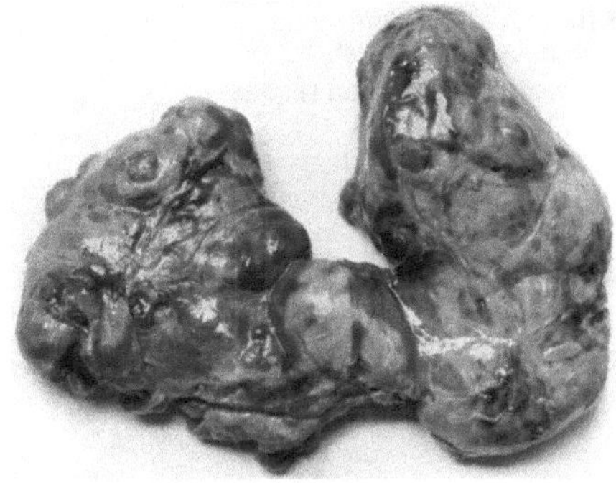

the removal is often not always adequate, small cysts may form, often reaching a diameter of 1 mm. Admittedly, in such circumscribed epithelial proliferations degeneration may set in again, evoking the same changes as in the original gland epithelium.

However, if the proliferation proceeds further, then gradually typical, sharply defined adenoma nodules develop, peculiar to common *Struma nodosa* or nodulous goitre (Fig. 64). Here, the adjacent, more or less atrophic, thyroid gland lobules are compromised by the growing nodules, so that the remnants of the gland tissue often perish completely. The nodules are then encased in thick capsules of pure connective tissue. There are atrophic or normal-sized glands that are suffused with numerous small nodules, so that it is often difficult to find the remnants of the original glandular lobules.

These types of cases mark the transition from the atrophic to the *goitrous cretin thyroid gland*, that is often quite markedly enlarged and frequently even hugely enlarged (Fig. 70). Since they lead not uncommonly to breathing difficulties and give cause for surgical removal, it is no coincidence that this form has been studied particularly from the surgical aspect (E. Bircher, Hotz, Wydler). However, in order to be able to evaluate the entity of cretinous goitre, it is essential to separate clearly adenoma nodules and original thyroid gland tissue (Wydler's so-called intermediate tissue). Unfortunately, E. Bircher's extensive material did not satisfy this demand.

The cretinous goitre, particularly in by far the greatest number of cases, is a nodular goitre (struma nodosa), as emerges very clearly from Wydler's investigations. Of his 106 cases, only two were purely diffuse goitres – all the others contained nodules and, of these, 90 matched pure *struma nodosa*, i.e., the enlargement was caused solely by adenoma nodules.

As to the nature of this goitre, it is mainly parenchymatous nodular goitre, i.e., trabecular, small-follicular, and tubular adenoma. Wydler found this type in 60 of his 106 cases, and combined with colloid nodules in a further 23 cases. Thus, epithelial proliferation in the nodules predominates by far, with solid epithelial cords often occupying great areas of the nodules. Issuing from these, through further differentiation, are short ducts or, more commonly, small, round vesicles (Fig. 71) which often hang together like chains, often even forming broad strands very similar to Langhans' proliferating goitres. Transitions into a malignant growth do in fact

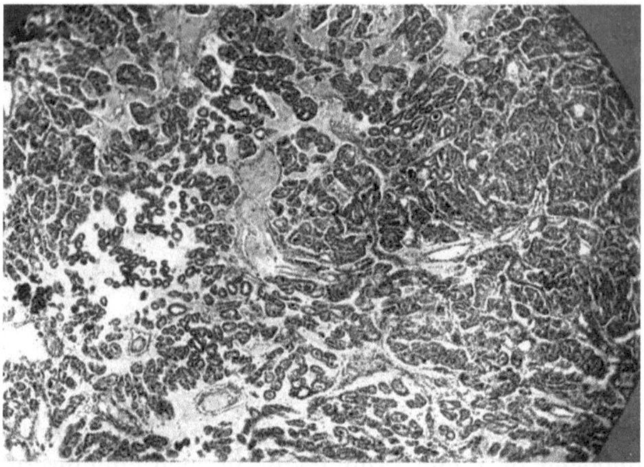

Fig. 71 *Struma nodosa parenchymatosa* of a 43-year-old full cretin (From Wydler (1926))

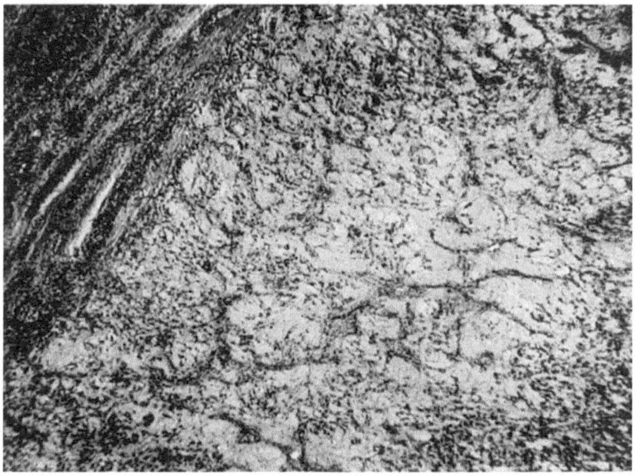

Fig. 72 *Struma nodosa parenchymatosa* with mucous degeneration of an 11-year-old cretin girl

occur – in four cretins I saw a *malignant epithelial goitre* of the common carcinoma type or proliferating goitre.

In the nodular epithelium then, the same degenerations often occur as in the epithelium of the cretin's atrophic thyroid glands. The above nuclear changes in particular are very often encountered (de Coulon, Wydler) and, like Wydler, I have very often seen severe levels of adiposis. This can even be more marked than in the surrounding thyroid gland tissue. Mucous degeneration of the epithelium also occurs (Fig. 72). I have asked myself whether the mucous accumulation could be the expression of a particular metabolic disturbance, as, for example, in myxœdema of the skin, but so far I have been unable to obtain any definite grounds for this interpretation, since mucous degeneration is not at all uncommon in the goitre of non-cretins either.

Regressive changes in the stroma are very common in the parenchymatous nodules of the cretin goitre, such as hyaline degeneration with secondary adiposis and calcification, with the fat and lime depositions occurring primarily in the area around the blood vessels. The calcification often transforms a nodule into a stone-hard mass; here and there, genuine ossification is associated with the calcification.

Far more rare than the parenchymatous nodules are the colloid nodules, which occur unadulterated only seven times in Wydler's material; although in 23 cases they are found in conjunction with parenchymatous nodules. The colloid content of such nodules can be significant, with congestion of the content leading to the tearing down of the septa and coalescing of the vesicles. The colloid presents varying consistency and, accordingly, stains more darkly or lightly with eosin. Thin colloid may also contain pale vacuoles. The epithelium varies in height and is always cylindrical over the cushion-shaped bulges where regeneration of small vesicles takes place through proliferation and pinching off. The stroma of such nodules shows overall less tendency to hyaline transformation and other regressive processes than does the stroma of the parenchymatous nodules; also, the colloid nodules as a rule remain smaller.

Thus, Wydler's finding, that the 'intermediate tissue' – the thyroid gland tissue remaining between the nodules – exhibits more or less pronounced degeneration, as is characteristic of the cretin's atrophic thyroid gland, is significant. This degeneration is not only the consequence of pressure on the part of the expansively growing nodules, but occurs also in places removed from the nodules that are no longer subject to pressure (Wydler). *Therefore the original thyroid gland tissue behaves in the same manner in both the reduced and the enlarged nodular cretin thyroid gland*, hence both forms are based on a common denominator. The nodular, by far the most common form of cretin goitres, differs from the atrophic thyroid gland only by the presence of larger nodules.

The *extremely strong vascularisation of the cretin goitre* should be mentioned. According to Wangensteen's investigations, the afferent arteries are often hugely enlarged so that they look like big trunks. In several cases, the inferior thyroid artery reaches a diameter of 9 mm (normally about 3 mm). Sclerotic changes, early onset in non-cretin goitres also, occur in arteries of every calibre, but particularly in the larger and medium branches – a very common feature. However, besides the arteries, the capillaries often show quite considerable enlargement; Wangensteen describes giant capillaries with a diameter of 0.029 mm lying in the lobules of the atrophic thyroid gland.

Furthermore, in the atrophic intermediate tissue of the nodular goitres, *clumps of lymphocytes* are not uncommonly found, often in the form of lymph follicles. Wydler found these collections of lymphocytes sometimes in the capsules and septa of the nodules and sometimes in the intra- and interlobular stroma. Their occurrence indicates that in this situation, the nodular cretin goitre behaves like other goitres and does not occupy a special place, as von Werdt thought. The infiltrations of lymphocytes are most probably the result of a rapid breakdown of glandular cells from the pressure of the nodules, assuming toxic or bacterial-toxic damage is not present (e.g. in iodine treatment or infections).

If we survey the totality of the changes described so far, and attempt to estimate the performance of such a thyroid gland, there can be no doubt that this is a *functionally poor quality organ*. It is, for example, impossible to imagine that such a high degree of degeneration of the epithelium as found in many atrophic and sclerotised glands permits normal secretion. Thus, clinical signs of *hypothyroidism* are regularly encountered in such cases, often reaching a most severe level.

The low biological value of atrophic thyroid glandular tissue is confirmed by its examination in Gudernatsch's tadpole test. While the effect of a normal thyroid gland is expressed in a restriction of growth and an acceleration of development, M. Branovacky found only a slight hint of growth limitation and a weak effect on development (five cases). In a further case from Branovacky-Pelech, the atrophic intermediate tissue of a cretin nodular goitre showed itself to be somewhat more active, particularly in the sense of a pronounced restriction of growth.

In the nodular cretin goitre we can certainly ask ourselves whether the degeneration of the original thyroid gland tissue is not offset by the newly formed tissue of the adenoma nodules. However, we know that the adenoma nodules are capable of preparing a secretion that is seen to be effective in both the tadpole test and Asher's rat test (sensitivity to lack of acid – Graham, Wegelin and Abelin, Hara, Branovacky) and can at least be partially absorbed by the organism. The best examples of this are the cases of so-called toxic adenoma, which show clear symptoms of hyperthyroidism. What is the situation in cretins?

According to de Quervain, the goitrous cretin (as opposed to the cretin with an atrophic thyroid gland) usually possesses a competitive edge, evident either in the physical or intellectual sphere or in both. Since the intermediate tissue in such cases often presents the most severe form of atrophy, we are almost persuaded to ascribe at least part of the gland's function to nodules with which the extremely rich blood supply of such goitres may be related. For example, Wangensteen interprets the extraordinary size of the supplying arteries as being a compensatory mechanism – maximal blood supply to a poorly functioning organ allows retrieval of maximum secretion.

If you examine the content of effective substance in the nodular tissue by the tadpole test, it shows only a weak effect or none at all (Dubois), or a slowing of development and a weak restriction of growth (M. Branovacky). That development cannot be promoted through cretin goitre but may even be slowed, is, perhaps, to construe a *dysthyrosis* in the sense of a change in the quality of secretion. In a further case from Branovacky-Pelech, the nodular tissue showed itself to be active both in relation to promoting development and in growth restriction. The iodine content of such nodules is small.

This therefore confirms that the thyroid gland of the cretin in both its atrophic and its goitrous forms is less able to perform at widely varying levels. In general, the functional insufficiency is more strongly pronounced in the atrophic thyroid gland than in the goitrous gland.

However, there are rare cases of cretinism where we encounter not a nodular goitre but a *diffuse* goitre (Scholz, Hotz, Doubler, Klose and Hellwig, Wydler). Almost always these are in young cretins, usually during childhood or puberty. The histological picture of such goitre usually matches *Struma diffusa parenchymatosa* (Fig. 73), of a small-follicle, very colloid-deficient type, (seldom a *Struma diffusa colloides* dominated usually by a very strong polymorphism of the vesicles with cushion-shaped and papilla formations), which is strongly reminiscent of a Basedow

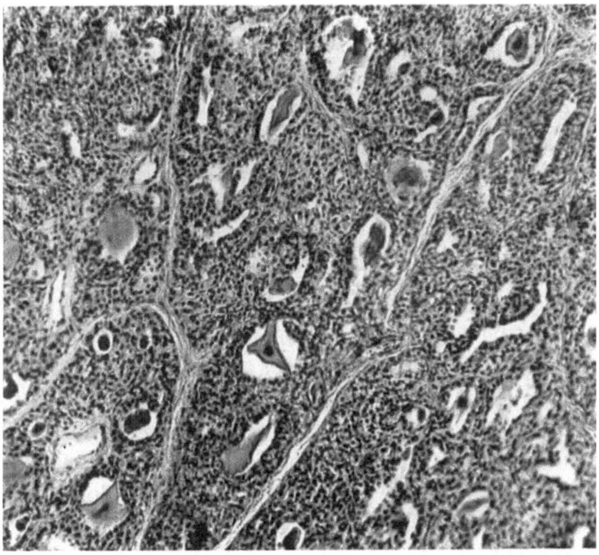

Fig. 73 *Struma diffusa parenchymatosa* of a 7-year-old cretinoid boy

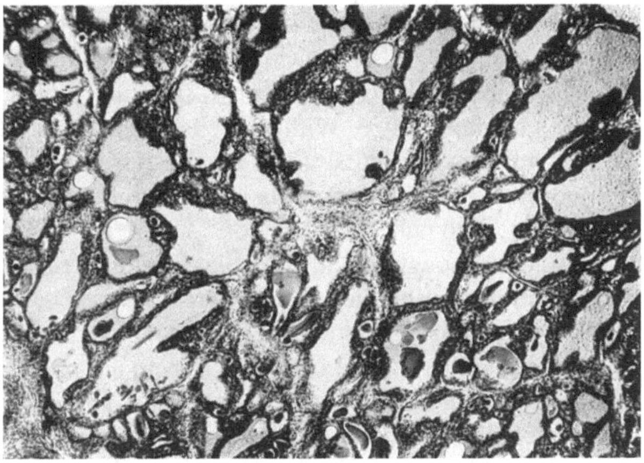

Fig. 74 *Struma diffusa colloides proliferans* of an 11-year-old cretinoid girl

goitre (Fig. 74) in many cases. Admittedly, this diffuse proliferation of the thyroid gland tissue is present in a pure form only extremely exceptionally – usually smaller nodules have developed as well in such goitres, histologically often mimicking the thyroid gland tissue type. Wydler, for example, records only two pure, diffuse goitres in his material but, on the other hand, 14 combined forms. Among the latter he mentions three diffuse colloidal goitres – one with parenchymatous nodules and two with colloidal nodules. Hotz saw a colloidal goitre on four occasions, but these were a small-follicle type.

In such goitres, a functional inferiority is not immediately obvious from the histological picture. Indeed, given the Basedow-like picture, you could even ask yourself whether there was not increased activity of the thyroid gland.

Hotz talks of a stimulus situation and increased secretion, and traces the successful outcome of a thyroidectomy in such cases back to a reduction of the goitre. Clinically, we are usually dealing with physically milder cases; growth restrictions and other physical symptoms are often less pronounced, and cyclic disturbances reminiscent of thyrotoxic effects (Doubler) are even found here and there. Admittedly, in the intellectual sphere, there may be total dementia. I have seen a *Struma diffusa et nodosa parenchymatosa* in a 29-year-old cretin, 145 cm tall, who could not speak at all. In other cases, the mental disturbance is negligible – we are dealing more with cretinoids.

However, it is still important to emphasize that in such diffuse goitres, the signs of a partial degeneration of the glandular epithelium are not lacking, as Wydler also points out. The nuclear changes are often very pronounced; more severe fatty degenerations also occur and, besides lobules with larger colloid-containing vesicles, these were markedly atrophic in Wydler's colloid goitres. It is therefore likely that, in these diffuse goitres too, only a portion of the gland tissue is functioning properly. However, it must be conceded that such histological pictures occur also in goitrous patients who clinically present only very mild symptoms of hypothyroidism or are euthyroid.

The cretin's diffuse goitre is therefore differentiated, by its almost fully parenchymatous character, from the diffuse goitre that occurs in goitre regions free of cretinism such as Holland, Danzig and most endemic regions of North America, that is predominantly or exclusively diffuse and that is often simultaneously small-nodular colloidal goitre. With this characteristic, it aligns itself with the diffuse parenchymatous goitre that forms the rule during the first decade of life also among euthyroids or mild hypothyroids in the Berne endemic region, and is often maintained right up to puberty.

Thus, even though the diffuse goitres among cretins also represent an exception, their occurrence still indicates that *there is no typical thyroid gland finding in cretinism*. Degenerations can indeed deform the entire thyroid gland into a virtually rudimentary organ, but, on the other hand, there are proliferation processes that seldom lead to a diffuse goitre but usually to a nodular goitre, creating a highly variable histological picture. We cannot speak of a specific cretin goitre (E. Bircher). This fact must be considered in any case in an attempt to explain the pathogenesis of cretinism.

In all the diversity of form, however, there remains one common feature, namely, the *tendency of the glandular tissue towards degeneration with the frequent outcome being atrophy and sclerosis*. This degeneration can set in early, as demonstrated in Schlaginhaufer and Wagner von Jauregg's observation: in the normal-sized thyroid gland of a 4-year-old cretin boy they found the most severe nuclear changes, described also by de Coulon and Getzova. Similarly, MacCarrison found atrophy and sclerosis in a cretin boy child whose age was unfortunately not recorded, and I too have seen pronounced epithelial degeneration and increase in connective tissue in cretin siblings aged 7 years and 10 years, and also in a 10-year-old boy and a 9-year-old girl whose growths were markedly retarded. Degeneration of glandular epithelium can therefore set in during the first decade.

Since the thyroid gland shows similar changes in old age (Clerc), we could describe glandular atrophy in the cretin as premature regression, *Senilitas praecox*, admittedly with circumscribed regeneration of the epithelium leading to the nodule formation that occurs also in the nodular hyperplasias and adenomas of old age.

Finally, we mention that in the thyroid gland of cretins you often come across *nests of squamous epithelium*, often also forming branching strands. These are probably nothing more than abnormal differentiations of the thyroglossal duct, which was in a position to provide stratified squamous epithelium along its entire course. Furthermore, Getzova has on occasion seen branchiogenic derivatives such as *dispersed aggregations of parathyroid cells* and remnants of the *ultimobranchial body* in the cretin thyroid gland. She suspects that the premature atrophy of the thyroid gland tissue promotes the preservation of the ultimobranchial remnants of the gland. In any case, they are more easily found than in a normal-sized organ.

2 Parathyroid Glands

The epithelial corpuscles (parathyroid glands) of cretins show in size, number and histological structure no deviations from the norm (Bayon, Scholze, Getzova, Schlaginhaufer and Wagner von Jauregg, E. Bircher, Wegelin), thus proving that they are totally self-supporting organs, independent of the thyroid gland. Also, during severe atrophy of the thyroid gland, you do not see any compensatory enlargement of the parathyroid glands. The oxyphilic cells that increase in number with age are in no way augmented, so you cannot talk of premature aging of the parathyroid glands. In the odd case, they are almost totally absent. Likewise, the appearance of colloid-containing follicles is rare. In any case, the parathyroid glands show no approximation to the thyroid gland type.

The clinical picture also corresponds with this morphological behaviour, since the function of the parathyroid glands is only rarely disturbed (Pineles), and de Quervain never saw the classical picture of parathyroid inadequacy among Swiss cretins.

Admittedly, cretins in the Himalayan region behave differently – MacCarrison quite often encountered the scenario of 'nervous cretinism', i.e., signs of tetany and of a spastic cerebral diplegia among children. Autopsy of one such case revealed that the parathyroid glands were completely absent. Whether they had never formed or whether they had secondarily decayed could not be determined. However, MacCarrison's statement that he had found marked fibrosis in the parathyroid glands of artificially cretinous rats supports the idea of secondary loss. Recently, nervous disturbances like those described by MacCarrison have been observed by Simons among the cretins of Sumatra.

3 Thymus

Since autopsy material available so far has usually involved cretins aged 30 years and over, we must also take into account the physiological involution characteristic of this age group. In addition, accidental involution may occur during illness, as

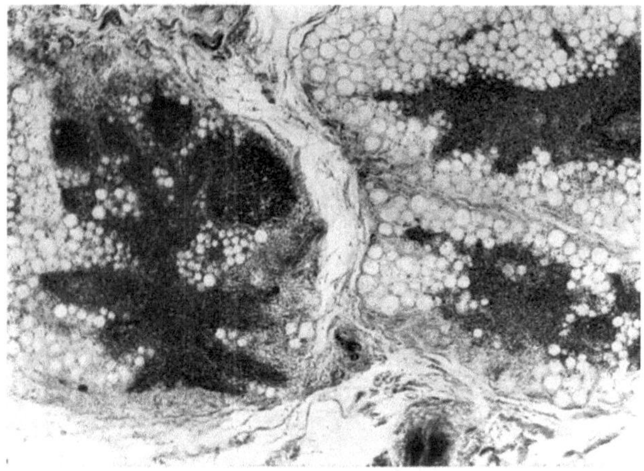

Fig. 75 Thymus of a 19-year-old cretin; marked involution; replacement of the cortex by fatty tissue

drawn to our attention particularly by Hammar. However, we also have to consider the latter form of involution among younger cretins, so that actually only those cases where death has occurred through accident or through very rapid onset illness can reveal the true picture of the thymus.

Unfortunately, the usable material is extraordinarily sparse. The 4-year-old child autopsied by Schlaginhaufer was rachitic; another illness went unreported. That particular thymus was small – only a few remnants were imbedded in the adipose tissue and connective tissue. In a 12-year-old cretin, Scholz saw a large thymus 'of regularly homogeneous parenchyma'. I found very small, microscopically markedly regressed thymus glands (Fig. 75) in a 19-year-old cretin who had died of acute influenza, a 22-year-old with glioblastoma, and in a 29-year-old who died on the day following thyroidectomy. A 17-g thymus only became available from a 26-year-old woman who had died of post-partum haemorrhage. However, microscopically it was already heavily permeated with adipose tissue and revealed only small lobules. It contained very big, necrotic, and often calcified Hassall's corpuscles. The same picture, although to a very severe degree, was revealed by the thymuses of juvenile cretins who had suffered chronic consumptive diseases.

Even greater was the regression in most of the over 30-year-old cretins. As a rule, only narrow medullary strands, with a few often markedly adipose Hassall's corpuscles, were to be found by microscope in these cases. The sole exception was the thymus of a 49-year-old woman who had died the day after excision of a Langhan's proliferating goitre.

In this case, the thymus was well maintained, weighed 17 g, with no microscopic signs of involution. It presented a wide cortex throughout, and a well-developed medulla with numerous, mostly necrotic and partially calcified Hassall's corpuscles, whose diameter was mostly 150–200 μ.

Even today a final opinion on the thymus condition in endemic cretinism is not possible. Although it appears that in most cases premature involution of this organ takes place, the last mentioned case shows that the involution may not occur right into the fifth decade, so that it is quite correct to talk of a persisting thymus. Admittedly, the grounds for this escape our knowledge. In any case, a restricting influence on the part of the genital organs cannot be the only cause, for otherwise, given the frequency of gonadal hypoplasia, thymus persistence would have to occur much more often.

In congenital athyrosis the thymus is generally small, wasting away to a premature, probably accidental involution. However, developmental restriction is not impossible in the odd case. Also, according to information from most researchers, thyroid gland removal in young animals led to thymus involution; only a few found subsequent enlargement of the thymus.

4 Hypophysis

The familiar close connections between hypophysis and thyroid gland have recently been confirmed and consolidated by the detection of thyrotropic hormones in the anterior lobes of the hypophysis. This proves that the anterior lobe of the hypophysis has a high-level influence on the thyroid gland, and that via the thyroid gland it develops an effect on metabolism as well.

As the investigations initiated by Rogowitsch and Stieda demonstrated, absence of the thyroid gland can evoke changes in the hypophysis, and therefore we cannot be surprised that the hypophysis, too, differs from the normal structure in endemic cretinism. It presents an enlargement involving only the anterior lobes. In my earlier material (*Handbuch von Henke-Lubarsch*, vol. 8), 20 out of 24 hypophyses were hyperplastic and, in cases studied since then, 9 of 11 hypophyses were hyperplastic. While the normal hypophyseal weight averages 0.6 g, the weights of cretins' hypophyses reached 0.7–1.8 g, indeed in one of B. Nièpce's cases 2.42 g. Generally, the enlargement in youthful cretins is more significant than in the aged, which can probably be explained by regression in old age. Yet the expansion of the *sella turcica* indicates that there was previously a considerable hyperplasia of the hypophysis; indeed, with shrunken hypophyses this can even reveal the original state.

Attracting attention histologically, particularly in the frontal parts of the anterior lobe, are broad strands of big cells rich in protoplasm, strongly reminiscent of gravid cells (Fig. 76). Sometimes they are just as large, with the fine, eosinophilic granulation of gravid cells. Then again, other cells have a more homogeneous protoplasm, slightly basophilic in places, and these are somewhat smaller, resembling more the transitional cells between the chief cells and the basophilic cells described by Kraus. Often you also find typical basophilic cells distributed among these strands, while eosinophilic cells are rare, occurring in greater numbers only in the lateral portions of the anterior lobe. The finest example I saw of this structure was in a 39-year-old male cretin (Fig. 76). However, there are also cases where these big cells are sparse, and the small chief cells with pale protoplasm predominate. In older cretins, over 50 years, the proportions once more approach the norm, with the chief cells being

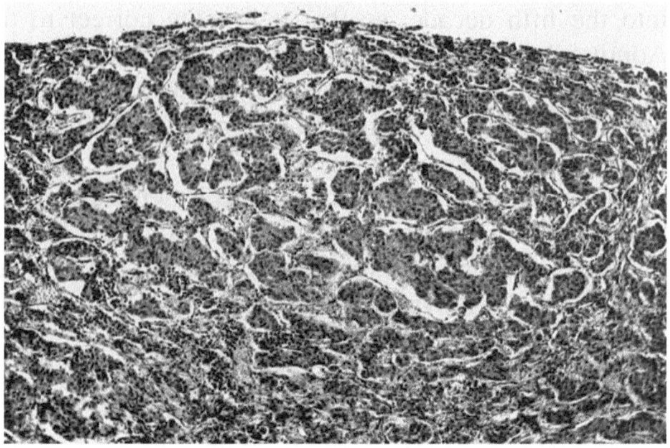

Fig. 76 Adenohypophysis of a 39-year-old cretin; broad strands of large chief cells

small and the eosinophilic cells being more numerous. In younger cretins, the basophilic cells are rather less frequently found than normal.

It remains to be mentioned furthermore that nuclear irregularities occur in the big cells of the anterior lobe. These are often reminiscent of those in the thyroid gland epithelium, e.g. abnormally big nuclei, sometimes clumped or swollen, sometimes also square or jagged. Similarly, the protoplasm can appear vacuolated or shredded, which can, however, probably be traced back to the influences of terminal illness. I have only occasionally seen colloid-containing vesicles, or concentrically layered blocks of calcium. The stroma is delicate, the capillaries often enlarged. In odd cases, I found small, chief cell adenomas with poorly-defined borders.

In the intermediate zone, there are colloid-containing fissures and vesicles in varying quantities and sizes, and in the posterior lobe the familiar strands of basophils occur occasionally. The pigment content of the glial cells of the posterior lobe varies within broad ranges; it is sometimes quite small among elderly cretins; among younger cretins, on the other hand, it is quite considerable – there is no hard–and-fast rule.

In the great majority of cases therefore, the cretin's hypophysis shows a *hyperplasia of the anterior lobe*, primarily involving the chief cells. This picture corresponds with the changes to be found in congenital athyrosis and *cachexia thyreopriva* in the hypophysis (Wegelin), and probably has its origin in inadequate function of the thyroid gland. Naturally, we will have to pose the question: how does the hypophyseal hyperplasia arise? Berblinger sees the authoritative influence in the metabolic change brought about by the hypothyrosis, and I, too, regard it as conceivable that metabolic products arising from athyrosis or hypothyrosis cause the hypophyseal chief cells to hypertrophy. Berblinger rejects a compensatory hyperplasia of the hypophysis in poor-quality thyroid glands, because the same hypophyseal changes are to be found in the total absence of the thyroid gland as are to be found in mild hypothyrosis, and because the hypophyseal change is not eliminated by substitution therapy with thyroid gland. The latter hypothesis is correct, because I too was able to determine the increase and enlargement of the chief cells in a case of *cachexia thyreopriva* that had been treated for years with thyroid gland preparations. However, in that particular case, the result of substitution therapy was incomplete. Since the thyroid gland and the anterior lobe of the hypophysis are growth glands, I consider it not impossible that in the case of a thyroid gland breakdown, a certain compensation comes about on the part of the anterior lobe of the hypophysis, and the big cells, which resemble gravid cells, generally enable physical growth, while without this assistance growth might have remained totally static. When growth is stimulated in thyroidectomized rats by adding anterior lobe of hypophysis to their feed (Larson), it demonstrates at least that the hypophysis can partially replace the thyroid gland.

You might also think that in atrophic thyroid glands a heightened need of thyrotrophic hormone would trigger hyperplasia of the anterior lobe of the hypophysis. However, this opinion is rejected because, in the total absence of the thyroid gland, i.e., omission of the downstream organ, the same change of the hypophysis comes to fruition.

I might therefore consider it likely that the big cells of the anterior lobe are the preparation site of Evans' growth hormone, for which there is an even greater need during pregnancy.

5 Pineal Gland

According to the sparse investigations in cretins so far, the pineal gland appears to be just as variable in size as in normal individuals. I have never encountered a definite enlargement. My own experience with seven pineal glands also supports the normal microscopic appearance – in particular I have always found a good development of the pineal cells, arranged in broad strands and clumps. The amount of *corpora arenacea* is often rather small, as has already been reported by Bayon. This was interpreted as a childhood condition, yet this is in no way a constant finding. In any case, according to the tissue picture, there are no signs of a disturbance of pineal gland function.

6 Suprarenal Glands

The suprarenal glands in cretins are somewhat smaller than in normal individuals. According to Schilf and Rössle, and Roulet, the mass of each suprarenal gland ranges between 11 and 14.5 g; among 25 cretins I find a minimum of 4.1 g, a maximum of 14 g and a mean mass of 8.8 g. The great majority of cases (17) had a mass of 8–14 g; in five cases it was 6–7 g; and in three cases 4.1–5.2 g.

Any kind of dependence of suprarenal gland mass on the degree of thyroid gland atrophy could not be determined, just as, according to Schilf, in normal dissection material there is no dependence of thyroid gland mass on suprarenal gland mass. Nor can fatal illnesses explain the weight reduction of suprarenal glands in cretins, since the mass of the suprarenal glands is generally independent of health and nutritional levels, and is barely influenced by illness (Schilf).

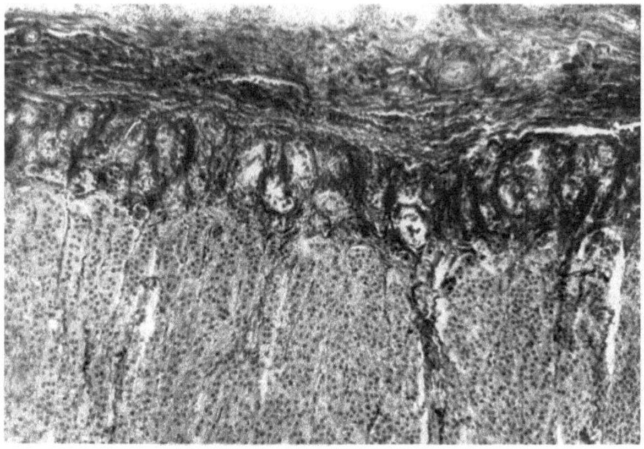

Fig. 77 Suprarenal gland of a 37-year-old cretin; sclerosis of the *Zona glomerulosa*

The simplest explanation seems to me: *the low weight of the suprarenal glands is a sign of general disturbance of growth among cretins*, for, by and large, there is a parallel between suprarenal gland mass and stature. The two lowest weights (4.1 and 5 g) were, for example, found among cretins 125 and 128 cm tall; the highest (13 and 14 g) in cretins of 144 and 147 cm. This agrees with the results of Schilf who, in his large sample from non-cretins, was similarly able to establish clear connections between suprarenal gland mass and stature.

The macroscopic appearance of the *cortex* is not uniform – sometimes it is evenly yellow, sometimes grey or greyish-brown with interspersed yellow flecks. The microscopic behaviour also corresponds with this. In the majority of cases, especially in sudden or rapid-onset death, the fat content is indeed substantial, but there are also cases with low fat content where usually only a few circumscribed areas have undergone marked fatty degeneration. As a rule, fat deposition is by far the greatest in the *Zona fasciculata*, the outer layers being more commonly preferred, yet the *Zona glomerulosa* can also be very rich in fat, while fat deposition is usually rare in the *Zona reticularis*.

The structure of the cortex usually does not deviate from the norm. I have seen only a few cases of more or less severe sclerosis of the *Zona glomerulosa* with shrinkage or atrophy of the epithelial strands (Fig. 77). In the *Zona fasciculata* of older cretins, nodular hyperplasia occurs here and there, the cells usually having a very high fat content, while the *Zona reticularis* is often very rich in lipofuscin even in adolescent cretins.

The *medulla* is always well developed, often markedly so; I have never encountered hypoplasia. In odd cases, abnormally large nuclei, occasionally very rich in chromatin, have attracted my attention because they also occur elsewhere in the suprarenal medulla, and possibly could be regarded as a sign of hypertrophy or incomplete regeneration. In freshly fixed material, the chromium reaction of the medullary cells is often strikingly positive so that the adrenalin production would therefore not be reduced. I have often encountered the familiar infiltrates of lymphocytes and plasma cells, especially at the border of the *Zona reticularis*. These might relate to a localised tissue breakdown.

Apart from the diminutiveness that parallels the general growth disturbance, the cretin's suprarenal gland is therefore a well-built organ that probably also performs its functions normally.

The comparison with the suprarenal glands of congenital athyroids produces corresponding behaviour, in that with an absence of thyroid gland the suprarenal glands are mostly well developed, and only the *Zona glomerulosa* sometimes presents premature sclerosis.

7 Gonads

The development of the sexual organs is defective among cretins in general with, however, very marked individual variation. This is usually easier to determine anatomically in male than in female cretins.

7.1 Male Gonads

As earlier authors have intimated, the *testes* are smaller than normal, and occasionally in younger cretins, prior to their 25th year, they can show a high degree of underdevelopment. For example, the testis of a 19-year-old cretin matched that of a 2-year-old normal boy (Fig. 78).

Similarly, the testes of a 22-year-old cretin were completely infantile (mass 6 g). The canaliculi were lined by a single-layered epithelium without a lumen, the *membranae propriae* thickened, hyaline, and the interstitial cells were almost totally absent. The connective tissue proliferated and was rich in cells, and concentrically layered balls of calcium lay in isolated canaliculi. However, since an infundibular glioma was present in this case, with compression of the hypophysis, it is highly

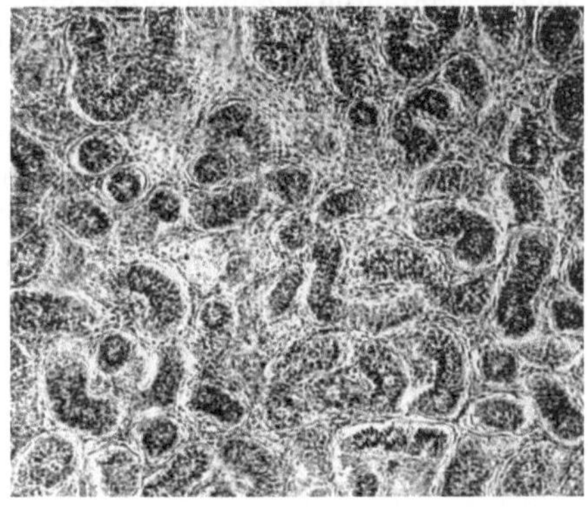

Fig. 78 Testicular hypoplasia in a 19-year-old cretin

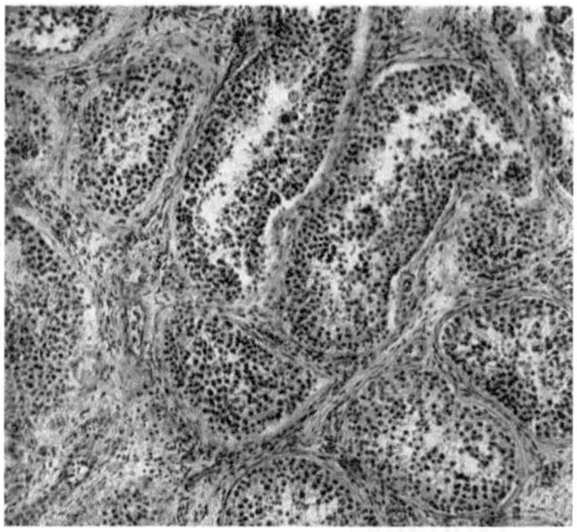

Fig. 79 Testicle of a 30-year-old cretin. Defective spermatogenesis

likely that the underdevelopment of the testis could be regarded in part as a diencephalic hypophyseal symptom. In a 20-year-old, the development stage of spermatocytes and spermatids had at least been reached, but the former were partially degenerated. The *membranae propriae* were thickened and hyaline in places, the interstitial cells had proliferated and undergone fatty degeneration and the intercanalicular connective tissue had proliferated somewhat. Weight of both testes was 22 g.

Many testes remain static at the infantile stage, others achieve a certain maturity around the thirties, leading to the formation of spermatazoa (Fig. 79). However, spermatogenesis is usually very conservative, often demonstrating its lack of completion by the appearance of numerous spermatids and naked heads of spermatazoa in the lumen of the canaliculi and also by the pyknosis of the spermatocyte nuclei. Other expelled cells have, to some extent, giant, clumped nuclei.

The *membranae propriae* of the canaliculi are often thickened and the interstitial cells sometimes proliferated, with marked fatty degeneration.

Among cretins of between 40 and 80 years the testes present a highly variable picture. You may find high-level atrophy and fibrosis, with total obliteration of a portion of the canaliculi and very marked hyaline thickening of the *membranae propriae*. Severe fatty degeneration of the remains of the epithelium and of the brown pigmented interstitial cells belongs in this picture, possibly arising directly out of the infantile underdevelopment, without the testis in question achieving maturity. In other cases, you will find a relatively well-maintained, semen-producing epithelium, admittedly usually with severe fatty degeneration and partial degeneration of the cells, with the *membranae propriae* also somewhat thickened, while the interstitial cells may have proliferated and show severe adiposis. Yet in one 77-year-old cretin a large number of sperm heads were present.

In exceptional cases, the cretin's testis can indeed stand comparison with the normal, both in relation to size and histological structure. In a 54-year-old cretinoid whose testis weighed 45 g, spermatogenesis was very well maintained, and his fathering of two children proved the functional proficiency of these gonads. The cretin therefore, at least in the milder grades, is no way always as sterile as Bayon has maintained.

In two cases, I have observed on the left side an undescended testicle with complete fibrosis and slight proliferation of the interstitial cells, while the right side presented a fairly well-developed testis.

The testes of cretins show therefore absolutely no uniform picture. Relatively frequently they remain at the *puerile level* or show *atrophy and degeneration to the point of fibrosis*. When they do mature, *spermatogenesis is almost always very sparse*, and only very rarely does the semen-producing epithelium reveal itself at the height of its ability to perform.

Direct dependence of testis development on the condition of the thyroid gland is not apparent, for even in very severely reduced thyroid glands the testes may be relatively well developed, and vice versa. Neither does stature reveal a firm relationship, even though generally the better-developed testes belong to cretins whose growth is not severely restricted (stature 140–150 cm).

The *rest of the male gonads (epididymis, seminal vesicle and prostate)* are almost always reduced as well, by hypoplasia or atrophy of the testis. I encountered prostate hypertrophy on three occasions, in 69–77-year-old cretins whose testes were usually still well maintained. The *penis* is small and flaccid as a rule, although in exceptional cases has been found unusually long (Wenzel brothers and Thieme).

7.2 *Female Gonads*

The *ovaries* of cretins at puberty were described by earlier authors (B. Nièpce, Eulenburg and Marfels, Bayon) as surprisingly small, whereas Langhans and I found normal-sized or slightly enlarged ovaries, with the latter offering the picture of the so-called small-cystic degeneration. After menopause, the atrophy is usually very severe – the difference from the norm often quite striking.

Histologically a reduction of the organ is often barely discernible. Schlagenhaufer and Wagner von Jauregg found a well-developed germinal epithelium and numerous primordial follicles in the ovaries of a 4-year-old cretin girl; in the pubescent ovary you can encounter all stages of maturation and regression of the follicle. At most, the number of primordial follicles in individual cases seems to be quite small. The image of small-cystic degeneration (Fig. 80) is evoked by numerous nonruptured Graafian follicles, many of which have already lost their epithelium and are partially, or totally, collapsed. The stroma of the outer cortical layers is often surprisingly poor in cell content, and may even show small calcium deposits. In the vicinity of the atretic follicles there are often aggregations of markedly adipose theca-lutein cells. There is usually an abundance of *corpora albicantia* and *corpora fibrosa*, and neither have I seen them in the post-menopausal ages, an indication that follicles had once matured and some ruptured here too.

That ova are also capable of fertilization in milder levels of cretinism emerges from repeated observations of definite pregnancy.

In two cretins aged 26 and 30, both of whom had died shortly after giving birth, I found a typical corpus luteum of pregnancy, in addition to a large number of

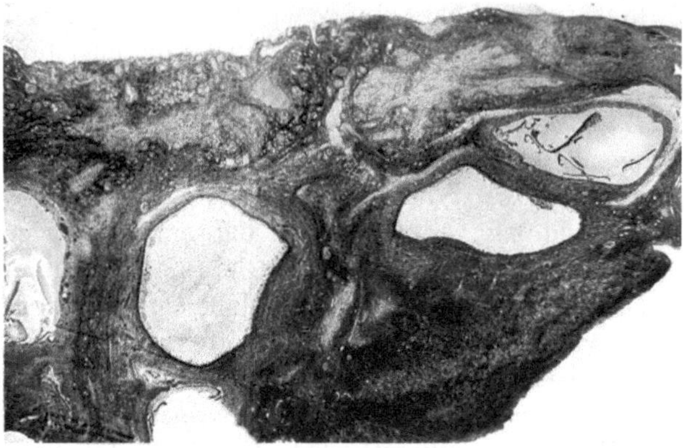

Fig. 80 Small-cyst degeneration of the ovary of a 28-year-old cretin

Graafian follicles – here as well, was a certain similarity to a small-cystic degeneration.

In many cases, the *uterus* remains infantile (Scholz), with the small size of the body quite striking in comparison with the length of the cervix. However, the body of the uterus can also reach normal size and develop a mucosa, indicating a completely normal functioning. For example, in a 28-year-old cretin I found a typical, premenstrual swelling. Admittedly, the periods are usually weak and irregular; however, it is incorrect to deny the occurrence of menstruation (Bayon). In some cases, even, the menstrual flow is very heavy (Thieme). Should pregnancy occur, the uterus shows completely normal growth and labour does not appear to be disrupted. On the other hand, the mother is often at great risk due to the narrowness of her pelvis.

Characteristic changes of the *Fallopian tubes* and *vagina* are absent, while the *vulvae* are usually small and flaccid.

In exceptional cases the *breasts* are large, and rich in fat (Thieme); usually however they remain hypoplastic – small and flat like the breasts of a child. Histology shows the very small, glandular lobes, consisting, for the most part, of lacteal ducts with few branches, imbedded in rich, connective tissue with few cells. Should a pregnancy ensue, however, milk let-down will follow as in a normal woman, and so you have the picture of a successfully lactating breast histologically as well, as I was able to ascertain in the two cases mentioned earlier.

The female cretin's gonads thus frequently reveal a certain hypoplasia, but at least as far as the mucous glands are concerned, they are rather less limited in development than are those of the males. The question of whether the relatively common small-cystic degeneration of the ovaries is a result of heightened hypophyseal anterior lobe function (E. Kraus) will only be resolved by further clinical and experimental investigations.

The sexual organs of cretins therefore experience a developmental limitation, as is familiar following premature thyroidectomy in humans and animals. There is also a tendency to presenile atrophy and sclerosis in the testicles, while the ovaries often remain in a long-term state of small-cystic degeneration, as in congenital athyrosis.

8 Nervous System

Since endemic cretinism had for a long time been considered a mental illness, it is understandable that information about brain anomalies is fairly frequently found in the earlier literature. However, that literature should be evaluated with even more caution because, back then, the notional boundary of cretinism was completely ambiguous, and accordingly all possible conditions relating to imbecility or idiocy were lumped together. Wagner von Jauregg has already quite rightly pointed out that common idiocy must be clearly distinguished from cretinism, which differentiation sadly does not apply throughout Scholz and Zingerle's extensive material. Meticulous separation has happened only very recently.

8.1 Meninges

Deviations from the normal state occur with roughly the same frequency as in non-cretins. In older cretins, the dura and arachnoid mater are not uncommonly thickened – the latter especially forming a white mist over the sulci, while, in my experience, juvenile cretins have extremely delicate meninges. As opposed to Scholz and Zingerle, I must emphasize particularly that firmer adhesion between the dura and the cranial vault is an extremely rare exception (of 34 cases I found it only once – in the frontal region). I have never, ever, encountered any adhesion between the pulpy meninges and the cortex. Nor can I corroborate the fibrinous pachymeningitis mentioned by those authors. Admittedly, I once saw *pachymeningitis haemorrhagica interna* and, twice, *meningitis tuberculosa* among cretins. An increase of cerebrospinal fluid is found only in older cretins whose brains are already atrophic.

8.2 Brain

The brain of cretins is by no means as small and underdeveloped as you could be led to assume from many accounts in the older literature. Scholz has already stressed this, and I can totally confirm it.

Scholz found brain weights between 1103 and 1300 g in his material from adult cretins. In one case, age unknown, this even reached 1698 g. A heavy weight 1393 g in an 11-year-old cretin is also remarkable. Low weights between 1000 and 1100 g were noted by Eulenburg and Marfels, Betz and Bayon, while His recorded a weight of 1492 g. The data from Scholz and the other authors are based on a brain freed of leptomeninges; mine, on the other hand, include leptomeninges with the following brain values. When comparing values it is therefore necessary to reduce mine by 50–60 g. Furthermore, express emphasis is given to all the various factors that complicate a precise determination of the weight of the brain – sectioning of the medulla

Table 5 Average weight of the cretin brain (26 cases)

	Normal, after Rossle and Roulet			
Age (years)	Male	Female	Male cretins	Female cretins
20–40	1393 g	1245 g	1321 g (4 cases)	1294 g (5 cases)
40–80	1318 g	1213 g	1288 g (11 cases)	1262 g (6 cases)

Table 6 Maximum and minimum weight of brain

Age (years)	Male cretins	Female cretins
20–40	1170–1485 g	1165–1450 g
40–80	1050–1505 g	1110–1350 g

oblongata at different heights, varying blood content, 'living' and *post-mortem* brain swelling and œdema. Brains with gross changes (glioma, meningitis) have been excluded from the evaluation.

Our values are directly comparable with those of Rössle and Roulet, since they too are based on weight of brain plus meninges. It follows that in the male cretin the average weight remains clearly below the norm, while, remarkably, the average values lie above the norm in females. The difference between the sexes, usually recorded as 100–150 g in the norm, is therefore significantly smaller among cretins, only 25–30 g. However, obviously, no binding conclusion can be drawn from such a small number of cases, since the range is not insubstantial either.

Apart from that, among cretins as among normal people (Rieger), brain weight shows a *certain correlation with body size*, in that – admittedly not in every case – in pronounced dwarfism (120–140 g) lower weight values predominate, whereas with greater body length (over 140 g) brain weight also increases. This might support the argument that, among cretins too, the brain obeys the general laws of growth and *a priori* does not remain static. The following summary shows the relationship between brain mass and stature.

Table 7 Relationship between brain mass and body length

1. 47 years	Male	123.5 cm	1050 g	14. 59 years	Female	143 cm	1280 g
2. 56 years	Female	125 cm	1260 g	15. 34 years	Male	144 cm	1485 g
3. 44 years	Female	128 cm	1110 g	16. 56 years	Male	144 cm	1432 g
4. 30 years	Male	132 cm	1180 g	17. 38 years	Female	145 cm	1165 g
5. 35 years	Male	134 cm	1170 g	18. 29 years	Female	145 cm	1450 g
6. 36 years	Female	134 cm	1310 g	19. 45 years	Male	147 cm	1505 g
7. 40 years	Female	135 cm	1185 g	20. 54 years	Male	147 cm	1320 g
8. 51 years	Male	135 cm	1210 g	21. 56 years	Male	147 cm	1290 g
9. 57 years	Male	138 cm	1065 g	22. 26 years	Female	151 cm	1360 g
10. 75 years	Male	138 cm	1175 g	23. 77 years	Male	151 cm	1250 g
11. 49 years	Female	140 cm	1350 g	24. 69 years	Male	152 cm	1470 g
12. 70 years	Female	141 cm	1300 g	25. 46 years	Male	155 cm	1400 g
13. 51 years	Female	142 cm	1275 g	26. 39 years	Male	155 cm	1450 g

Where the earlier literature often describes the cretin brain as misshapen, this is definitely incorrect. Cerebral asymmetries (B. Nièpce, Scholz, and Zingerle) are reported to be common, likewise an abnormally small cerebellum by comparison with the cerebrum. Particular deficiencies of cerebral convolutions or special types of convolution have never attracted my attention. Microgyria is a very rare exception (Scholz and Zingerle). Current experiences render Fodéré's strongly emphasized hardness of the brain (contradicted by the abnormal softness claimed by other authors), a chance finding.

Hydrocephalus internus is said to be a very common occurrence in the cretin brain (Wallmann, Rösh, Guggenbühl, Nièpce, Stahl, Lombroso, Ferrus, Virchow, Scholz and Zingerle). However, I cannot support the finding, since of my 29 cases (apart from two cases of tubercular meningitis) only 14 showed a mild enlargement of the lateral ventricle, usually involving the posterior horn; enlargement of the other ventricles was even more rare. Anomalies of the ependyma and plexus are uncommon – the former may present a mild sclerosis in older cretins but only quite rarely is it granulated. Small cysts can be encountered here and there in the plexus.

Macroscopically therefore, the cretin brain shows absolutely no characteristic finding. The most that can be said is that, with greater restriction of growth in general, there is usually a related diminution of brain size.

Microscopic investigation of the cretin brain has taken a major step forwards in recent times. Admittedly, Scholz and Zingerle (1909) had already given a description of multiple changes, including delving into individual cases. They interpreted those changes as a mixture of degenerative processes with a distinct limitation of development varying in proportion and intensity. The principal site of these changes was found in the cortex and expressly conceded a certain similarity with many idiot brains. However, the investigation was unsatisfactory because it did not draw a sufficiently sharp dividing line between cretinism and common idiocy. Above all, however, there was an urgent need to tackle the question of the finer structure of the cretin brain using the newer microscopic techniques.

At my instigation F. Lotmar took on this problem, and studied various sections of the brain in 14 cases from the endemic region of the Berne canton. Changes were detected in the *cerebral cortex* that were admittedly isolated to a certain extent and not seen in all cases over a long time. However, the totality of the changes are of considerable importance as developmental restrictions in cell and fibre structure. Often architectural deviations in the laminar structure were found to a greater extent but never in a more gross form. These deviations were expressed as a reduced thickness of the ganglion cell content, and as a reduced average size of the ganglion cells in certain layers or sub-layers. Less commonly, the cortex was thinner overall, with individual layers expanded or thinned, or less distinctly defined, than in normal cases, with the ganglion cells tending to form colonies here and there. Purely localized anomalies were noted in individual cases – ectopic ganglion cell collections in the molecular layer with transition into the external granular layer (Fig. 81); giant glial cells in the molecular layer; disorientated or deformed pyramid cells and atypical,

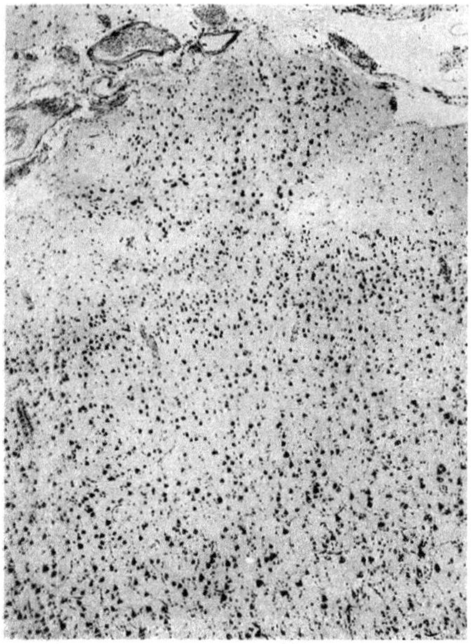

Fig. 81 Ectopic granular cell aggregation in the molecular layer of the cerebral cortex, merging into the outer granular layer (From Lotmar (1933))

giant pyramidal cells in Layer III (Fig. 82). Such changes are signs of more gross regression, already demonstrating a developmental restriction in the 5th–6th foetal month. In Lotmar's opinion, the cortical anomalies are, in any case, sufficient to interfere strongly with higher brain function, so that the mental state characteristic of cretins has therefore a certain morphological support.

Developmental restrictions also arose in the *cerebellar cortex*, in the form of a retained superficial granular layer with Purkinje cells (Fig. 83), and also isolated sub-pial, or deeper-lying Purkinje cells (Fig. 84), which were often hypoplastic or deformed.

The timing of this disturbance must be placed at the junction between the second and final third of the foetal period. In addition, bi-granular Purkinje cells were found, their genesis probably occurring within the foetal period as well. And finally, in several cases, there was a lack of medullary fibres in the granular layer, in the Purkinje layer and in the deep molecular layer, as well as a sparseness of parallel fibres in the deep molecular layer.

In addition to such obvious limitations in development, however, the cretin brain also shows extensive chronic regressive changes, involving mainly pigment atrophy, and adiposis of the ganglion cells that fits a honey-combed cell alteration in Nissl pattern. Lotmar stresses that these processes cannot adequately be explained either by the individuals' age or by the illnesses leading to their death, and therefore to blame the cretinogenic noxious goitre would be in the sense of a reduction of the cells' ability to resist. Pseudo calcium concretions, found quite often in the pallidum and cerebellum of cretins, with a marked tendency to calcification, are, in Lotmar's opinion the expression of a characteristic metabolic disturbance among cretins which might be particularly hypothyroid or dysthyroid.

Fig. 82 Deformed pyramidal cell in the deep third cerebral cortical layer (From Lotmar (1933))

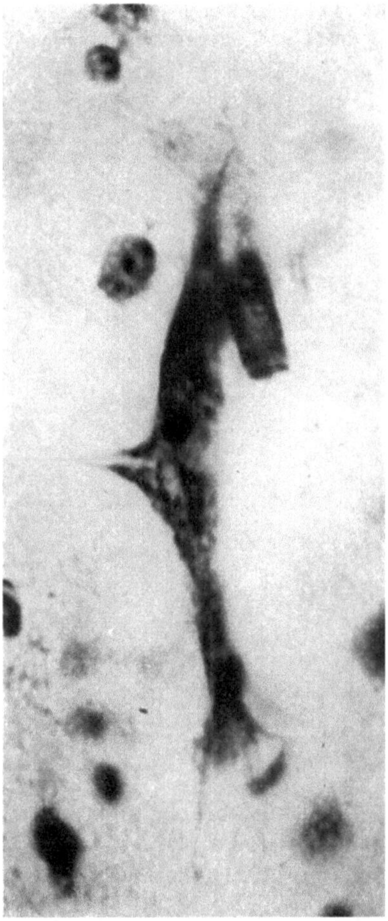

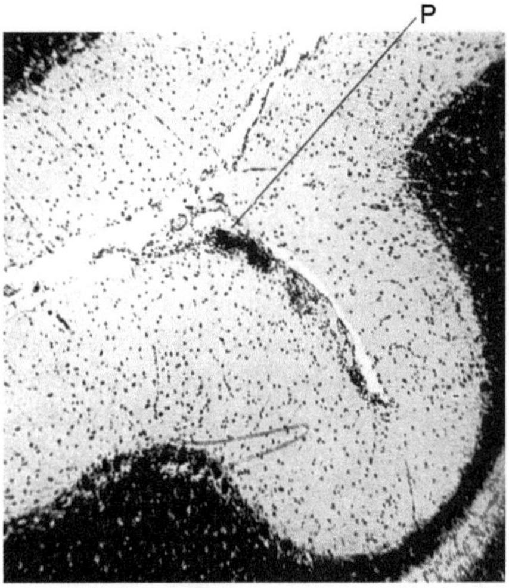

Fig. 83 Remnant superficial granular layer, with loose layering of the granules to some extent. Purkinje cell indicated by 'P' (From Lotmar (1931))

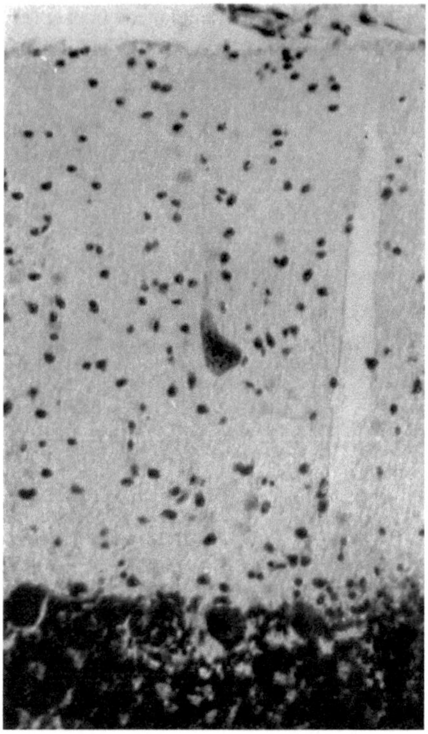

Fig. 84 Markedly ectopic Purkinje cell (From Lotmar (1931))

It clearly emerges from Lotmar's studies that the cretin brain shows, on the one hand, developmental restrictions whose period of activity can be fairly precisely determined, but, on the other hand, the brain tends toward degeneration. Both aspects show a broad similarity, even partial agreement with the brain findings that stem from congenital absence of thyroid gland (congenital myxœdema). Here too, there are architectural disturbances in the cerebral and cerebellar cortices (Fig. 85), fatty degeneration of the ganglion cells, and pseudo calcification in the pallidum and dentate nucleus, out of which there emerges again the extant relationship of endemic cretinism with undoubted athyroidism or hypothyroidism (Lotmar).

It would naturally be interesting to determine whether the severity of the brain changes depends on the degree of atrophy of the thyroid gland. However, Lotmar's material is insufficiently extensive to resolve this issue, since, in the majority of cases, only a few parts of the cortex could be investigated, and the individual's age and complicating illnesses can play a role in the ganglion cell changes. Thus, in the first instance, sufficient material must be harvested from youthful brains. Here we are only pointing out that the cretins' mental capability in no way parallels thyroid gland illness. However, we must always be mindful that, in dissected material, the microscopically detectable thyroid gland atrophy represents an endpoint, often probably only a form of scar tissue, whereas we know nothing about the appearance and function of the thyroid gland during the most important developmental periods of the cretin brain.

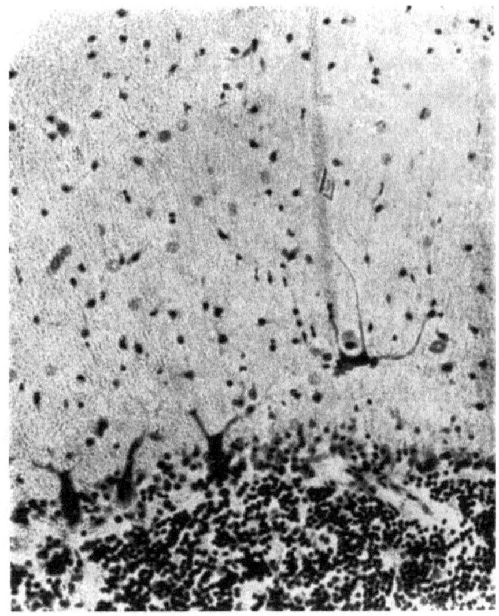

Fig. 85 A case of congenital athyrosis; an atypically shaped Purkinje cell is imbedded in the molecular layer (From Lotmar (1929))

8.3 Spinal Cord

In my material I have been unable to confirm the severe atrophy of the spinal cord described by earlier authors (Ackermann, B. Nièpce, Eulenburg and Marfels, Bayon). Admittedly, the ganglion cells, like those of the cerebral cortex, can be noticeably small and rich in lipofuscin granules, while the Nissl aggregations do not attain their normal size either. Thus, the spinal cord appears to have been subjected to similar influences as the brain.

8.4 Peripheral Nerves

Changes in the peripheral nerves are a rare exception among cretins. Scholz mentions that multiple neurofibromas were present in two cases from Schiffner. The aggregations of endoneurial growths and vesicular cells in the lymphatic spaces, described by Langhans, are not at all characteristic of cretinism and other functional disorders of the thyroid gland. As Langhans and his students later recognized for themselves, they are totally normal structures.

9 Musculature

The musculature of cretins is generally not very powerfully formed, but microscopically it shows no coarser changes. In older individuals, or in those who have died after a protracted illness, there may admittedly be varying degrees of atrophy, with proliferation and linear alignment of the sarcolemma nuclei, in addition to a clustering of brown pigmentation in the vicinity of the nuclei. This, however, has nothing to do with cretinism as such. According to my investigations, the same is true of the adiposis first found by Langhans in two cretins, and traced back to lower body temperature and deficient oxidation. Firstly, this fatty degeneration does not regularly exist among cretins, and secondly, as my student Surbek demonstrated, it is found also among the most varied of illnesses and even among healthy individuals, and is primarily dependent on nutritional status. It certainly does not have any kind of significance in muscle function, and, when Langhans traced the slowness and powerlessness of cretins' movements back to this fatty degeneration, he was incorrect.

I would still like to mention that, in cretins who have died suddenly, the glycogen content of the musculature can be quite significant – probably due to the thyroid gland's deficient glycogen storage function.

Again, the occurrence of mucus in cretins' muscle spindles, as determined by Langhans, is important; with similar findings in congenital athyroidism, this points to an anomaly of metabolism.

10 The Skeleton

The general restriction of growth, the particular proportions of body parts, the facial features and the motor disorders in cretins are all simply outward signs of multiple changes occurring within the skeletal system. Consequently, a more detailed analysis reveals a multitude of alterations in the form of the individual bones. For their origin and classification in the state of cretinism, development is the determining factor, able to be followed up not only purely anatomically but also radiographically, and differing from the norm in a characteristic manner.

In severe cases the skeleton's *general restriction in growth* is expressed as pronounced dwarfism. Not once, by the twentieth year, was a body length of one metre found (B. Nièpce, Wagner von Jaurreg). Flinker saw a 27-year-old Jewish male cretin only a metre tall; and Scholz a 26-year-old of 103 cm; Eggenberger saw a 62-year-old cretin woman of only 110 cm. Admittedly they usually, though often belatedly, reach a length of 120–160 cm: the higher values being predominantly cretinoids. Among my subjects I cannot find any case with a stature below 120 cm. In 41 cases, the youngest 19 and the oldest 77 years, the following divisions appeared:

123–130 cm	7 cases	141–150 cm	17 cases
131–140 cm	11 cases	151–155 cm	6 cases

Obviously the restriction in growth occurs long before the twentieth year – from the second year on, according to Diviak and Wagner von Jauregg. In the endemic region where most of the children are short, it is generally not very remarkable. It does become clearly apparent when seen in comparison with children who are growing up in areas that are free of cretinism. Those differences are quite considerable – among children between seven and ten, for example, they amount to 10–30 cm or more.

Physical proportions are similarly determined primarily by the skeletal components. Even from cursory inspection the length of the torso and the size of the head stands out in comparison with the short limbs – a ratio approaching that of a child's body. According to Flinker, the body proportions should actually *be* those of a child, and it can be explained as a simple growth restriction, while other authors, who have recorded precise measurements –some from living subjects, others from skeletons – have obtained somewhat different results.

H. Bircher, who was probably the first to delve more deeply into this question, came to the conclusion that the relationship between lower limbs and body length in both normal and cretin individuals is the same, and does not approximate in cretins to a long torso atop short legs. Scholz, however, could confirm this detail for only a portion of his cases; in others the legs were too short in relation to total body length. Moreover, in comparison with normal total body length, among cretins he found the upper arm too short, a somewhat lengthened forearm, a surprisingly long femur, and a less-shortened, or normal, lower leg.

While Dieterle regarded cretinism as being proportionate dwarf growth, E. Bircher regarded the cretin skeleton as disproportionate. The growth disturbance was totally irregular and did not follow a pattern, which is why there were marked differences between individual parts of the skeleton. The trunk and lower limbs should be relatively overlong in relation to body length, with the lower leg relatively shorter than the thigh, while the upper limbs were retarded in growth – the reduction involved mainly the upper arm, while the forearm seemed rather too long.

Finkbeiner's measurements, restricted solely to the skeleton, revealed that cretins' limbs are relatively too short, so that the cretin type approximates micromelia. The lower limb in particular, and mainly the lower leg, shows surprisingly short length. The upper limb divisions are less disproportionate. Patellae, hands and feet are small. The asymmetry of the cretin skeleton is insignificant and, apart from the greater length of the right leg, match asymmetries in normal people.

Finkbeiner's values therefore confirm the impression of surprising brevity of the limbs in comparison with total body length, and thus a certain similarity with the child state, particularly when you consider the size of the head. However, according to Gamper's very recent comparative investigations we cannot speak of pure child proportions, because the cretin, when compared with a child of similar size, has too large a head, too short a trunk, limbs relatively too long and a much larger transverse diameter.

10.1 Development

Despite Stahl and B. Nièpce's observation of a persisting spheno-occipital synchondrosis in adult cretin skulls, Virchow's tenet on the premature synostosis of cretin skull bones for a long time held the power of a dogma, which H. Bircher also supported, evidenced by his not wanting to include an 18-year-old dwarf from the endemic region as a cretin because of his open epiphyseal joints. Virchow had actually found a synostosis of the bones of the cranial base in a newborn child with a saddle nose (1856) and believed, though with certain limitations, that he had found an explanation for the defective brain development in cretins. Admittedly, he protested later (1883) against having explained cretinism purely from this synostosis. His concept however lost any grounds when Weygandt and Bayon (1904) demonstrated that Virchow's newborn cretin was actually chondrodystrophic – the converse of Virchow's teaching proved correct.

Premature synostosis had indeed been recorded in odd cases (His, Klebs, Hanau, Ziegler), with even elderly cretins presenting still-patent cartilaginous joints. However, only Langhans (1897), with a much larger sample, could emphatically assert that so far no premature ossification of cartilaginous joints had been demonstrated in any cretin. 'The bones modelled in cartilage grow very slowly in length, the epiphyses remain low, ossification proceeds very slowly, the epiphyseal nuclei of ossification appear very late, and the epiphyseal discs are retained long beyond the normal termination'.

Even when ossification of the cartilaginous joints has already occurred, the bony trabecula that replaces the cartilage stands out much more noticeably than normal. A significant disturbance of periosteal growth does not exist, according to Langhans.

Langhans has thus emphasized not only the restriction of endochondral ossification of the diaphyses, but also the belatedness of the formation of the centres of ossification in the epiphyses of long bones. His exposition has been comprehensively confirmed since then, both through anatomical investigations (Bayon, Breus and Kolisko, Stoccada, Wegelin) and also by radiography (Hofmeister, von Wyss, Dieterle, E. Bircher, Wydler). The cartilaginous joints (Figs. 86–88) can be retained right into the fourth, fifth and even the sixth decade.

In a 20-year-old cretin I found the upper part of the intersphenoidal synchondrosis extending over 6 mm with a thickness of 1–2 mm (Fig. 89), whereas normally ossification of this cartilaginous joint begins at birth and can retain only remnants of cartilage up until the thirteenth year (Virchow). However, while Dieterle is of the opinion that the relationship between epiphyseal ossification and longitudinal growth of the diaphysis is parallel with the norm, E. Bircher emphasizes also here the irregularity of the disorder, in that the ossification centres of the epiphyses and bones of the upper limb joints, for example, experience greater restriction in occurrence and growth than do the centres of ossification of the lower limbs.

That a certain irregularity in the growth disturbance does actually exist is revealed by both Stoccada's and my own anatomical investigations. These show that the spheno-occipital synchondrosis, that normally disappears around the twentieth year, remains longer, and is more often retained than the joint cartilages of the limb bones. The synchondrosis can be found still complete or partially so, even into the sixth decade (Fig. 90) (Bayon, Stoccada, Wegelin). There are also irregularities in the disappearance of the cartilaginous joints of the limb bones; for example, in the tibia

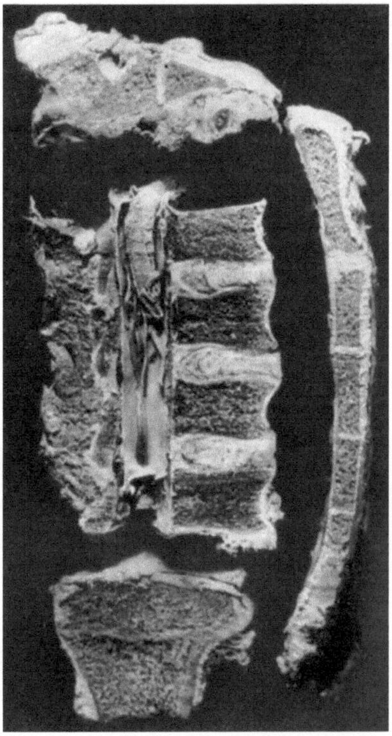

Fig. 86 Cranial base, sternum, vertebrae, and proximal epiphysis of the tibia of a 30-year-old cretin

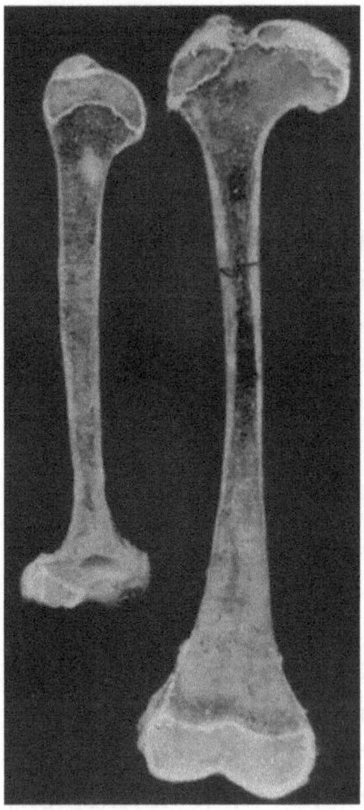

Fig. 87 Humerus and femur of a 20-year-old cretin. Cartilaginous discs retained. Femoral head partially cartilaginous

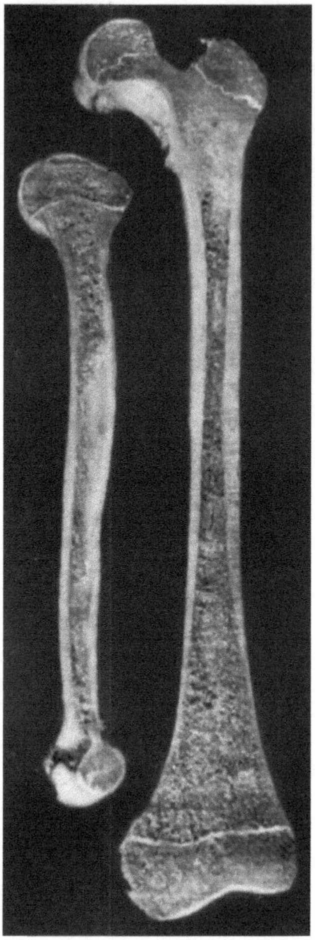

Fig. 88 Humerus and femur of a 30-year-old cretin with retained cartilaginous discs

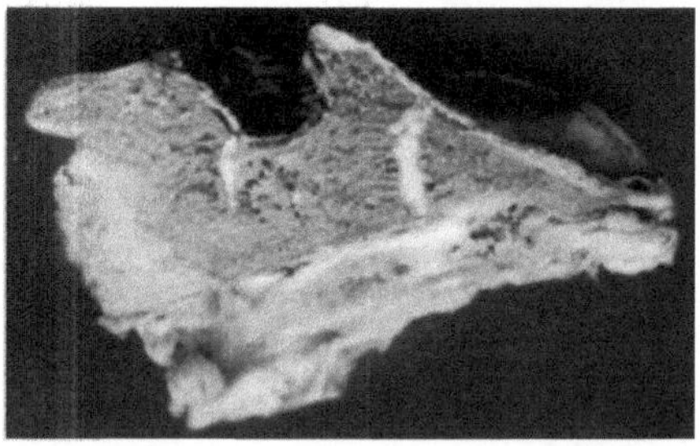

Fig. 89 Retained spheno-occipital and intersphenoidal synchondroses of a 20-year-old cretin

of a 34-year-old cretin I found the complete, distal epiphyseal disc, while the proximal disc was only partially retained. Normally, the distal disc ossifies first. In a 56-year-old cretin, Bayon saw a complete cartilaginous disc in the distal end of the radius, while other epiphyseal discs in radius, ulna and femur were merely suggested.

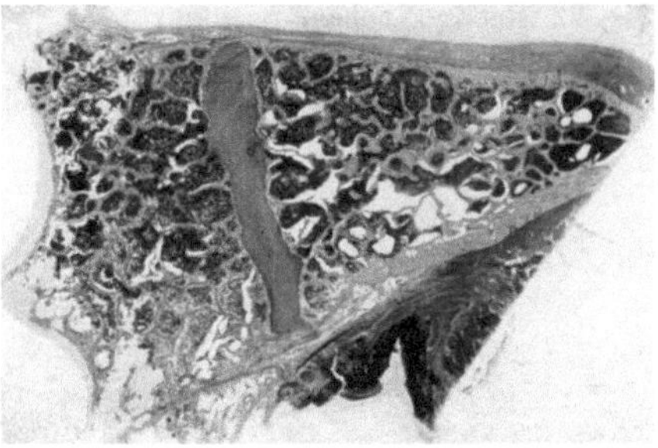

Fig. 90 Spheno-occipital synchondrosis of a 57-year-old cretin. *Left*: sphenoid bone; *right*: occiput

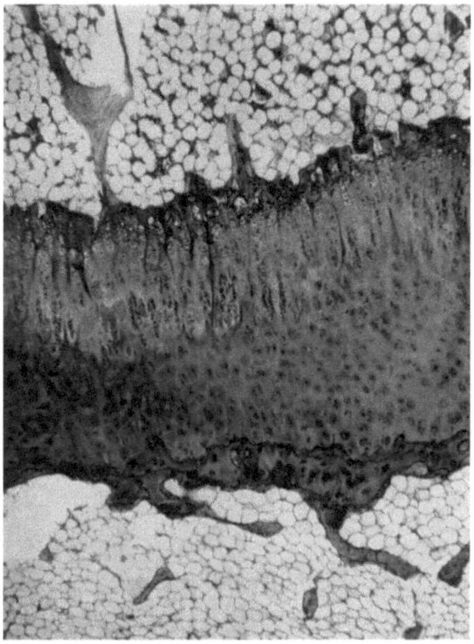

Fig. 91 Distal epiphyseal disc of the femur of a 20-year-old cretin

Similar differences were also described by Breus and Kolisko, and by Looser. Like Langhans, they pointed out cartilaginous vestiges in flat bones (ilium, scapula).

The histological relationships in the cartilaginous joints have been clarified by my student Stoccada, who examined the spheno-occipital synchondrosis in particular, but other epiphyseal cartilage as well. The cartilage itself, from whose proliferation longitudinal growth of the bone depends, usually displays well-formed, parallel columns of cells (Fig. 91) in juvenile cretins and the zone of calcification is also always detectable. In older cretins you may of course miss any cartilage cell proliferation, or it is present only as very short columns of cells. Particularly striking, however, is the small number and irregular division of the primitive marrow cavities, which are often completely cut off from the cartilage by a thin layer of bone.

Finally, an uninterrupted plate of bone may form on both sides of the cartilage disc (Fig. 92). An insufficiency of the marrow in the destruction of cartilage is

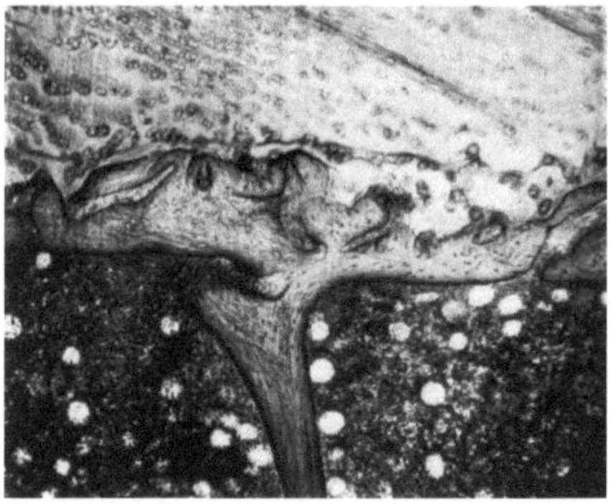

Fig. 92 Retained spheno-occipital synchondrosis of a 44-year-old cretin. Bony trabeculae at the margin of the dormant cartilage

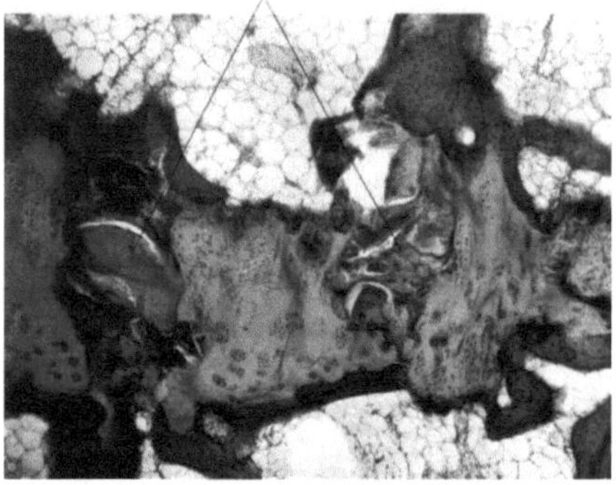

Fig. 93 Distal epiphyseal disc of the femur of a 30-year-old cretin

therefore probably the main feature of growth restriction, yet cartilage proliferation must also be deficient, since with complete, even though delayed, ossification, bone length, and consequent total body length remains below the norm.

Dr. E. Bircher has spoken of a 'delayed calcification of osteoid tissue'. It must be emphasized particularly that calcification of the newly-formed bone sets in immediately and appears, at least histologically, absolutely normal.

Growth disturbances in the epiphyses of the long bones, principally femur and humerus, are also significant, for here the ossification proceeding outward from the bone nucleus seems to be not merely slowed but often totally irregular in its completion so that, according to the radiographic picture, we have to assume ossification outward from different sites (E. Bircher, Läwen). Added to this there are the processes of degeneration and softening in the cartilage (Fig. 93) that occur in localized areas also in normal individuals, even during the foetal period (Hintzsche), but here these processes have often risen to immeasurable levels. For instance, in the cartilaginous head of the femur of a 10-year-old cretin, Lang found liquefaction holes with aggregations of mucus and areas of more marked basophilia of the ground substance, with strands of fibres and enlargement of the cartilage cells. Corresponding with this, radiography revealed poorly defined clear zones (Roth). Looser has

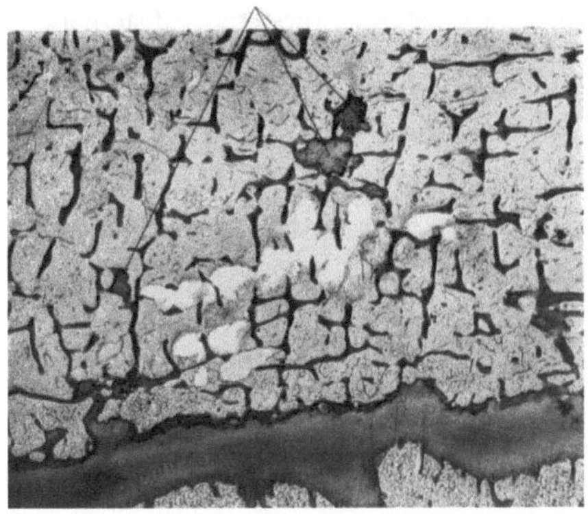

Fig. 94 Distal epiphyseal disc of the femur of a 20-year-old cretin

observed very severe disturbances. Between scattered clumps of bone he found highly degenerated, fibrously and mucilaginously degenerated cartilage, with disintegrating cavities and invading vessels. Here, ossification is completed probably not from one central, unified nucleus outward, but from various adjacent marrow canals. Finally, the markedly fissured cartilage can collapse and crumble under functional loading, causing the formation of free articular bodies and high-level deformation or atrophy of the bony heads (Looser, Klar, Haumann, von Seemen). Probably such depredations and ravages of the cartilage are possible only because its replacement by solid bone tissue takes place in a totally inadequate manner, and the growing cartilage is nourished completely inadequately by diffusion from the surface. However, if the ossification does materialize on a larger scale, you can still find remnants of cartilage enclosed within the bony trabeculae of the epiphysis (Fig. 94) for a long time afterwards, or it may be that the bone will also contain large, irregular islands of cartilage.

Stoccada has further demonstrated that the ossification disturbances of endemic cretinism are essentially the same as those of congenital and postoperative athyrosis, with only quantitative differences (Figs. 95 and 96).

This agreement is especially surprising when you compare the bones of adult cretins with those of athyroid people of roughly the same age (Looser, Knaggs, personal observations). I have, for example, seen mucous softening similar to that described by Looser and Lang, in the epiphyses of an athyroid young woman of 19 years, except that in this case ossification was even more severely retarded.

Growth restriction of the cretin skeleton is expressed moreover not just in endochondral bone but also in intramembranous bone, since, for example, the bones of the cranial vault are retarded in their surface growth. Closure of the anterior fontanelle is delayed; relatively often the frontal suture is totally or partially retained; and, not uncommonly, sutural (wormian) bones are found in the cranial sutures. Very rarely does a synostosis come into being in the region of the cranial vault (Vrolik, Lombroso), which again contradicts any influence by the skull on the brain.

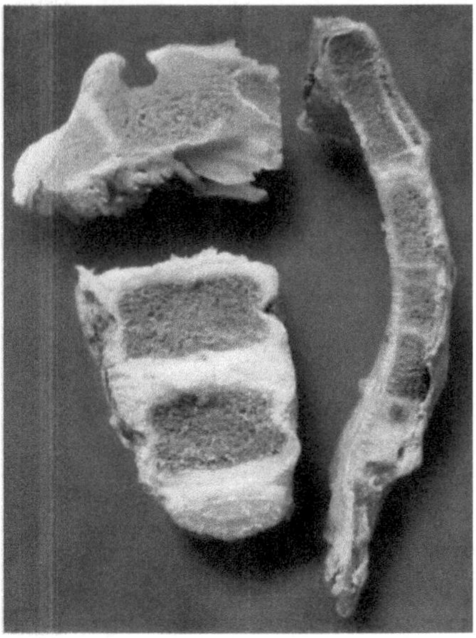

Fig. 95 Congenital athyrosis in a 19-year-old female: cranial base, vertebrae and sternum

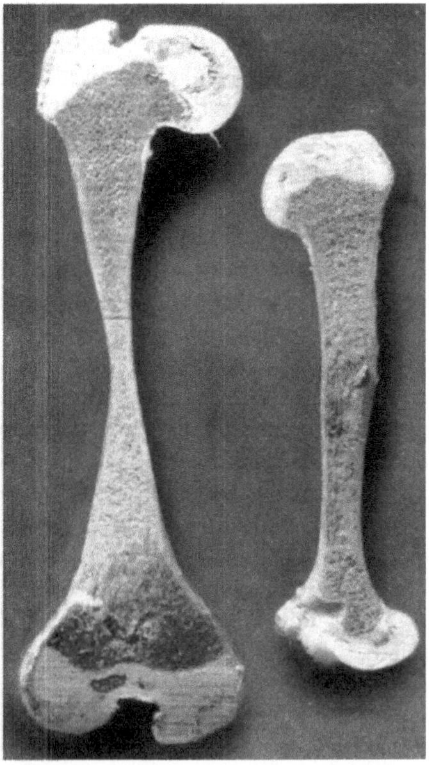

Fig. 96 Congenital athyrosis in a 19-year-old female: femur and humerus with cartilaginous epiphyses

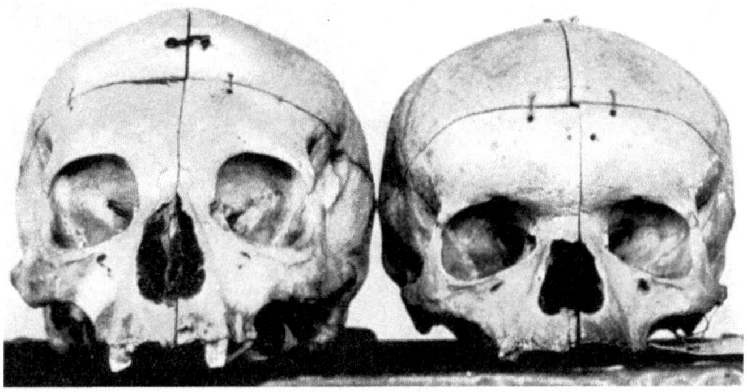

Fig. 97 Two cretin crania with very broad, sunken roots of the nose

Fig. 98 Cranial base of a 25-year-old cretin with patent spheno-occipital synchondrosis; clivus very short and steep; broad *sella turcica*

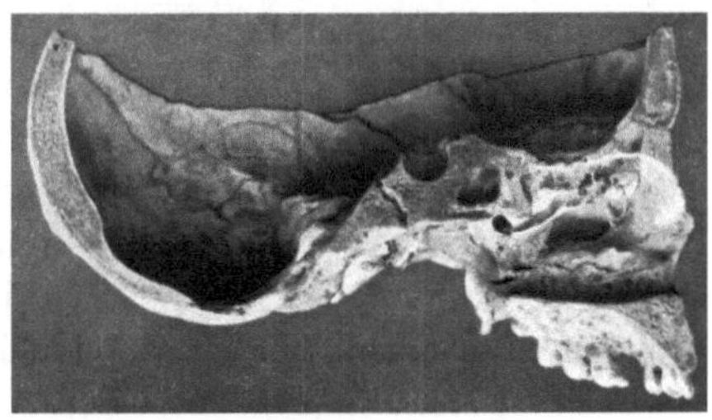

10.2 Bone Form Relationships

Once ossification has progressed to completion among cretins with greater or lesser delay, thus terminating growth, the disorders in endochondral ossification still leave their clear traces behind, in the bone's form. Gross variations are recognisable merely by the naked eye, or with use of radiographs, others can be determined only by using anthropological methods of measurement. At this point, cretin osteology cannot be dealt with in detail; accordingly, I refer the reader to the meritorious works of Scholz, E. Bircher and Finkbeiner, and my own compilation in Henke-Lubarsch's manual. Only a modicum is discussed here.

The cretin's skull is usually brachycephalic, which, offhand, in the Alpine region results from their belonging to the alpine population. However, pronounced dolichocephalic types also occur. In my experience, asymmetries are no more prevalent than among non-cretins, and particular thickness of the vault occurs only in a low number of cases. The most remarkable feature is the reduction in length of the cranial base – its origin lies in the defective growth of the spheno-occipital synchondrosis and its outcome is the deep contraction of the root of the nose (Figs 97 and 98).

The *clivus Blumenbachii* is, in many instances, shorter and steeper than normal, and the foramen magnum too shows a marked anterosuperior inclination. Çorresponding with the enlargement of the hypophysis, the *sella turcica* is also noticeably wide and deep (Fig. 98).

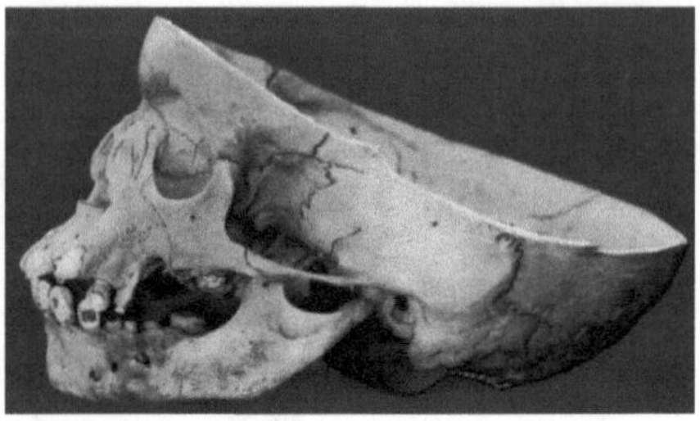

Fig. 99 Skull of a 24-year-old cretin. Pronounced prognathism

The most striking feature when observing the facial bones is the width and deep position of the root of the nose (already commented on by the Wenzel brothers), and the related, abnormal breadth of the interorbital septum. Facial breadth exceeds facial height, for both the external nasal bone and the maxilla are short, and in many cretin skulls there is also marked prognathism (Fig. 99).

The skeleton of the *trunk* is borne by the vertebral column which, in the dwarf cretin, participates in the general growth disorders in a totally characteristic manner. The vertebral bodies in particular are abnormally short, often almost flat, and roughly disproportionate to the thick intervertebral discs, which are often almost the same height as the vertebral bodies (Fig. 86). Like Breus and Kolisko, I too have seen inadequate fusion of the individual vertebrae in parts of the sacrum. The same is true of the sternum (Fig. 86), where individual segments of the body are often still separated by cartilaginous joints (Langhans, Stoccada, Wegelin). The ribs are generally slender.

10.3 Upper Limbs

In the scapula, which is broad and, according to Finkbeiner, often concave, you not uncommonly still find cartilage on the medial margin of the body, as well as in the coracoid and acromion.

The latter may still be joined to the body solely by cartilage. On the clavicle too, you can still find cartilaginous ends in the adult (Bayon).

The deformity called *Humerus varus* by E. Bircher and *Axilla vara* by Finkbeiner is frequently seen (Figs 100 and 102) in the humerus. This deformity is expressed by a reduction of the angle between head and shaft, giving the appearance of the head having slid down on the medial side of the diaphysis. Consequently, the tubercles stand high, with the greater tubercle often lying in the same plane as the highest point of the joint surface. Incidentally, it stands to reason that this change in form is brought about by the loading on the epiphysis that has remained cartilaginous for a long time, especially during the child's crawling stage. The most remarkable feature of the radius is its often-pronounced curvature with its convexity towards the ulna; according to Finkbeiner, the shortness of the carpal bones and, in the hand, the dominance of the third digit ray over the second is characteristic (?)

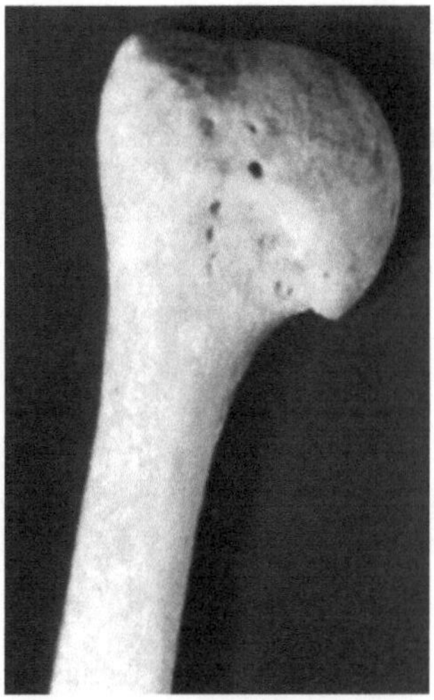

Fig. 100 *Humerus varus* in a 63-year-old cretin woman

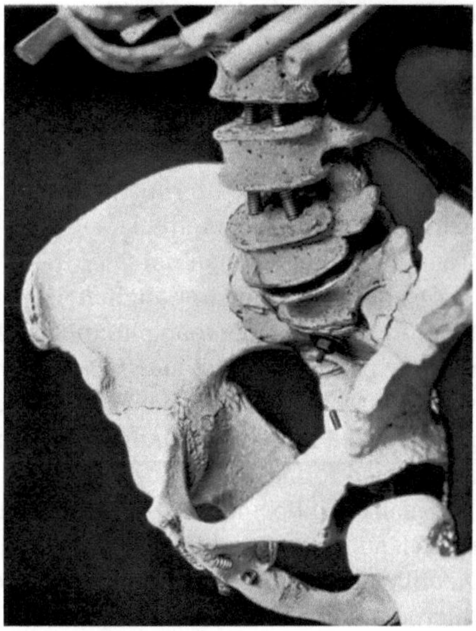

Fig. 101 Pelvis of a 57-year-old cretin. Cartilage retained in places, with bony convolutions; cartilage of the iliac crest retained

10.4 Lower Limbs

P. Müller has alluded to the generally narrowed pelvis and others (Breus & Kolisko, H. Bircher, Bernard, Scholz) have confirmed this. At the acetabulum there are articular cartilage remnants or bony bulges in places, separating the three pelvic bones (Fig. 101).

Furthermore, the iliac crest is often cartilaginous. Moreover, Breus and Kolisko emphasize that the cretin pelvis does not simply have an infantile character, but is still spreading in the later years of growth.

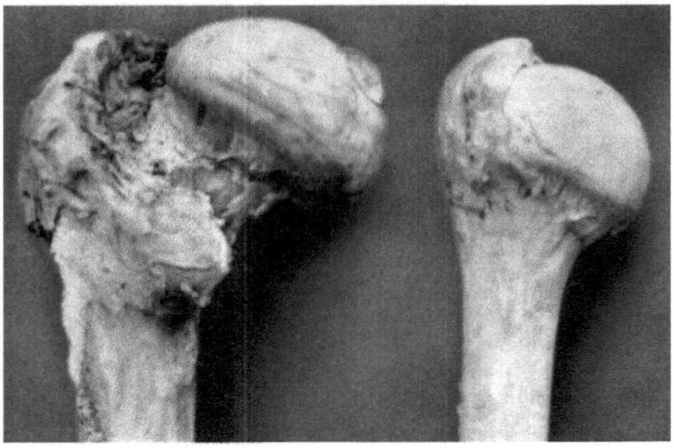

Fig. 102 Femoral and humeral heads of a 20-year-old cretin: femoral head flattened, with a short neck; *Humerus varus*

In the femur, Klebs has already noted the flat, quasi-compressed form of the head (Fig. 87), subsequently described by others as well (H. Bircher, Scholz, Roth, Klar, Looser). Often, the head sits like a mushroom atop the short, squat neck (Fig. 102) although it may also have a normal shape. More often a *Coxa vara cretinosa* occurs (E. Bircher, von Seemen), with not only the angle between neck and shaft reduced but there is also a posterior curvature of the head. These types of deformation are explained probably by the displacements to which the cartilaginous, often softened epiphysis is subjected by loading. On them, to a great extent, rests the shambling gait of the cretin. Tibia, fibula and foot bones do not differ very markedly in shape from non-cretinous material.

Overall, according to Langhans' and my own experience, the bones of cretins are far more often slender than plump, which allows the development of growth in girth, running parallel with reduced growth in length (Fig. 103). There are always cases with remarkably plump bones as well, which is why Finkbeiner differentiates a gracile and a massive type, mistaking the latter (observed only in men so far) as an age-related form.

Finally, Finkbeiner has made the important discovery that the bones of cretins present numerous primitive features reminiscent of those of certain Polar populations, Neolithic pygmies and, indirectly, the Neandertals as well. We will come back to the interpretation of these characteristics of the cretin skeleton.

11 Joints

In recent years *Osteochondritis deformans juvenilis* and *Osteochondritis dissecans* have been observed relatively frequently in juvenile cretins (de Quervain, Scabell, Reich, von Seemen).

This has led to hypothyroidism being considered as a factor that, at least, favours the emergence of these diseases. The hip joint and the knee joint are considered the

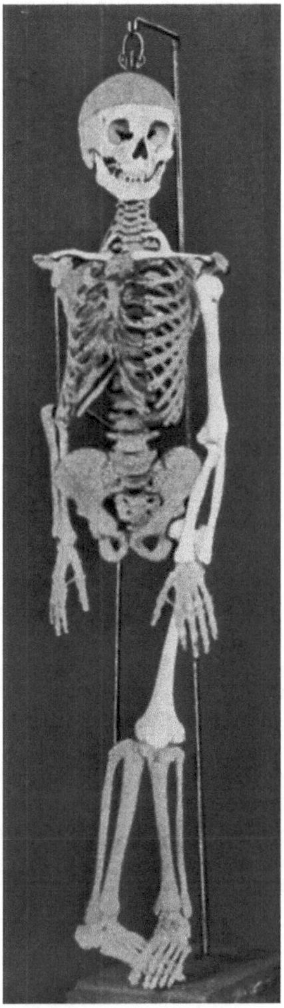

Fig. 103 Skeleton of a 57-year-old male cretin: gracile bone structure

prime sites. The disturbances in epiphyseal ossification mentioned above were standard for pathogenesis, with the degenerated cartilage collapsing, and fragments detaching, to eke out their lives once more as free articular bodies. With some justification, Looser points out that here there is usually no primary *arthritis deformans*, and Lang too emphasizes the difference from *arthritis deformans* in that the cretin's femoral head lacks the vascular and osseous structures that predicate the basal articular cartilage layer. Thus von Seemen speaks of *osteochondropathia cretinoidea* or *osteoarthrosis hypothyreotica*, and Haumann of *osteopathia cretinosa*. It must be stressed that in all cases inflammatory changes are completely absent and so there is no justification for the term 'osteochondritis'. It should be replaced by *osteochondrolysis dissecans*.

In older cretins you can find changes here and there, again especially in the hip joint and the knee joint, which correspond with *arthritis*- (or, better: *arthropathia*)

Fig. 104 *Arthritis deformans* of the femoral head with major cartilaginous defect of a 29-year-old cretin

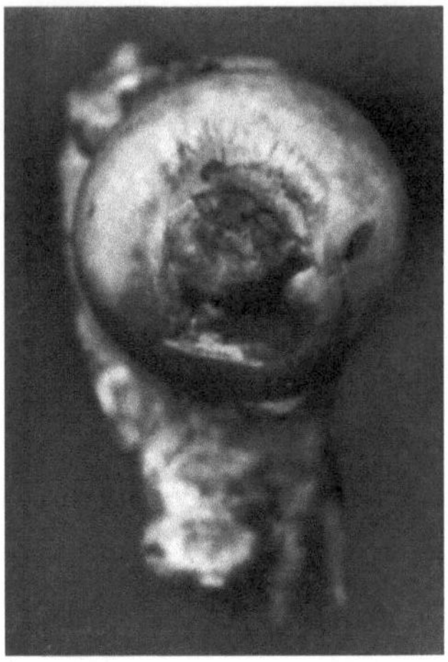

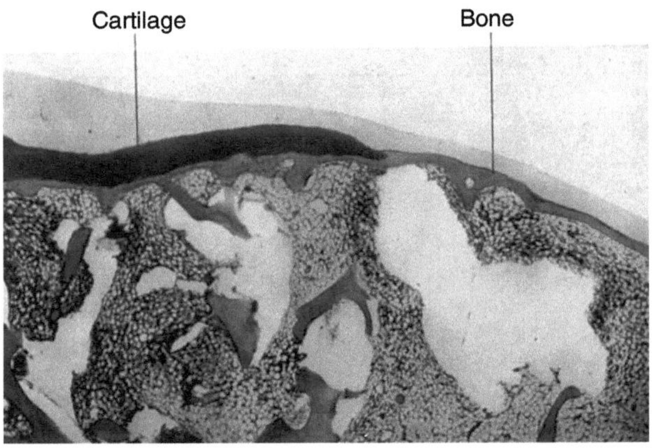

Fig. 105 *Arthritis deformans* of the femoral head of a 28-year-old cretin; cartilage atrophy

deformans atrophica. This mainly involves relatively extensive surface defects in the articular cartilage (Fig. 104), arising only after epiphyseal ossification. On the femoral head they are encountered mainly around the Ligamentum teres, and at the distal end of the femur especially at the condylar level. The articular cartilage is always thinner towards the defect; finally it disappears, and is replaced by a bony lamella that lies somewhat deeper than the bordering articular cartilage (Fig. 105).

Besides these changes arising on the free articular surfaces, there are often small protuberances and tori on the rim of the articular cartilage, as in common *arthritis deformans*. However, such excrescences appear to be no more common in cretins than in non-cretins, and the same is true of the cartilage defects that, according to Beitzke, may also regularly be encountered after the fiftieth year among non-cretins. However, it is highly likely that the defective function of the thyroid gland also favours the emergence of such wear and tear on cartilage.

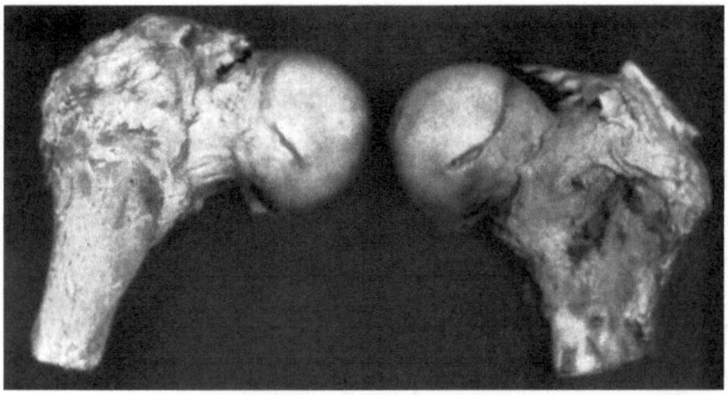

Fig. 106 *Arthritis deformans*: anterior aspect of the femoral head with deep cartilaginous furrows of a 29-year-old cretin

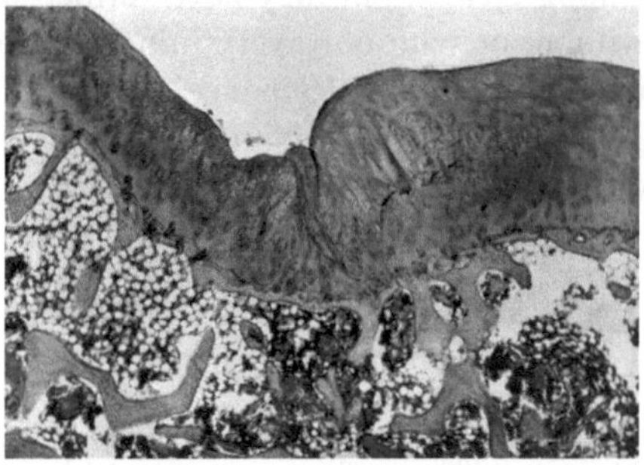

Fig. 107 Cartilage furrow in the femoral head of a 29-year-old cretin; thickening of the *spongiosa* deep to this

Apart from that, deforming articular alterations can of course also develop on the basis of the ossification disorders of the heads of bone described above (Looser); for it is clear that the mechanical stress on such malformed and partially softened epiphyses is quite different from the stress on a well-formed and well-ossified head of a bone. In regard to the softening process in the cartilage preparatory to the ossification, I would, for example, like to go back to a remarkable groove structure that I saw in the articular cartilage of both femoral heads of a 28-year-old cretin (Fig. 106). From the microscopic view these grooves must have arisen through compression of the cartilage. In particular, the cartilage in the groove shows converging columns, rich in cells, with the basal substance unravelling. The bone located beneath has adapted to the new mechanical relationships through the formation of supporting pillars (Fig. 107).

12 Teeth

Delayed dentition and delayed dental transition are quite common occurrences in severe cases of cretinism (Cerletti and Perusini, E. Bircher, Diviak and Wagner von Jauregg, Mayrhofer). In rare cases the dental changeover does not even occur. If you visualize the analogous situation in congenital absence of a thyroid gland, it may immediately become clear that this is a consequence of defective function of the thyroid.

Anomalies in the position and form of the teeth are quite common among cretins, as is enamel hypoplasia (Scholz, Kranz, Schenkel). Eggenberger describes a locking bite which he ascribes to growth restriction of the mandible and maxilla.

In the opinion of various authors (B. Nièpce, St Lager, Scholz, Bayon, E. Bircher, Kranz, Eggenberger) cretins are quite particularly predisposed to dental caries; Eggenberger in particular draws the latter disease into a causative relationship with endemic hypothyroidism. I do not consider this correct, because totally different factors can come into play here – food characteristics, for example. Moreover, Mayrhofer even found an astonishingly high number of caries-free dentitions among cretins, and Stahl too mentions a cretin dentition without any caries. The most recent studies by Schenkel do indeed confirm the frequency of caries among cretins, but they have further shown that the rarer type of somatic cretins without or with only very minor intellectual defect show an extensively reduced incidence of caries. Schenkel explains this simply by the later onset of the cretinogenic noxious agent, with brain and teeth consequently being better developed and, on the other hand, by better dental care in those who are cretins only physically.

13 Skin and Subcutaneous Tissue

The myxœdema often encountered in juvenile cretins (always encountered, according to Cerletti) is found primarily in hands and feet, as well as the face, particularly eyelids, cheeks and lips. On several occasions, a characteristic accumulation of fat was described in the supraclavicular fossa (Bayon, Wagner von Jauregg). After puberty the skin swelling usually disappears, giving way to a wrinkly, dry, scaly skin that is easily creased. But you can still encounter definite myxœdema in older dwarf cretins as well. It should disappear at around 40 in women, according to Cerletti. The skin shade is usually pale yellowish to brownish. The scalp is usually thick and coarse, severely wrinkled to an abnormal degree, and often shows the characteristics of *Cutis verticis gyrata* (Jadassohn).

The histological skin changes found so far are negligible in nature. I have personally found an increase in connective tissue cells in the upper layers of the dermis and especially in the papillary layer, as well as a certain swelling and pale staining of the collagen fibres, and a reduction of the elastic fibres. The pigment content of the basal cell layers was usually fairly heavy, as correspondingly was the number of chromatophores in the papillary layer. On the other hand, like other authors (Langhans, Bernard, Bayon, Schlagenhaufer, and Wagner von Jauregg) I have never seen mucin or similar substances. I have, however, never had the opportunity of examining any samples of myxœdematous facial skin from juvenile cretins. It is therefore quite possible that in the fresh state a heterogeneous, possibly mucous infiltration takes place in the skin, disappearing again later.

On the other hand, Schlagenhaufer and Wagner von Jauregg found a characteristic basophilic substance in cretinous dogs, deposited in the dermis, especially around the sebaceous glands, and significantly reduced after nourishment of the thyroid gland. However, since this substance did not display all the reactions of mucus, it could not be identified definitively as mucin. I have personally seen a mucus-like substance totally lost in the skin, in three young, cretinous dogs. It is noted, however, that in the myxœdema of congenital athyrosis also mucus or mucus-like deposits had rarely been found.

The *hirsuteness* of cretins shows certain characteristics. Male scalp hair is usually bristly; beard and moustache thinly sown. In both sexes of dwarf cretins, the axillary hair and genital hair are very sparse – the former may be absent entirely.

I found the *glandular appendages* of the skin always well maintained, even though rather small; the same is true of the apocrine glands of the axillae.

Finger nails are described as short, cracked, brittle and thick by Eggenberger and Zangerl. Furthermore, white flecks are said to occur not uncommonly in the finger nails, but these are certainly unrelated to cretinous degeneration.

14 Ear

The fact that the percentage of hard-of-hearing cretins and deaf-mutes is higher in the region of endemic cretinism than elsewhere, and the hearing problems themselves, have provided the impetus for numerous specialized examinations of the entire auditory system of deaf-mutes and cretins (cf. Nager).

As regards the *external ear*, it is often noticeably thickened through myxœdema, but, according to Wagner von Jauregg and my own observations, it rarely shows so-called signs of degeneration, such as swollen ear lobules, pointed ears or a rolled-up helix. Scholze found these in 40% of his cases, although it is suspected that these included cases of common idiocy, where such deformities are known to occur particularly often.

The *middle ear* is probably the most commonly altered and the most severely afflicted. The mastoid process is often small; in many cases, it lacks a cavity. As for the bones, according to Nager and M. Meyer, the endochondral bones of the capsule of the labyrinth are completely normal, while the periosteal capsular layer, which borders the tympanic cavity, shows a very marked thickening, particularly on the promontory, thereby causing a narrowing of the fenestra. The roof of the tympanic cavity is also thickened. It can therefore be concluded that the pathological process takes place mainly post-embryologically although still in the initial years of life; its beginnings can extend right back into the late foetal period. In later life, the bony overgrowth can progress further, even to the formation of exostoses. The endosteal layer of the semicircular canals can likewise present hyperostoses.

Other changes involve the ossicles, which are plump and enlarged; the periosteal part of the stapes especially is thickened. The mucous membrane of the tympanic cavity is similarly thickened with the sub-epithelial connective tissue proliferated and interspersed with fat and mucous tissue. However, the latter is derived from foetal stroma that only incompletely degenerates (Habermann, Alexander, Manasse, O. Meyer, Nager).

The *inner ear* frequently exhibits an anomaly of the cochlea in the form of a columnar, hyaline band that is found between the organ of Corti and the membrane of Corti (Oppikofer, Siebenmann, Schlittler, Mayer, Nager).

Thus in endemic cretinism there are primarily disturbances in the region of the middle ear that impair conductivity. Yet the middle ear can also be completely normal, as demonstrated by a case from our material examined by Siebenmann. Goitrous deaf-mutes and cretins in the endemic region might therefore not always offer the same finding, and there should be even more stringent differentiation between these two groups. Furthermore, it must always be borne in mind that part of the central hearing difficulty in cretins may have its underlying cause within the auditory centre (H. Bircher).

If we include the situations obtaining in congenital athyrosis for comparison, in the very few cases examined so far, the auditory organ has been found to be remarkably normal apart from an incomplete ossification in the endochondral and periosteal capsular layer of the labyrinth (Siebenmann, Nager). In a further case (27-year-old woman), dissected in my institute and examined by Siebenmann, the labyrinthine bones and the inner ear were normal; there was only a minor, acute inflammation of the middle ear. However, it remains to be seen whether the hearing organ is normal on a regular basis, and whether a drastic difference between thyroaplasia and endemic cretinism exists at this site.

15 Circulatory System

Among cretins, the *heart* participates in the general growth disorders and is, accordingly, small. On several occasions I have encountered hearts weighing only 170–200 g among cretins of 19–38 years old, and among old cretins too the weight usually remains below 300 g. There is often a strong brown pigmentation. Under the influence of valvular defects and extracardial diseases (pulmonary emphysema, contracted kidneys) this may also lead to mild hypertrophy and enlargements, although more often we are dealing only with a terminal dilatation of the right side of the heart. Findings recorded in the literature about cardiac behaviour are quite contradictory; however, the majority of authors describe the heart as being small.

Mild fatty degeneration (usually only speckled adiposis) of the muscle fibres is often detectable histologically, although, in the main, this might stem from the terminal illness. Inflammatory infiltration and connective tissue calluses are rare, and must similarly be traced back to diseases that inherently have nothing to do with cretinism. On the other hand, it is probably no coincidence that lipofuscin appears precociously in greater quantities at the nuclear poles of the muscle fibres, indicating early wear and tear at a relatively young age.

Sclerotic changes of the cardiac valves seem to be no more strongly developed than among non-cretins of similar age. The same is true regarding the frequency of endocarditis and valvular insufficiency.

Also, *arteries* in general show no particularly pronounced tendency toward sclerotic changes. These are of course common among older cretins, to the same degree as in non-cretins. In younger cretins, arterial behaviour is not uniform. Indeed, like Bayon, I have seen a slight or relatively severe sclerosis in the odd 20 to 25-year-old cretin, with the aorta presenting thick, severely adiposed lamina, while other cretins of similar age showed completely normal arteries; and older cretins, between 30 and 50 years, presented only a mild degree of sclerosis. Therefore, it cannot be suggested that cretinism leads regularly to premature arteriosclerosis. The same is true moreover of congenital athyrosis, where the findings are similarly highly variable.

In order to study the influence of thyroid gland deficiency on the development of experimental arteriosclerosis in rabbits, my research student, Miss Rösli, fed cholesterol to thyroidectomized animals. However, no clear difference in the severity of arterial changes could be established from the control animals. Therefore, we can hardly talk of a significant proportion of hypothyroidism or athyroidism being involved in the development of arteriosclerosis. Possibly it is different with arterial calcification, which had been observed by von Eiselberg, Pick and Pineles in thyroidectomized goats and sheep; although this probably does not match human arteriosclerosis.

15.1 Capillaries

Since the introduction of capillary microscopy in the living, the state of the capillaries among cretins has been the object of many investigations. The honour falls to Jaensch, Wittneben and Hoepfner for having pointed out the frequent occurrence of restrictions in capillary development –the so-called *Archicapillaren* – among cretins and goitrous individuals (Fig. 52). Even though the same restrictions had been found in other mental disorders, for example, in pure cerebral idiocy, a dependence of the capillary structure on thyroid gland function was nevertheless assumed by several authors (for example Stefko and Glagolewa) whereas, according to Jaensch and Hoepfner, the altered capillary structure represented only an equivalent of thyroid gland disorder.

Admittedly, the investigations, carried out by Gehri on a large sample of cretin material, did show that there was no characteristic capillary picture for hypothyroidism, and that normal or insignificantly changed capillaries are found by way of exception even in severe cretinism. Nevertheless, the capillary picture in roughly 67% of cretins is markedly changed, and in 33% moderately changed, with a correlation between the severity of capillary anomalies and thyroid gland atrophy being clearly recognizable. On the other hand, there is no correlation with restriction of body growth. Among non-cretin idiots and other purely cerebral diseases, the deviations of capillary formation were to some extent even more severe than in cretinism. Also, Bock has often evaluated the arcuate capillaries in thyrogenic dwarf growth and imbecility, and emphasizes that they are in no way specific for endocrine disorders. Luchsinger obtained the same results with regard to endemic hearing difficulty and deaf-mutism. Here, too, the capillary restrictions are absolutely not a regular appearance. Nevertheless, in the endemic form they appear significantly more often and in greater severity than in common labyrinthine deafness and inherited degenerative deaf-mutism. Thus the formation of cutaneous capillaries among cretins as far as we know is not totally dependent on hypothyrosis, but up to a certain level goes its own way.

16 Blood and Blood-Forming Organs

The majority of cretins present certain anomalies in the formation of *blood*, which is, in turn, dependent on the activity of the blood-forming organs. Here, we shall consider only the morphological findings – the rest is found in the section on pathological physiology.

According to E. Kind and Wälchi, who examined a large number of cretins, there is often a reduction in the number of erythrocytes, although elevated numbers can also occur. In spite of this, enhanced regeneration does not happen, so Wälchi assumes that there is an adaptation of the blood to low metabolic requirements. The total white blood cell count was usually over 7,000 (no units provided). Kind was able to determine an increase of lymphocytes in 73% of cases, while Wälchi found variations in lymphocyte numbers in the majority of cases to be within the normal range. The eosinophilic leucocytes are fairly commonly increased (in 33–50% of cases), likewise the basophils. The phagocytic ability of the leucocytes shows no deviation from the norm (Aeschlimann).

There is thus no typical haematological picture for cretinism, although the main features show a good match with the changes seen in athyrosis.

The same is true for the blood cell production sites. According to Stoccada and my own observations, the *bone marrow* is indeed always red in the bones of the base of the skull and the torso (vertebrae, sternum, ribs, and pelvis), but in the long bone diaphyses and epiphyses there is often a premature conversion into yellow marrow. Nevertheless, in the odd case I have found normal behaviour in the femur, namely, red marrow in the proximal part of the diaphysis and yellow in the distal portion. Microscopically, the abundance of eosinophilic myelocytes and leucocytes usually stands out; furthermore, here and there lymphoid follicles with germinating centres are detectable (Stoccada). The number of megakaryocytes is somewhat lower than normal. Apart from that, a very marked fat cell infiltration is often recognizable, both histologically and macroscopically, in the red marrow, so that the cell-forming activity of the bone marrow is, therefore, on the whole a lot less vigorous than the norm. Admittedly, this is a lot more energetic in congenital athyrosis.

The *lymphatic glands* have normal size and structure; a swelling is found only during local infectious processes or during systemic illnesses of the blood-forming organs, for example, leukaemia. This is true also of the lymphatic apparatus of the digestive tract, only occurring more strongly in juvenile cretins. Only once have I encountered the pronounced pattern of *status lymphaticus* in a cretin (a 49-year-old woman with persisting thymus).

The *spleen* is usually small, its weight usually ranging between 35 and 120 g, exceeding this upper limit only during the type of general infection that would otherwise lead to an enlarged spleen. In juvenile dwarf cretins the spleen usually weighs less than 100 g, and with ageing there is often secondary atrophy. The follicles are normally big or small; the trabeculae are usually thickened into varying degrees of fibrosis. In the pulp a major haemosiderosis attracted my attention a few times, possibly indicating a certain sluggishness of the splenic metabolism with increased decline in erythrocyte numbers. Deposition of hyaline in the wall of the small follicular arteries occurs not uncommonly among cretins, but obviously has no specific character.

17 Respiratory Organs

The larynx shows growth delay in dwarf cretins, however, virtually never so severe that voice-breaking does not occur in men. No particular swellings stood out here, nor did ossification of the cartilage occur in advanced years. In goitrous cretins the trachea can be narrowed. The remainder of the airway presents no peculiarities.

The *lungs* too are normally formed, apart from a certain diminutiveness. With age, as in other individuals, they tend to emphysema.

18 Digestive Organs

18.1 Tongue

Enlargement of the tongue (macroglossia) has been observed in isolated cases among juvenile cretins; according to Bayon it is based on a proliferation of fatty tissue. I have never observed this personally.

Pharynx and *oesophagus* show no differences.

18.2 Stomach and Intestine

Several authors have often found these enlarged, and, according to Scholz, inflammation is quite common. The enlargement, which I too have often encountered, could be a consequence of stagnation of the contents due to the commonly found inertia of the gastric and intestinal peristalsis. In a 38-year-old cretin male, I observed a megacolon that had led to a volvulus of the sigmoid colon which had its origin in a wrinkling at the transition of the sigmoid into the rectum. Peptic ulcers are rare – I saw one perforated duodenal ulcer and an ulcer scar in the stomach.

18.3 Salivary Glands

So far, no changes in size or in the histological structure have been detected.

18.4 Pancreas

Size and weight of the pancreas show quite significant variation among cretins. In several instances I found the weight very low (41–53 g), in others again so high (75–95 g), that you would speak of normal proportions among non-cretins (average weight in healthy soldiers 91 g, according to Rössle). However, when you take into account the small body size, the weight of the pancreas in such cretins appears to be surprisingly high. On one occasion, I even came across an enlarged pancreas weighing 155 g.

Histologically the glandular lobules are well formed, only rarely do you find fatty tissue replacing glandular tissue in places. The islets of Langerhans (Fig. 108) are usually abundant, and small or medium sized (150–250 μ); only exceptionally rarely are they particularly large (300–350 μ).

Their cells are often rather heavily impregnated with fat, while the remaining glandular cells reveal only a small fat content, or none at all. The demarcation from the surrounding glandular tissue is usually not very distinct. The insular apparatus is thus histologically well developed, but not unduly so. However, in view of the relative size of the organ, in many cases the total mass of the insular tissue in proportion to body mass could be considered elevated, which, perhaps, might be related to the deficient thyroid gland secretion.

In one case I found a discrete mass of splenic tissue, 5 mm in diameter, in the middle of the pancreas.

18.5 Liver

Liver weight among cretins usually ranges between 1000 and 1400 g – i.e., lower than normal. In one case it weighed only 670 g (29-year-old woman, 145 cm tall).

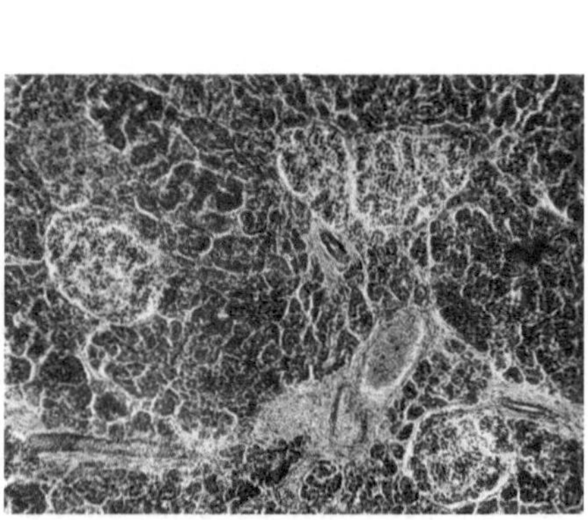

Fig. 108 Pancreas of a 20-year-old cretin: large islets of Langerhans

The lobular structure is unchanged. Very often there is fatty degeneration of the hepatic cells varying in both severity and extent; on the other hand, I have never come across great quantities of glycogen. Yet both of these can stem from terminal illnesses. Even in juvenile cretins a rather large amount of lipofuscin is often contained in the central cells within the lobule. I once also saw central lobular necrosis in a case of chronic tubulonephritis.

18.6 Gall Bladder

Only the not-very-rare cholelithiasis is mentioned here (Stahl, Eulenburg and Marfels, Bayon, Wegelin). In the Bernese cases, it usually involved mixed bilirubin-lime calculi and, on one occasion, pure-black pigmented calculi. Remarkably, these calculi were found only in males.

18.7 Peritoneum

The relatively limited growth of the abdominal muscles and the sluggishness of peristalsis favour the development of hernias among cretins. Their frequency has already been noted in the earlier literature and I have confirmed this. In addition to umbilical hernias, inguinal and femoral herniation also occurs.

19 Urinary System

The *kidneys* vary markedly in size and weight, ranging from 100 to 300 g. Their surface often presents foetal grooves. In individual cases you may find very minor fatty degeneration of the epithelium of the main components, occasionally also calcification of the epithelial cells. In the cortex, among older cretins, small, isolated patches of shrinkage often accrue; in exceptional cases, cysts also.

As for the more severe degenerative and inflammatory changes, I have only seen chronic tubulonephritis on two occasions, when the tubular epithelium showed turbid swelling and minor fatty degeneration, with many hyaline cylinders present in the lumina. The interstitium was infiltrated by swarms of lymphocytes – in one case leucocytes had also crossed over into the tubules. Since similar renal changes had been observed following thyroidectomies in animals, you could ponder the effect of a hypothyrosis in these cases – the more so as no other causes could be found for the nephritis. However, such cases are too infrequent for the hypothyrosis to be regarded as the sole factor. Clinically they conformed to a nephrosis.

In one case I saw a pyelonephritis after cystitis. However, diseases of the urinary tract are decidedly rare among cretins.

20 Further Anatomical Findings

In a perusal of the autopsy reports, it struck me that *malformations* of individual organs frequently exist among cretins. Among 42 cases, on three occasions I encountered club feet; Meckel's diverticulum three times, and one case each of hypospadia, cryptorchism and polycystic disease of the kidney and liver. By comparison, normal autopsy cases give one case of Meckel's diverticulum in 50 (E. Kaufmann), or 65 cases (Döpfner).

Due to the small sample size, obviously no far-reaching conclusions can be drawn from these data. However, should further observations confirm that malformations among cretins are more frequent than in other autopsy material, it might then be assumed that cretins are highly predisposed to disruptions in development, and especially inhibiting malformations.

Also of interest is the frequency of blastomas among cretins. Of my 42 cases of autopsy material 13 were tumescent, although I reserved judgement on diagnosing adenoma of the thyroid gland.

Malignant tumours were present in eight cases – on four occasions these involved thyroid tumours (two carcinomas and two proliferating goitres), one pharyngeal carcinoma; one carcinoma of the bladder, two cerebral gliomas and one lymphosarcoma of the ileum. I found the carcinoma of the pharynx and the lymphosarcoma of the intestine in the same individual.

The percentage of malignant tumours seems high (19%) at first glance. However, when you consider that four cases involved a goitrous thyroid gland, and that only two carcinomas were found outside the thyroid gland, in no way can you argue that cretinism induces a universal predisposition to cancer development. Also, when you add on the four cases of malignant thyroid tumours, this gives a percentage of only 15, which roughly corresponds with the incidence of cancer among the adult population of Switzerland. You would expect considerably more cancer cases among cretins if hypothyrosis were an actual cause of the cancer, and it is therefore a mistake to ascribe fundamental blame for the frequency of cancer in Switzerland (Bayard) to the hypothyrosis connected with endemic goitre. The very fact that goitre-free Denmark nearby, has a higher cancer mortality than Switzerland, makes such an assumption invalid.

Benign tumours were observed on seven occasions: three haemangiomas (liver, sternum and vertebrae), two lipomas (intestinal), one chondroma of the lungs and one leiomyoma of the uterus. In two cases the haemangiomas were found alongside malignant thyroid tumours. Since, with the haemangiomas and also the chondroma, we might assume a congenital malformation as the basis of the tumour, then here too, as with the deformities, we could imagine a specific predisposition among cretins. However, the numbers available are still far too small to provide any kind of conclusion.

Tuberculosis among the cretins who were autopsied in Berne does not play a particularly major role, since among 42 cases, I found signs of tubercular infection in only seven—five of them in the form of a latent pulmonary and hilar tuberculosis, to some extent with a calcified primary complex. In one case there was a tubercular spondylitis of the lumbar vertebral column with carry-over into the meninges. Only two cases showed haematogenic metastases (in the meninges, hip joint, suprarenal glands and hypophysis). This is a confirmation of the data from B. Nièpce, who likewise only rarely found tuberculosis among cretins.

I have never seen signs of *syphilis* among cretins, whereas Cerletti suspects that congenital syphilis could play a certain role in the pathogenesis of cretinism by enhancing hypothyrosis in the foetus and in young children.

21 Lifespan and Diseases of Cretins

Finkbeiner calculated for 100 cretins that their *average age* is significantly lower than that of the total population where they live (30 years for cretins, compared with 35 years (males), or 38 years (females), in the Swiss population[1]). Scholz too reports that cretins have a relatively brief lifespan, while Cerletti thinks that they seldom reach 50.

Among the 42 cretins of my autopsy material, the various age groups are as follows:

Death in	Male	Female	Total
2nd decade	2	–	2
3rd decade	3	3	6
4th decade	5	5	10
5th decade	4	2	6
6th decade	7	3	10
7th decade	1	3	4
8th decade	3	1	4

The average age for all 42 cretins was 46.3 years (46.2 years for the men and 46.4 for the women), so that the values are far below that of the current average life expectancy of the total population. However, the instances of death during childhood are missing and, since it cannot be assumed that cretins have no childhood mortality, my data cannot possibly give an accurate picture of the lifespan of cretins. Nevertheless, they are sufficient to show that many cretins can reach quite a high age, particularly when they are under institutional care (see page 31), and it is therefore quite likely

[1] These values have been obsolete for a long time. In the period 1901–1910 the average life span of the Swiss population was 49 years (male) and 52 (female); during 1921–1930, 58 years (male) and 61 (female).

that statistics for a larger sample would show that the cretins' lifespan currently does not differ much at all from that of the rest of the population.

The summary of the *causes of death* is as follows:

Pneumonia (including viral pneumonia)	4	Wound infections after trauma and surgery, peritonitis following herniotomy	6
Pneumonia following thyroidectomy	3	Perforated duodenal ulcer	1
Pulmonary emphysema	2	Myeloid leukaemia	1
Cardiovascular disease	5	Tubercular meningitis	2
Urological disorders (nephritis and cystitis)	3	Cancer of the thyroid gland	4
Prostate hypertrophy	2	Carcinoma of other organs	2
Exsanguination in childbirth	1	Cerebral glioma	2
Puerperal infections	3	Suicide	1

Thus, besides the malignant goitres, acute infections (pneumonia, wound infections, puerperal infections) primarily play a substantial role, for cretins possibly have a reduced resistance to such infections. Yet, for example, the peritonitis observed on two occasions after herniotomy can also be traced back to the indolence of cretins when faced with incarcerated hernias.

In any case, in my opinion, no conclusion can be drawn that cretins are generally less resistant, and therefore die earlier than other sections of the population (H. Bircher). It is remarkable, for example, in my material that in only two instances did tuberculosis lead to death and that, as highlighted above, tubercular foci were rarely found among the Berne cretins. This contradicts the accounts of Allara and Scholz that tuberculosis among cretins is surprisingly common. Evidently it depends very much on the environment where the cretins grow up. Maffei, for example, is of the opinion that cretins are 'on average very healthy' – they come through the common childhood illnesses with flying colours, and only rarely are they taken ill with epidemic ailments. As causes of death among older cretins he names primarily stroke, tuberculosis, and œdema. It has already been discussed that cancer is not particularly common among cretins.

In my autopsy material, besides the illnesses quoted as causes of death, there are of course, a whole series of other ailments mentioned. These are to be regarded as secondary findings, or to have favoured the onset of the fatal illness. However, I have been unable to recognise any characteristic connection with cretinism.

In any case, the current statistical material is still too small for us to claim, with any certainty, that cretinism achieves for itself an enhanced predisposition for other illnesses, and behaves, in this sense, in a life-shortening manner. Where a greater mortality actually does exist among cretins as opposed to the rest of the population, it is probably, as Scholz correctly points out, caused for the most part by poor nursing and the level of care afforded these creatures. Added to this is the mental sluggishness that is often connected with bodily neglect and lack of cleanliness, since hygiene is, of course, not taught to cretins.

22 Cretinism in Animals

Undoubtedly, in an endemic area, cretinism would also occur in animals. Von Hanseman even saw a cretinous jackal with a large goitre in the Berlin Zoo, although this would have been only an isolated case.

So far, the endemic form has been observed with any certainty only in dogs (Cerletti and Perusini; Schlagenhaufer and Wagner von Jauregg; Dexler; von Kutschera; Bayer) and it occurs in the same way in different populations. It is expressed as in humans, both in the intellectual and in the physical sphere. The animals are mentally blunted, very sluggish, and unsteady in their gait. Affective movements are totally lacking. They are physically striking due to their plumpness. Facial structure, as in humans, is distinctive– mainly due to the broad, deep-set nose, which is related to a corresponding foreshortening of the muzzle. The skin is very thick and flabby, in great floppy folds, and the tail that is always tucked between the back legs is bald, or quite deficient in hair.

The metabolism of such a dog is clearly limited – they eat very little, drink almost nothing or not at all and excrete very small quantities of faeces and urine. Their hearing ability is defective (Schlagenhaufer and Wagner von Jauregg).

Remarkably, there is usually no significant deviation of any kind in the behaviour of the thyroid gland of these animals. In Schlagenhaufer and Wagner von Jauregg's cases, gland size corresponded roughly with the norm, and, microscopically too, the picture gave no suspicion of a reduction in function. The well-formed vesicles bulged with colloid; the epithelium was low, but without any signs of degeneration; and the connective tissue had not increased. Nevertheless, the thyroid glands in these cases must have been functioning quite inadequately, because thyroid gland nourishment led to a favourable influence on the mental and physical behaviour of these animals, beyond all expectation. Likewise, the myxœdematous skin changes mentioned earlier were, for the most part, eliminated by organ therapy. In Cerletti and Perusini's case involving a 6-month-old puppy, the main feature was a colloid goitre that also contained isolated sclerotic portions with small follicles and degenerated epithelium.

The thyroid gland of cretinous dogs therefore appears to behave differently from that of human cretins. An atrophy has still not been found among dogs, although a personal observation revealed that cretinous dogs can present high-grade goitre at least shortly after birth.

Through the kind offices of Professor Kottmann, I received from Mr A. Hess in Berne a litter of four 5-week-old, rough-haired fox terriers of healthy parentage. The first three litters from these parents were completely normal; the fourth litter for the first time included a goitrous puppy. The puppies of the fifth litter were very severely retarded in growth, markedly dull and lethargic and all were goitrous. The head was short; the root of the nose broad and deep-set and the incisor teeth had erupted in only the biggest and relatively liveliest of the pups (Fig. 109). The smallest of the four siblings could neither stand nor walk, lay totally immobile on its belly, was totally apathetic and emitted only gentle, quavering noises (Fig. 110).

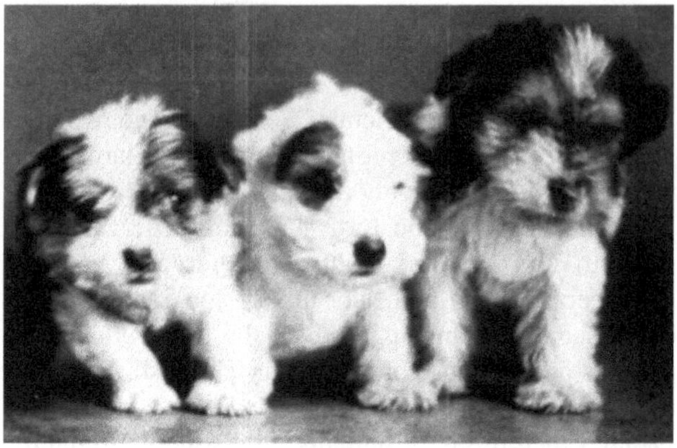

Fig. 109 Cretin puppies; 5 weeks old (No. 1–3)

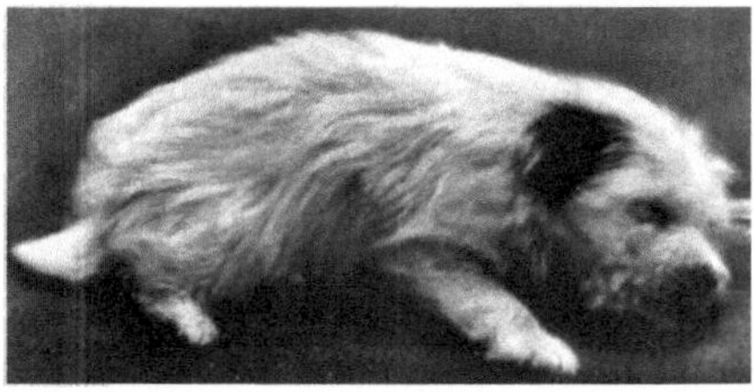

Fig. 110 Cretin puppy No. 4; 5 weeks old

Of the other three pups, two, somewhat bigger, could walk unaided, but were otherwise very dull as well. All three had a large, hard goitre and suffered increasing dyspnoea. Two pups died within the first few days, a third was in a very bad way and was euthanased with chloroform. Only the fourth, biggest and somewhat more lively puppy (on the right in Fig. 109) which could walk well, could already bark, and had only a small goitre, remained alive. With the administration of iodised cooking salt the pup continued to develop very well. The goitre clearly regressed. This pup was sacrificed at 4 months old. Subsequent litters from the same parents produced no further goitres, even though special prophylactic measures were not undertaken.

Dissection of the first three pups revealed a very large, bilateral, diffuse goitre (Fig. 111) with no distinct compression of the trachea; and furthermore, a lobular pneumonia; with some degree of atelectasis of a few areas of the lung and enlargement of the right side of the heart and, in one case, the left half as well. The thymus was not enlarged. The intestinal canal contained parasites (*Taenia canina* and *Ascaris mystax*).

22.1 Histological Finding

In all three cases the goitre showed a uniform structure, namely, a very marked polymorphism of the vesicles, with many cushions and papillae and a fairly tall, cylindrical epithelium (Fig. 112).

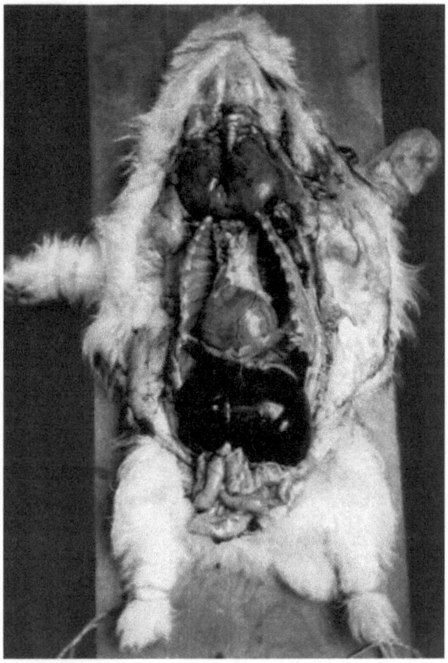

Fig. 111 *Struma diffusa parenchymatosa* of a 5-week-old cretin puppy (No. 3)

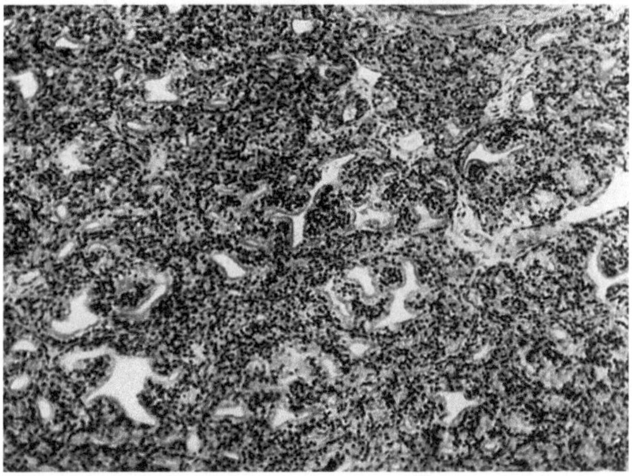

Fig. 112 Thyroid gland of a cretin puppy (No. 4): *Struma diffusa parenchymatosa*

In addition, there were also shorter and longer tubules and solid, undifferentiated masses of epithelium with polyhedral cells. The nuclei were round, rich in chromatin and regular in size. The protoplasm was usually pale, finely vacuolated, but not adipose. Colloid was present in trace amounts only, in two cases; in the third it was very sparse, partially granular, mostly very thin and eosinophilic. The connective tissue stroma was generally delicate. Therefore, this was a *Struma diffusa parenchymatosa* that, with its abundance of epithelium, its vesicular polymorphism, cylindrical

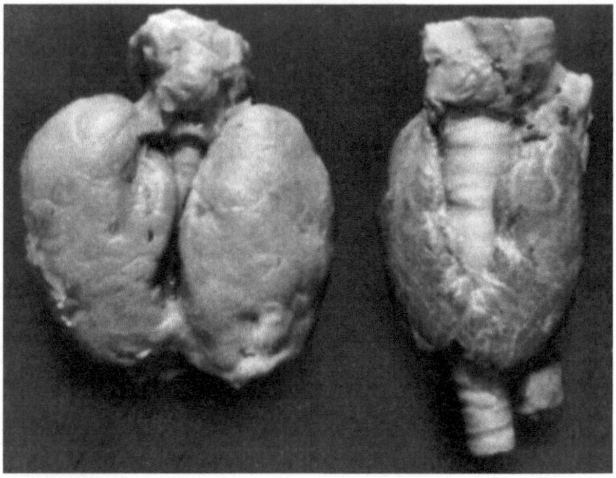

Fig. 113 *Struma diffusa* in cretin dogs. *Left*: a 5-week-old puppy; an animal 4 months old, treated with iodised salt

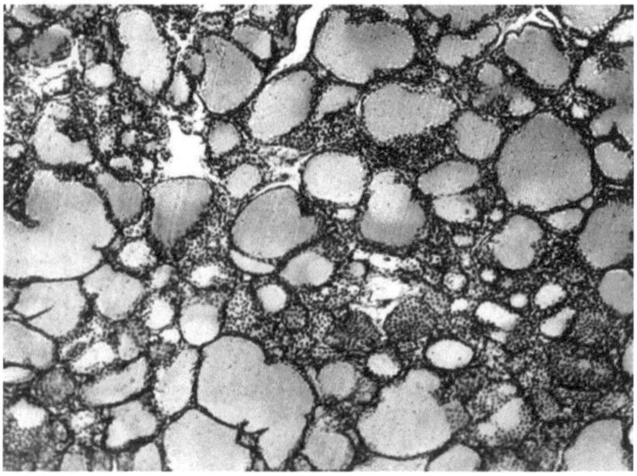

Fig. 114 Thyroid gland of a young dog (No. 1): this animal was previously cretinous, before treatment with iodised salt. Subsequently, the goitre diminished (*Struma diffusa colloides*)

epithelium and colloid impoverishment, was reminiscent of a genuine human Basedow's goitre.

Examination of the other organs yielded nothing remarkable, apart from a lobular, fibrinous pneumonia, and a mild fatty degeneration of the myocardium, skeletal musculature, and liver. In particular, the basophilic masses in the skin, described by Schlagenhaufer and Wagner von Jauregg, were not found.

In the *normally developed animal that had been sacrificed at 4 months*, the thyroid gland was significantly smaller than in its younger siblings (Fig. 113). The other organs were normal; *Ascaris mystax* was in the gut.

The histological picture of the thyroid gland was quite otherwise. The lobules overall comprised roundish, oval or slightly sinous vesicles with flattened epithelium; the latter were plump and filled with thick, eosinophilic colloid (Fig. 114). The undifferentiated epithelial masses had completely disappeared; the septa between the alveoli were narrow throughout – thus, the typical picture of a *Struma diffusa colloides*. The other organs presented no remarkable histological findings.

It follows from these observations that the *clinical picture of canine cretinism can be related to a congenital goitre*, which coincides with certain discoveries in humans. Fodéré had already described the nut-sized goitre as a characteristic of neonatal cretinism, while Diviak and Wagner von Jauregg found a congenital goitre in at least a portion of their cases of cretinism in children. It is, of course, possible that the goitre does regress again and that the symptoms of cretinism therefore similarly disappear, as my experiment demonstrated with the fourth dog, which became completely normal with iodised salt. Thyroid gland treatment can have this effect too, and when Schlagenhaufer and Wagner von Jauregg found thyroid glands rich in colloid, that had not enlarged, in their cretinous dogs, in at least two of these animals earlier thyroid gland nourishment was responsible.

MacCarrison wanted to study cretinism in rats as well, particularly the offspring of animals that had been administered a filtrate of fecal emulsion as drinking water for several months. These cretinous rats were characterized by very stunted growth and curvature of the spine. One would have to concede however that it would probably be quite difficult to find all the symptoms of cretinism in such rats.

23 Summary

If we survey the morphological findings in typical cases of endemic cretinism, they are as follows:

In the *thyroid gland* that is probably goitrous at birth, i.e., diffusely hyperplastic, the glandular epithelium decays into premature degeneration, even total decline in some cases, so that in the very first decade there can be a severe atrophy and sclerosis of the entire organ, with hypothyrosis the implicit consequence. In many cases, regenerative epithelial proliferation takes place in the damaged organ leading to the formation of nodular hyperplasias or real adenomas. Thus, a very large nodular goitre can often develop. It usually however has a parenchymatous character with little secretory activity. The glandular tissue between the nodes can, to a large extent, decay.

The *endocrine glands*, which are correlated with the thyroid gland, are often influenced in structure and function by the hypothyrosis. The *anterior lobe of the hypophysis* almost always presents a probably compensatory hyperplasia with increase and enlargement of the chief cells, which show similar changes to those of pregnancy. The development of the *generative glands* is restricted, as is the development of the other sexual organs; and the secondary sexual characteristics are curtailed, or at least retarded. The testes of cretins at puberty often show premature atrophy and sclerosis. Also, probably in the majority of cases, *thymus* development remains below normal and the thymus tissue tends toward premature involution. On the other hand, the *suprarenal glands* are well developed, only rarely showing sclerosis of the glomerular zone. The *parathyroid glands* and the *epiphyses* do not deviate from the norm.

In the *brain*, which is usually unchanged macroscopically, there is a frequent occurrence of developmental disorders, whose origin must be traced back to the foetal period. In addition, there are chronic regressive changes, indicative of premature depletion and metabolic disturbances.

Disorder in the area of the *skeleton* is very pronounced, with both growth and development of the bony system experiencing fairly major restriction. Also, at the onset of functional loading, the restriction carries the seeds of regressive changes which can lead to severe deformations in the cartilaginous epiphyses and, further, to joint diseases. Likewise, development of the *teeth* is retarded and, not infrequently, impaired. The *skin* of juvenile cretins is, as a rule, myxœdematous, but shows signs of premature ageing.

The oligocythaemia very often present in the *blood* is matched by the tendency of the *bone marrow* to premature conversion into yellow bone marrow, while the *lymphatic tissue* is generally well developed although not hyperplastic.

The organs of the *circulatory* and *digestive systems*, as well as the *kidneys*, often remain somewhat below normal in size, but otherwise show no regular changes.

In the *auditory apparatus*, in deaf-mute cretins and cretins who are hard of hearing, there are changes primarily in the middle ear and, more rarely, an anomaly of the cochlea.

Thus, the changes in the organs, apart from those of the thyroid gland, are mainly restrictions in development, together with premature degenerative and involutionary processes. This may explain the characteristic fusion of childlike and geriatric features in many cretins.

Cretins die, frequently in advanced years, of a wide range of illnesses. Tuberculosis and cancer are not particularly common among them.

Cretinism also occurs in dogs. In these animals, as far as current knowledge goes, the thyroid gland is altered in the sense of a congenital, diffuse parenchymatosed goitre. Early administration of iodine or thyroid gland nourishment may remedy the symptoms of cretinism, with the thyroid gland transforming into a diffuse colloid goitre.

Chapter 7
Pathological Physiology

As we said at the beginning, during the early decades the study of cretinism was confronted with the confusing impression that cretinism on the one hand was bound geographically to those regions of most severe goitres, while on the other hand a large number of cretins do not present goitre. Initially, the clinical relationship linking cretinism with *cachexia thyropriva* discovered by J. and A. Reverdin, Th. Kocher and P. von Bruns in particular, and the myxœdema described by English authors, redirected research for the last 50 years in the direction of the thyroid gland. The fact that a normal thyroid gland had not been found in a single cretin demonstrated that cretinism is in actual fact a thyroid gland problem to a great extent. The non-goitrous cretin turned out to be a person with an atrophic thyroid gland. This atrophy showed the same geographical spread as did the severe endemic goitres. Transitions between thyroid gland atrophies without goitre, and those with goitre, are fluid, and occasionally, within the same family, we find one child stricken purely with thyroid gland atrophy, and the others stricken with cretinous feeble-mindedness with goitre and atrophy of the remnants of the thyroid gland. We therefore had to broaden the idea of goitre endemic disease into that of *endemic thyropathy* encompassing both endemic atrophy of the thyroid gland and the endemic goitrous enlargement of it. Admittedly, that still did not solve the problem but simply defined it more sharply. Thus, in cases of partial and total thyroaplasia unrelated to endemic disease, their nature allows us to define the anatomy and physiology of the individual without a thyroid gland or with isolated remnants, and to compare this with the situation in cretins. As shown in Chap. 6, there was agreement in the essential features, which justified regarding cretinism pathologically and physiologically as a problem of internal secretion. However, there were also differences in the two scenarios, posing the question whether cretinism suffered exhaustion within the concept of hypothyrosis. The view of cretinism that assumes damage of the *entire organism* caused by the still-unknown noxious agent of goitre and, in cretinism and endemic deaf-mutism, sees parallel outcomes of a general degenerative condition with relatively severe damage to the thyroid gland, posed that same question. While Kocher, Moebius and, later, Langhans and von Eiselsberg can be considered the fathers of the purely endocrine approach, the other approach is definitely attributable to

J. Dennison et al., *Endemic Cretinism*,
DOI 10.1007/978-1-4614-0281-7_7,

Virchow, but traces back particularly to Ewald and H. Bircher, and is championed today by E. Bircher and, in part, by Scholz and – in overconfidently expanded form – by von Kutschera.

The problem will not be solved by incontrovertible claims about their nature, nor by merely theoretical deliberations, but it must be tackled by the currently available and constantly improving clinical and laboratory methodologies, with the methods themselves being compared for reliability both in the laboratory and in the clinic. In analyzing the results, it should not be forgotten that the loss of function, whatever its nature, begins to exert its influence on cretins and on congenital athyroids even during intrauterine life, continuing throughout the developmental years, and even persisting throughout life, in contrast to the postnatal damage to the gland. This process leads, on the one hand, to damage very early in development and is therefore irreversible, but, on the other hand, it allows the organism time to enlist the aid of certain protective and compensatory mechanisms. Thus, within individual cretin examples, the process is not completed in precisely the same manner either anatomically or chronologically, so that the pathological–anatomical and the pathological–physiological behaviour of the individual types will also show differences. We are, therefore, far removed from the simple, highly conspicuous conditions yielded by animal experimentation; and the behaviours are also more complex than the relatively straightforward pathological events that we encounter in our *clinical* comparative material, thyroaplasia, and postoperative *cachexia thyropriva.*

In the future study of cretins we should not – as happened all too easily in the past – focus on isolated findings, but, if at all possible, we must carry out studies of larger series, thereby reassuring ourselves in the clinical diagnosis of cretinism. In this area there remains, as a warning, the error of Virchow, who was so critical elsewhere, involving a chondrodystrophic skeleton that he had considered a cretin, which was classified conclusively only by examination of a larger sample.

Wherever we go, the investigation of the pathological physiology of cretinism comes across *one* difficulty that we have not yet mentioned. We still know too little about the *normal* physiology of the thyroid gland. Indeed, physiology affords irreplaceable work through animal observation, and pathological physiology cannot do without this means of research. However, the great ideas and isolated groundbreaking discoveries have flowed out of the clinic into normal physiology. We mention only the new direction given to thyroid gland physiology by the detection of *cachexia thyropriva.* Our current perception of the thyroid gland as an essential organ is based on the observations of J. and A. Reverdin, T. Kocher, P. von Bruns and Horsley; through the project of his student, Grundler, P. von Bruhns was the first to explain the disease process of *cachexia thyropriva* as the breakdown of thyroid gland function. When we became involved in research into cretinism 18 years ago, after many years of work in other areas of thyroid pathology, most physiologists dismissed ideas of a plurality of thyroid gland secretions. Today, evidence for the accuracy of this conjecture, then based on clinical considerations, is increasing. At that time also, the possibility of a dysfunction was almost unanimously rejected by physiology, and the clinical supporters of dysfunction could not produce any evidence for this purely-intuitive opinion. However, both the investigation of

Basedow's disease and the investigation of cretinism then compelled us, and still compels us, to hold on to this possibility despite Gley and Pézard's notion of differentiated threshold values, without it bringing us any closer to the explanation of certain phenomena. What we emphasized in 1921 remains true today: the study of cretinism is just as important as the study of Basedow's disease in research on thyroid gland function.

Ostensibly you could be justified in reproaching us for moving so much in a circle with this approach that it might turn into a vicious cycle. We are basing thyroid gland physiology on the observations of cretins, and then, from this physiology, we aim to interpret cretinism as a functional disorder of the thyroid gland. The reproach would be justified, if our ultimate aim were to arbitrate on thyroid gland problems based on cretin observations. It fails when the study of cretinism defines the problem for us, and when the solution itself is sought in conjunction with means beyond our knowledge of cretinism. Here morphology and pathological anatomy are imperative as a foundation, and as a control mechanism – of which we have been aware since the period of our tutelage under Langhans. It is a special privilege for us to be able to address and investigate these questions in the company of Wegelin, Langhans' pupil and successor.

When, in the following pages, we present a brief synopsis of our results so far, we have to point out, at the very outset, that we are still in the middle of the work, and that an expanded clinical investigation of the nervous system and of the circulatory relationships should only now be considered. In the interests of clarity, we shall be circumspect in referring to the old and the contemporary literature in this area. Discussion about other approaches and research results are found in individual papers by myself and my students, while the paper by Gamper and Scharfetter offers the reader a lucid and objective orientation on the most important points.

We begin with the area of *metabolism.* Scholz, in his highly meritorious works, deals in particular with *albumen* and *salt metabolism.* He comes to the conclusion that cretin metabolism is to be described as very sluggish. He found an astonishing parallel with myxœdema but not with actual (experimental) athyrosis. It is to be noted that Scholz determined most of his comparative values not from his own research but extracted them from the literature. Under the term 'myxœdema', there is no distinction between cases of spontaneous myxœdema in adults and myxœdema with congenital thyroaplasia. Experimental comparative values relate to dogs and rabbits, and are, in this respect, not directly comparable. Finally, Scholz's own experiments were undertaken on just three cretins so that, even here, universal applicability of his observations is limited.

Parallel investigations following thyroid gland nourishment led to the discovery that, in nitrogen metabolism, cretins appear to behave differently from myxœdematous patients but similarly to those individuals suffering from Basedow's disease. From this, Scholz does not conclude a principal contrast between myxœdema and cretinism, but rather that myxœdema lies beyond cretinism. We will enlarge on this significant observation later. In any case, should the small number of observations here likewise give a universal validity to the results?

In recent years, much greater significance has been accorded to *carbohydrate metabolism* in the form of analysis of *basal respiratory metabolism*. This investigation admittedly encountered difficulties among many cretins because its execution required a certain measure of understanding on the part of those being investigated. It can thus be undertaken only by medium and low-grade cretins, and often even there it requires long, intensive practice until the subject is ready to lie motionless, breathing calmly, for 10 min. Values recorded during the first examination are often unusable, and we also, while using all prudent measures, have to take into account that it is only exceptionally that we will be able to determine the actual resting metabolism, and, as a consequence, we usually obtain values that are too high. Nevertheless, the unreliability of an initial investigation is also observed often enough among the mentally healthy. It is generally recognized that individual values can range between plus and minus 10% even in normal thyroid gland activity; *group values*, on the other hand, must align themselves more narrowly around the standard values on which the determinations are based, in order to be regarded as normal.

In a table from our clinic published in 1926, in goitrous individuals without clinical functional disorders we found the precise mean value corresponding with the normal standard of 0% with the usual plus and minus distribution. Among goitrous cretins, on the other hand, there was a mean value of *minus 8%*, with a distribution from minus 39 to minus 9; and among cretins without goitre, a mean value of *minus 11%*, with distribution from minus 29 to 0%. As grouped values therefore, these values are below the norm, even when individual distribution values border on normal.

Among cretins, the basal metabolism is therefore on average decreased, though not as markedly as in myxœdema and postoperative *cachexia thyropriva* where, according to the literature and our own findings, values of minus 40–50% are found. For the most severe cases of cretinism we may assume the likelihood of a greater lowering of basal metabolism, since, given the state of torpor, the clinically estimated oxygen requirement will be even lower. However, as already discussed, the relevant values are unobtainable since investigation is not possible among most cases of Type III. Of significance is the fact that the basal metabolism decreased on average also among the goitrous cretins, but still somewhat less than among the non-goitrous individuals (Table 8).

People have also attempted to obtain a criterion from *blood examination*.

After Mendel and Leichenstern had found a proliferation of lymphocytes in thyroid gland deficiency in 1893, T. Kocher and his students plus, at Wegelin's suggestion, Miss Kind, in 1908 again took up these investigations, and detected leucopenia and a reduction in neutrophilic leucocytes in favour of lymphocytes, among cretins. Niderberger's examination of material from our clinic demonstrated that the mean value in a large series deviated little from the norm, but that, in both Basedow's disease and in cretinism, a relative increase in lymphocytes is not uncommon. Wydler's subsequent examination of a sample of cretin material three times the size from our clinic demonstrates that the lymphocyte numbers among cretins *with* goitre for all three grades show normal means, whereas among cretins without goitre (including dwarf cretins), they are considerably raised, at the expense of neutrophils. We reproduce Wydler's compilation in Table 9.

Table 8 Clinical thyroid function and basal metabolic rate

Basal metabolic rate					As a percentage									
	–	–	–	–	+	+	+	+	+	+	+	+	+	+
Groups	30–39	20–29	10–19	0–9	0–9	10–19	20–29	30–39	40–49	50–59	60–69	70–79	80–89	90–100
Basedow's goitre					...	....	....	....	....	...	.	..	..	.
(hyperthyroid-						....	....	.	..					
ism)							...							
Goitre without			....	....	....	.	.							
functional			....	....	....									
disturbances				....	....									
(euthyroidism)				....	....									
				...	....									
					...									
Goitrous cretins	..	...	....	....	....									
			....	....	....									
				..										
Cretins without		..	..	....										
goitre				.										

Table 9

	Mean value				
Grade of cretinism	I	II	III	Mean total	Number of cases
Haemoglobin[a]					
Goitrous	110.60%	111.18%	115.69%	112.49%	96
Without goitre	–	95%	103.3%	99.1%	10
Red blood cells					
Goitrous	4.48 Mill.	4.59 Mill.	4.417 Mill.	4.49 Mill.	85
Without goitre	–	4.35 Mill.	4.47 Mill.	4.44 Mill.	7
White blood cells					
Goitrous	7870	8390	7557	7939	85
Without goitre	–	7040	8380	7997	7
Neutrophilic leucocytes					
Goitrous	63.7%	65.7%	67.53%	65.64%	86
Without goitre	–	55%	47.6%	51.3%	7
Lymphocytes					
Goitrous	30.25%	31.14%	26.15%	29.18%	86
Without goitre	–	43.5%	47.8%	46.65%	7

[a]We are inclined to trace the relatively high haemoglobin values in part back to the instability of all standard solutions

The frequent studies undertaken in our clinic since then confirm Wydler's data. We must conclude from this that, in spite of the relative lymphocytosis in dwarf cretins, no characteristic indicators arise from blood morphology. The relative lymphocytosis is actually such an ambiguous phenomenon that we cannot draw any conclusion from it.

As Fonio and Wälchli have ascertained, cretins, on the other hand, show a tendency to *acceleration of blood clotting*.

The analysis of *sedimentation rate of the red blood cells* is repeatedly offered as the criterion of thyroid gland function. Investigations undertaken at our instigation by Shein, in both Basedow patients and in cretins, show however that this investigatory criterion is unusable for differential diagnosis. Both in hyperfunction and hypofunction of the thyroid gland we found a tendency to accelerated sedimentation, not only among cretins but also in congenital athyroid individuals.

Investigation of the *dispersion grade of blood albumen bodies* appeared to offer better prospects of usefulness. Walder undertook this at our instigation, aided by a refined Kottmann reaction, on ordinary goitres, Basedow patients, and cretins of various types. In fact, he was able to demonstrate a stronger browning in dwarf cretin serum than in normal serum, and the serial progression in browning grades – from dwarf cretin serum to goitrous cretins to ordinary goitre to normal sera – corresponds with our clinical perceptions of the behaviour of thyroid gland function. Evidence that stronger browning corresponds with a *coarser dispersion* has still not been produced and, in the opinions of experienced chemists, the methodology contains no small sources of error. We therefore dispensed with drawing any broad conclusions from Walder's findings.

More reliable is the *analysis of the individual fractions of albumen bodies in the blood by weight determination*. This was undertaken on our cretin material by F. Starlinger. These investigations showed that among cretins there is an absolute and relative proliferation of fibrinogen, and that there are the following stages towards normal values:

Full cretin – nodular goitre with predominant parenchyma –; half-cretin – nodular goitre with preponderance of colloid –; normal condition.

Two important conclusions can be drawn from these investigations:

Firstly, the clinically euthyroid goitre patients exhibit an alteration that lies on the line of cretinism.

Secondly, this alteration is found both in goitrous cretins and in goitre-free cretins.

Also, even if these deflections are not very great, yet the investigations may assume that endemic thyropathy as such exercises an influence on blood albumen composition, and that this influence is most strongly pronounced in the cretin.

Reduction of *phagocytic performance of leucocytes* in the cretin is, according to the investigations undertaken in our clinic by Miss Aeschlimann, as small as in the congenital athyroid individual, in contrast to the findings in the animal freshly parted from its thyroid gland. This investigatory principle therefore appears to be of significance only in *acute* thyroid gland failure. Also, in 10 years post-operative myxœdema cases, despite the further existence of the myxœdema there is no demonstrable reduction of phagocytosis. The methodology is described in *Endokrinologie* **12**(2) (1933), and in de Quervain and Abelin, *Handbuch der biologischen Arbeitsmethoden*, Chapter VIII, p.1597.

Certain disorders show the *ion relationships* in the blood of the cretin. According to the investigations carried out in our clinic by Saegesser, the *calcium values* remain normal while the *potassium* level is reduced and hence the Ca/K ratio. This finding therefore is of interest to us because, in euthyroid goitre patients, there is a slight reduction in potassium level. This could be designated as a unique phenomenon of endemic thyropathy, the more so since it is found in both goitrous and non-goitrous cretins.

Peculiar, and still requiring explanation, is the fact that potassium is slightly reduced in the Jod–Basedow Phenomenon and – admittedly less clearly – in true Basedow. The former finding would be explainable insofar as the Jod–Basedow Phenomenon also appears in the frame of endemic thyropathy, whereas this is not the case with true Basedow. According to these investigations, no connection between blood potassium level and thyroid gland function appears to exist. The question, whether such connections are present via endemic thyropathy, must be left open, unless a larger case series is studied in the meantime.

The *iodine distribution* in cretins constitutes a significant chapter. According to Marine and Lenhart, a normal thyroid gland contains 1–5 mg iodine per gram dry weight. The latter value is to be regarded as a seldom-attained maximum; the lower limit is not always achieved in goitre-free regions either.

For non-goitrous glands from the goitre-depleted Jura, in 1905 our student Aeschbacher found 0.844 mg/g dry weight, i.e. 5.47 mg on average per thyroid gland, though with marked age differentials. Baumann in Germany found 0.68 mg in a gram of dry substance, with 4.31 mg for the whole gland; Lunde and Wülfert in Norway recently obtained an average of 2.9 mg/g in thyroid glands from Bergen, and minimum 1.5 mg for thyroid glands from Oslo, with an average total value of 10.8 mg for Bergen and 9.86 mg for Oslo. If we take the total weight of thyroid glands into consideration, we arrive at an average content of 7–10 mg in a normal gland.

As demonstrated by numerous analyses both from earlier times and from our clinic, euthyroid goitres show a very different iodine content. Saegesser found variations from 0.19 mg right up to 3.8 mg/g of dry substance, with an average value of 1.9 mg. Baumann found the iodine content in goitre to be lower than that of normal thyroid glands – Oswald, conversely, higher. Eggenberger assembled a data series from various countries, showing that, on average, it was lower than the normal total content. No general rule can be established and there are probably marked individual variations, quite apart from the fact that in many cases statistical reliability is obfuscated by previous iodine treatment of goitre; the considerable influence exerted on the iodine content by the age range of the sample; and, in autopsy material, by the preceding illness.

Six cretin goitres gave an average of 0.21 mg/g; 19 cretin goitres from Wydler's statistics an average of only 0.095 mg/g. In this latter series, from the weight of removed goitre tissue, there was a total iodine content of around 5 mg; if you include the remnants of the goitre, you obtain roughly the iodine content of a normal thyroid gland.

It follows from comparison of the values just presented that neither the percentage nor the absolute iodine content of a thyroid gland allows any opinion on its function, and that an opinion is possible only with simultaneous consideration of the histological structure, and is, even then, only conditional. At most, we can establish that, in a bigger investigative series, the cretin goitre is significantly more iodine-deficient than in correspondingly formed euthyroid goitres, although in individual cases the same values can be found.

Saegesser has attempted to determine whether a functional evaluation of the glands is possible based on the composition of iodine content from the alcohol-soluble (so-called inorganic) and alcohol-insoluble (organic) fraction. This demonstrated that the higher the basal metabolism of patients, the lower the percentage portion of the alcohol-soluble fraction was found to be. Among normal thyroid glands the alcohol-soluble fraction was 2%; among true Basedow [Graves' disease] patients, without prior iodine treatment, it was 27.2%; among Jod–Basedow, 14.6%; while among the cretin-goitres an average 49% were found. There the alcohol-soluble fraction in the Asher–Streuli rat study was demonstrating a thyroxin effect, while the extract from cretin thyroid glands led to a reduction of basal metabolism. We will come back to the significance of these latter results.

Further information on iodine turnover is given by *analysis of the blood iodine level*. This was investigated in several of our cretins both with and without goitre by Smith. It showed a reduction of iodine level to around half, compared with control subjects living under the same conditions. Thus cretins excrete the artificially introduced iodine somewhat more rapidly than the control subjects, which is no longer

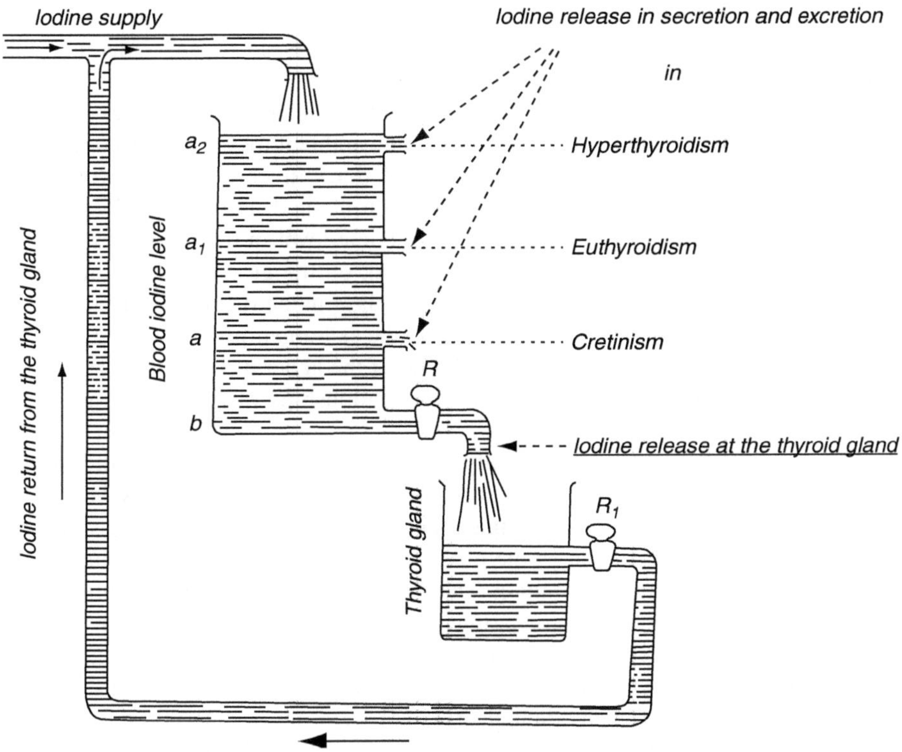

Fig. 115 Schematic diagram of an organism's iodine metabolism

attuned to very small quantities (5 mg) of iodine (Saegesser). They held their blood iodine level very constant. In so doing they take up just as much iodine in their food as do the control subjects, and eliminate just as much in the urine as the latter do.

When we compare these observations with Veil and Sturm's finding of an elevated blood iodine level in Basedow patients, we come to the conclusion that an automatic regulation of the iodine level probably exists – adjusting to the needs of the thyroid gland. The cretin thyroid gland releases little iodine-containing secretion and therefore has a low iodine requirement. Conversely, the iodine requirement of Basedow patients [probably the 'true' Basedow/Graves' disease patients – Editor] is high. In both cases, the blood iodine level is adjusted to these requirements by the organism, without worrying about the iodine quantity introduced to the body.

Figure 115 gives a schematic representation of these relationships.

The harder the thyroid gland works, the greater is its iodine metabolism; therefore, the wider the regulating taps R and R_1 are opened, the higher the blood, aided by an automatic swelling adjustment (probably outflow restriction in secretion and excretion), allows the blood iodine level to rise. This allows a certain level of pressure to be maintained in the blood to be delivered to the thyroid gland. The harder the turbines are allowed to run in an electricity generating plant, the higher you have to raise the level of the reservoir by closing the sluices, in order to maintain the necessary pressure.

As interesting as these results are, even more essential are the iodine levels in the blood of the control subjects. These are only comparable if they are carried out using exactly the same methodology. In a closed circulation with consequent prevention of loss due to evaporation, the iodine determination method used today gives higher values than previously. The constancy of the iodine level in the blood observed in investigations so far now requires reexamination, on the grounds of the improved method, apart from the role that the *hypophysis* plays in the regulating mechanism.

Application of the *Asher–Streuli method* to the examination of goitrous tissue, of thyroid venous blood, and of the venous blood of the general circulation (arm vein) gave us a major insight into the functional relationships of the thyroid gland in cretins.

The Asher–Streuli Method generally consists of feeding goitrous matter to the rat or injecting it into the blood serum, and then comparing its behaviour under reduced oxygen conditions, using a pneumatic pump. In normal rats, signs of oxygen deficiency appear as soon as the air pressure under the bell of the pneumatic pump drops to an average 300 mmHg. The signs then increase, until reaching death due to asphyxiation, should the experiment not be interrupted. Artificial hyperthyroidisation of rats by feeding them normal thyroid tissue, or thyroid extracts including thyroxin, or by thyroxin injection, leads to hypersensitivity towards oxygen deficiency with signs of asphyxia appearing at a pressure of 450–500 mmHg. The significance of this investigation was recently acknowledged from a different quarter, in particular the Bergmann Clinic, and the methodology has undergone an improvement, insofar as the air pressure is held constant while only the oxygen content is reduced, so that the oxygen concentration at which asphyxia occurs can be measured directly.

The original method, adapted to clinical requirements and carefully standardized by our students Hara and Branovacky, yielded valuable results, reproduced here from a 1922 table (Table 10).

It showed a gradation of biological activity of thyroid gland tissue from goitre in patients with Graves' disease downward: to euthyroid goitre, to diffuse colloid goitre, to nodular adenomatous goitre, and finally to the least-active cretinous goitre. Thereby the goitrous venous blood in Basedow patients was markedly active, in common goitre moderately active, and in cretins inactive. The same gradation, with a correspondingly lower activity, was found in brachial venous blood. Finally, of theoretical importance was the discovery that the brachial venous blood in high-grade dwarf cretins not only showed no activity, but rats injected with this blood were *less* sensitive to lack of oxygen than the normal control rats, or even the rats themselves *before* starting the experiment. This related to six cretins without goitre and one dwarf cretin with nodular parenchymatous (adenomatous) goitre. This observation again throws up the question whether or not at least a fraction of the thyroid gland activity involves *detoxification* (in the sense of Schiff; Horsley; Ballet and Enriquez; Burghart and

Table 10 Summary of Hara's and Branovacky's results

Type of goitre	Number of cases	Brachial venous blood	Goitrous venous blood	Goitre tissue
1. Basedow goitre	17	++	+++	+++++
2. Common goitre:				
(a) *Struma colloides diffusa*	9	+	++	++++
(b) *Struma colloides nodosa*	25	+	++	+++
(c) *Struma parenchymatosa diffusa*	5	+	++	+++
(d) *Struma parenchymatosa nodosa*	19	0 to +	+	++
3. Goitre in cretins:				
(a) *Struma colloides diffusa*	4	0	0	+
(b) *Struma colloides nodosa*	5	0	0 to +	+
(c) *Struma parenchymatosa diffusa*	1	0	0	+
(d) *Struma parenchymatosa nodosa*	27	0	0	+
4. Dwarf cretins:				
(a) *Struma parenchymatosa nodosa*	1	–	0	+
(b) *Without goitre*	6	–		
5. Normal thyroid gland	119	0		

0 Normal sensitivity of rats to a lack of oxygen

+ Elevated sensitivity to oxygen deficiency (A + corresponds to an average pressure difference of 40 mmHg)

– Reduced sensitivity to oxygen deficiency

Blumenthal; Moebius; Lanz; Blum etc.), or whether in cretin metabolism there is a *substance restricting thyroid gland function*. Further investigations by Branovacky showed that cretin blood and Basedow blood mixed *in vitro* neutralize each other in such a way that the mixture is ineffective in the Asher–Streuli experiment. It loses the metabolism-decelerating effect of the former, and the metabolism-accelerating effect of the latter. Investigations on thyroid gland implantation in cretins with atrophic thyroid glands showed that this neutralizing process had no need of a normal, functioning thyroid gland and probably acted via blood circulation in the healthy organ.

In 1932, in our clinic, Saegesser again took up the investigations of an antagonist (probably produced in these experiments) to thyroid gland secretion, and came to the conclusion that a lipoid, probably of the cholesterol type, had to be involved. Shortly before his first announcement about these experiments Anselmino and Hoffmann reported similar results to their investigations. Since then, reports have also come in of other antagonist substances – Blum on the catechin said to be formed in the liver, and Baló on a substance arising in the pancreas. The chemical nature of these substances is still not clarified.

The *behaviour of the liver* in cretins must also be of theoretical interest. Since thyroid gland secretion mobilizes liver glycogen, and since a particularly strong blood sugar level drop has been established (Csépai) in Basedow patients following insulin injection, you might theoretically expect a raised insulin tolerance among hypothyroid patients. Contrary to this expectation, animal experiments (rabbits, sheep, guinea pigs, rats, dogs) by various investigators demonstrated that thyroidectomy enhanced the blood sugar lowering effect of insulin. Accordingly, at our instigation, W. Lauterburg investigated the blood sugar curve in 11 cretins, and one case each of postoperative myxœdema, and congenital athyrosis, following administration of glucose. To some extent he found congruent deviations from the norm. Particularly remarkable was the abnormal reaction of seven of these cretins to subsequent insulin administration. This hypoglycaemia, found also in a non-cretin hypothyroid individual with a basal metabolism of minus 19%, accords with the animal experiments involving thyroid gland removal, and is probably explained most simply by a lack of the thyroid gland secretion that mobilizes the liver glycogen reserve. The insulin hypoglycaemia in Basedow disease would therefore occur because the liver, under the activating influence of the thyroid gland, had not stored sufficient glycogen. In the cretin however, the glycogen store was indeed available, but, because of a lack of thyroid gland secretion, it could not be mobilized quickly enough. You could also suggest that the insular apparatus in hypothyroid individuals is adjusted to the reduction of thyroid gland function, and consequently does not react to a sudden, large surplus of insulin. This explanation would be valid at least for chronic hypothyroid individuals, while, in experimental thyroid gland removal, the explanation of insulin sensitivity might rest simply on the breakdown of the thyroid–gland–liver relationship without the input of accessory mechanisms.

The *result of the pathological–physiological investigation of cretinism so far* is a *positive* one, insofar as all applicable methods of examination point to inadequate activity of the thyroid gland – both in cretinism *without goitre* and in cretinism *with* goitre. However, it is a *modest* one inasmuch as the number of practicable methods so far is small. Various methods from which we hoped for something practical have, on closer examination, shown themselves to be not useable or not sufficiently sensitive. In our laboratories over the last 15 years, much effort has been spent on paving the way for a pathological–physiological investigation of cretinism. We might expect a next step from the analysis of thyroxin and diiodotyrosine in the blood. However, we ought immediately to be sceptical, because we recall the difficulties raised already by the simple analysis of blood iodine level. We even hesitate to mention the seemingly self-explanatory postulate that results obtained according to elementary rules are to be interpreted as a balance sheet. A lot of printer's ink would be spared if the author and the reader would actually think numerically, rather than emotionally, when numbers come into consideration. I would emphasize once more that in future clinical-experimental work, sufficient cases should always be studied so that the randomness of one single observation can be discarded. Of course, that one case might offer a valuable suggestion. However, it is insufficient to establish legitimacy.

The question now is whether, based on current pathological anatomical and physiological knowledge, we can explain the picture both of goitre-free and goitrous cretinism as an inadequacy of the thyroid gland and *only* that, and whether certain details do not stand in contradiction of this view, requiring a different explanation. This will take place in the chapter on the pathogenesis of cretinism. Before that, however, we should deal briefly with a related question.

Can cretins present Basedow appearances? This question seems absurd since cretinism is actually the converse of Basedow disease. Nevertheless, we have followed it up for years because it is of great significance, not only for the pathology but also for the physiology of the thyroid gland.

It is known to have been discussed in detail initially by Sattler and later by Kaufmann. An initial possibility of the combination of hyperthyroid and hypothyroid phenomena is out of the question, namely the transition of a Basedow into myxœdema through spontaneous degeneration of the gland. The simultaneous spontaneous appearance of signs of both groups of illness is unproven. On the other hand, it is conceivable that, on the basis of a cretinism with goitre, secondary Basedow phenomena arise. The following observations belong in this group of events.

Investigations undertaken in our clinic by H. Doubler in 1920–1921 show that among young girls with diffuse goitre and mild physical signs of cretinism, a cardiovascular lability reminiscent of Basedow may be present at puberty. The question then is whether such phenomena can be traced back to a plurality of secretions, one available in insufficient quantity, the other in surplus, or whether a dysthyroidism is present, in the form of secretions totally differing from the norm. This has still not been resolved experimentally.

However, might it not be possible to explain such cases even based on the assumption of a single secretion, and without assuming a dysfunction? We commence from a concrete observation in our clinic, communicated by Wydler.

A 45-year-old, feeble-minded, typically cretin individual, hard of hearing, with a stammer, and mentally limited, suddenly began to exhibit Basedow symptoms: accelerated pulse rate 100, hand tremor, basal metabolism plus 18%. She presented a big, tri-lobed goitre, described histologically as a diffuse and nodular colloid goitre. In the nodular tissue, and in the intermediate tissue, there were numerous infiltrations of lymphocytes and, in places, infiltrations of leucocytes as well. In addition, there was atrophy of the thyroid gland tissue in the nodular capsule.

The iodine content of the goitre is unusually high for a cretinous goitre (0.067% of dry substance = 0.67 mg/g) and the Asher–Streuli rat experiment comes out markedly positive with the goitre substance.

The obvious assumption is that an inadequate thyroid gland during youth belatedly showed strong outgrowth with unusually strong resorption processes which, given the original cretinous foundation, evoked the unequivocal sign of a hyperfunction.

The observation that temporary Basedow-like phenomena appeared in a half-cretin in connection with iodine supplement belongs under the same heading. Evidently there are cretin goitres whose secretory reserve is mobilised in such a way that it triggers the pattern of a transitory increase in function. The rarity of such events alters nothing of their basic importance.

Chapter 8
Pathogenesis

In the preceding chapters we emphasised the close relationship of endemic cretinism with endemic goitre, and the morphological and physiological inadequacy of the cretin thyroid gland, and have been confronted repeatedly by the similarity with the changes due to athyrosis in the pathological anatomy of the other organs – it has been almost like drawing a red line through our statement. You might therefore think that the pathogenesis of endemic cretinism conveniently involves a simple formula, and that this formula must relate to thyroid gland insufficiency. However, when you delve deeply into the whole problem area, here and there you come across facts whose explanation, as we have shown time and again, is not so simple. Similarly, deriving these hard facts from functional disorders of the thyroid gland function creates difficulties. This is very clearly expressed in Gamper's recent critical discussion.

It is hard to believe that anybody can still seriously dispute the view that endemic cretinism in its pronounced and severe forms is, in the main, hypothyrosis. Ever since T. Kocher in 1892 first drew a parallel between *cachexia thyropriva* and so-called cretinism, clinical observations and morphological and functional investigations have, as we have seen, brought together so much material as proof that any doubt about the thyrogenic nature of the main symptoms of cretinism seems no longer appropriate. Despite this, we must examine the question once more, in greater detail, in this chapter.

The earlier-indicated deviations from the classical pattern of thyroid gland insufficiency, made familiar to us through congenital athyrosis, spontaneous myxœdema and postoperative myxœdema, can be summarised as follows:

1. In those cases of cretinism not extending back to earliest childhood, the longitudinal growth of the body is not always conspicuously disturbed – occasionally not at all.
2. Myxœdema is not always present.
3. The skin appendages are sometimes normally formed,
4. as are the sexual organs.
5. Besides the central disturbances, cretins with hearing disorders often show defects in peripheral sound conduction that we do not find in pure hypothyroids

J. Dennison et al., *Endemic Cretinism*,

DOI 10.1007/978-1-4614-0281-7_8, © Springer Science+Business Media, LLC 2011

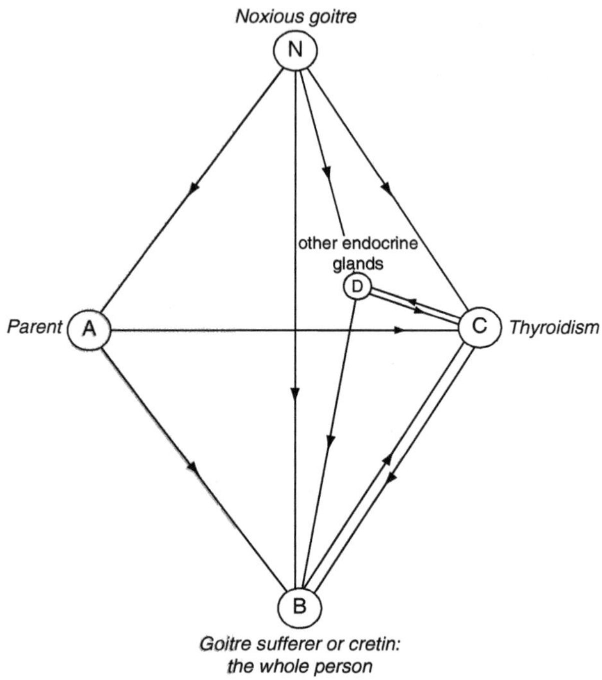

Fig. 116 Schematic representation of the relationship between the noxious goitre and cretinism

and athyroids. The speech disorder in cretins comes to light in a more conspicuous form than in pure hypothyroids who are capable of speech.

6. The mental anomalies show a greater diversity among cretins than in individuals with pure loss phenomena.
7. The dissociation of the somatic and intellectual symptoms of cretinism goes considerably further than the dissociation also present in congenital thyroaplasia.

People have attempted to explain these inconsistencies in different ways. The diagram in Fig. 116 helps us to separate clearly the various possibilities.

The NCB pathway from the noxious agent of goitre N, via the thyroid gland C, to the cretin B typifies the damage to the cretin body through the higher-level damage of the thyroid gland – *pure hypothyrosis*. First, we have to find out how far this takes us in explaining the deviations from the usual pattern of thyroid gland insufficiency.

For adult dwarf cretins, we must affirm unconditionally the presence of a hypothyrosis as being the main cause, even though insufficient on its own. The severe atrophy of the gland tissue, the loss of seasoned parenchyma and, above all, the degeneration of the epithelium make normal gland activity impossible, even when such tissue is still clearly effective in the tadpole test. We also know, both from experiment and from human pathology, that normal thyroid gland tissue, when it is quantitatively reduced beyond a certain level, no longer suffices for the maintenance of normal homeostasis. How much less so can glandular tissue that is not merely quantitatively reduced, but is highly degenerated as well, be responsible for normal function? Here, within the very framework of the histological picture, we have to consider not only the possibility of a hypothyrosis but also of a *dysthyrosis* in the sense of an incorrectly mixed or a quantitatively altered secretion.

Of course through regenerative epithelial growth, leading to the scenario of nodular hyperplasia or adenoma, a certain compensation can be created, with the functional effect, for example, of stronger physical growth, better maturation of the gonads, and disappearance, or non-development, of myxœdema. Thus it transpires that the goitrous individuals among cretins often present only relatively minor somatic hypothyroid symptoms (de Quervain–Wydler). Admittedly a total upgrade to normal does not materialise, because virtually all cretin goitrous adenomas are attuned far more to growth than to secretion, and, in spite of the often extensive vascularisation, resorption of adenoma secretion usually remains inadequate.

Yet how does the atrophy of the thyroid gland, characteristic of adult dwarf cretins, arise? Since, according to clinical findings, the first symptoms of cretinism appear right back in early childhood, at least between the second and third years, you would expect the thyroid gland to be changed by this age. But in what way? Unfortunately, the repeatedly-mentioned gaps in our knowledge remain unfilled. Even today, Schlagenhaufer and Wagner von Jauregg's 4-year-old cretin remains the youngest case to have provided accurate information about thyroid gland condition. That gland was normal in size, but showed marked degenerative changes in the epithelium.

What does a newborn cretin's thyroid gland look like? We do not know, and possibly we will not know for a long time, since it is always some time after birth before cretinism can be diagnosed with certainty. One thing that might be certain is that, at birth and just after, the thyroid gland is still not atrophic as a rule, but rather slightly goitrously enlarged; this is confirmed by clinical observations (Fodéré; Rösch; Diviak and Wagner von Jauregg). In the Berne goitre region we have never encountered an atrophic thyroid gland among neonates or infants, although one of us (Wegelin) has often seen nuclear degeneration in the *struma congenita*, very similar to that in cretin thyroid glands.

It is therefore generally likely that, in the initial stages, cretin thyroid glands present the picture of a diffuse, parenchymatous goitre, such as we find among first-grade cretins during later childhood. This is corroborated by the thyroid gland findings already reported in young cretinous dogs. One might also have been tempted, from the histological picture, to assume an augmented function, a *hyperthyrosis*, as Hotz did for certain child cretin goitres.

However apart from that, for such a labile, growing thyroid gland not to be needing to deliver more secretion than a normal gland, the quantity of secretion discharged from such a hyperplastic organ is always too little in relation to the needs of the downstream organs. This also corresponds with the clinical picture that supports the opposing view – of a hypothyrosis.

Thus it is very easy to assume that the thyroid gland of incipient cretins is indeed very premature, reacting probably even *in utero* to the needs of the rest of the organism by a goitrous enlargement. But then, however, under the influence of the noxious

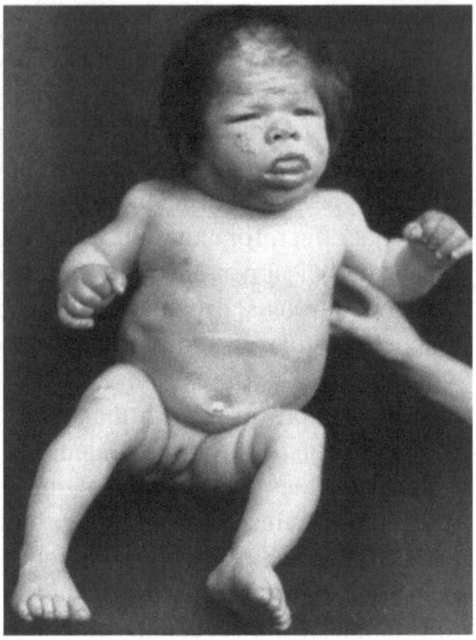

Fig. 117 Thyroaplasia in a 6-year-old child (surgically managed)

agent of goitre, a rapidly-progressing degeneration of the seasoned epithelium sets in – at higher levels of cretinism leading to atrophy and sclerosis during childhood.

And so we would have the following possibilities laid out schematically:

1. *Slight damage to the thyroid gland through the noxious agent.* Goitre-forming reaction of the gland, with good function. Goitre without cretinism.
2. *Moderate damage.* Goitre-forming reaction with functional disorder: (a) persistence of the goitre, cretinism with goitre; (b) secondary atrophy, cretinism without goitre.
3. *Major damage.* No beneficial reaction. Primary atrophy. The most severe cases of cretinism without goitre.

Given our sparse knowledge of the early changes in the cretinous thyroid gland, the following case is of interest.

A nine-year-old girl, daughter of a goitrous, hard-of-hearing mother, from a goitrous family, and coming from a goitrous region, shows signs of thyroid gland insufficiency from infancy onward. Exploratory surgery with simultaneous transplantation reveals, in place of the right half of the thyroid gland, a small vascular cluster that is carefully conserved; an absence of the isthmus; and atrophy of the left lobe, with the usual histological picture of severe cretinous atrophy. Subsequent intervention four years later, with the aim of a second transplantation, shows that the right lobe is now clearly recognizable, but it is also atrophic and histologically of the same quality as the left lobe was previously. Given the chronic goitrous environment, the mother's goitre, and the histological findings, this case was ranked as cretinism with atrophy, in the endemic thyropathy series. If, in this case, we are able to exclude a preceding hyperplastic phase, as little as we can in the other cases of cretinous atrophy that we examined, then given the high level of atrophy and the youth of the child, this does not seem likely.

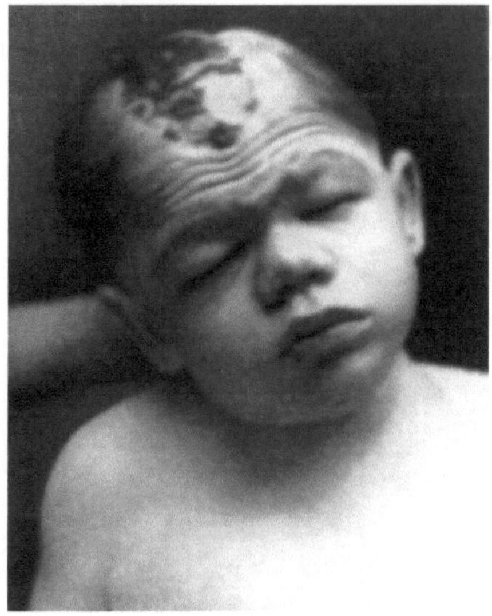

Fig. 118 Thyroaplasia in a 17-year-old male with congenital myxoedema (surgically managed)

In any case, besides the probably-more-common, primary hyperplasia, we must acknowledge the possibility of a primary, intrauterine or early-childhood atrophy.

Before we go into detail on the aetiology of these premature thyroid gland alterations, we must look at the question of what conclusions on hypothyrosis can be drawn from the rest of the anatomical findings in cretins. This includes not just individual signs but a consensus of the entire anatomical picture. Such an argument by analogy actually achieves greater probability only when this consensus is present as numerous points virtually right along a line. It thereby depends mainly on the comparable nature of the changes. Quantitative differences do not play a decisive role.

Since endemic cretinism first makes itself noticeable not in later life but during the early years of childhood, congenital thyroaplasia should be called on as the object of comparison, not the myxœdema or *cachexia thyropriva* of adults. Congenital athyrosis also qualifies, because in most cases it does not constitute total absence of thyroid gland in the strict sense of the word, but remnants of thyroid gland tissue remain at the base of the tongue, with a certain undeniable functional ability. Strictly speaking, this usually involves a dystopic hypoplasia and not a total aplasia – from a functional standpoint a more or less severe *hypo*thyrosis.

One of us (Wegelin) together with his former intern, Dr Olga Fischer, was able to examine two such cases, aged 19 and 27 years respectively. In the base of the tongue were roundish clumps of thyroid gland tissue with a diameter of 7–8 mm. The situation was the same in a two-day-old athyroid infant where the base of the tongue contained a thyroid gland of 2.5 mm. In another case of athyrosis however, examination of a series of sections revealed an absence of any thyroid gland tissue. This case involved a 20-day-old infant.

In addition to our own material, there are cases from the literature involving investigations of extrathyroid organs and organ systems (Bourneville; Langhans; Erdheim; Quincke; Maresch; Peucker; Schilder; Heyn; Bernheim-Karrer; MacCallum and

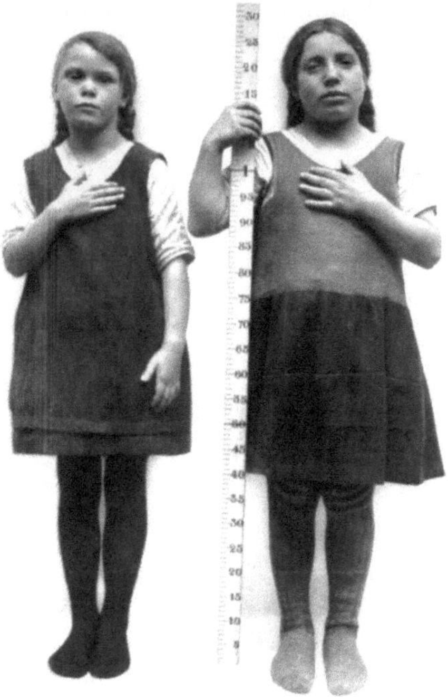

Fig. 119 *Right*: congenital myxoedema (dystrophic aplasia of the thyroid gland, surgically managed). *Left*: Normal sister, 6 years old

Fabyan; Dieterle; Marchand; Rössle; Zuckermann; Schultz; Schultze; Comte; Rocaz and Cruchet; Boyce and Beadles; von Siebenthal; Pennacchietti; E.J. Kraus etc.).

First of all, with regard to the system of *endocrine glands*, there is conformity between thyroid aplasia and cretinism simply in the behaviour of the *hypophysis*, characterised in both cases by enlargement of the anterior lobe with increase in and enlargement of the chief cells. Furthermore, there are similar changes in the *thymus*, which falls victim to a premature involution; and finally the gonads and their dependent sexual organs, since the secondary sexual characteristics of both the athyroid and the cretin are similarly restricted in development. In both disorders the *pineal gland*, the *parathyroid glands*, and the *suprarenal glands* exhibit normal behaviour as a rule; at most, a sclerosis of the zona glomerulosa of the suprarenal glands can set in relatively prematurely. Finally, there are no differences between thyroaplasia and cretinism in the *pancreatic islets* – characteristic changes being absent in both cases.

Conformity in the area of the *skeletal system* is quite extensive – you could almost say that the disturbances in cretinism are a diluted copy of athyroid changes. If you simply compare Figs. 86 and 87 with 95 and 96, you must concede that the same developmental and growth disorder is present, expressed particularly by inhibition of ossification. The same is also true of the microscopic subtleties, both at the cartilage–bone interface and at the epiphyseal cartilage, where the more recently discovered mucous centres of softening occur in exactly the same way. Also, the gross structure of the skeleton does not reveal pervasive differences, for even when frequent, irregular, disproportionate growth of individual body parts and bones occur among cretins, this feature is not totally foreign to thyroaplasia either, as one of our cases showed; only, because of the more severe growth restriction, the disproportion was less.

Bone marrow function is inhibited in the same way in thyroaplasia and cretinism, leading to a corresponding alteration of the *blood*.

Furthermore, the *skin* is affected in a similar manner. Even though myxœdema regresses as a rule among older cretins, histologically there is no essential difference in the skin and its appendages compared with thyroaplasia. Also, in the behaviour of the *teeth*, only gradable differences arise.

Finally, a further very important link in the chain of evidence is the *brain* whose alterations indicate totally comparable disorders of development, established fairly precisely (Lotmar) as arising during the foetal period.

Insofar as they do not deviate significantly from the norm, the morphology of the other body organs shows no drastic differences between cretinism and thyroaplasia. The sole exception is the *ear* which usually, although not always, shows strongly pronounced changes in cretinism, whereas in cases of congenital athyrosis – admittedly, so far only three have been examined, to our knowledge – it was always normal.

It is therefore conceded that the two scenarios – thyroaplasia and cretinism – do, generally, coincide, although not completely, and that cretinism, in its individual anatomical alterations and clinical symptoms, shows a much broader quantitative field of play and thus a greater diversity than the more uniform thyroaplasia. As already mentioned, this is demonstrated by the dissociation of symptoms where, for example, the mental defects of cretins do not run absolutely parallel with the physical developmental restrictions, or the somatic features are varyingly pronounced. A high-grade sclerosis of the thyroid gland may for example combine with a relatively minor testicular hypoplasia, or even, within the skeletal system, we see a quantitatively dissimilar behaviour of the individual parts where, for example, bone growth in the base of the skull is particularly strongly inhibited while the limb bones show roughly normal longitudinal growth.

We are not lacking in *attempts to explain* this remarkable situation. For one thing, the time of onset of the hypothyrosis is important, because the thyroid gland is in the front line of control of differentiation, and we also know that this thyroid gland activity is not uniformly and simultaneously asserted in all tissues and organs, but according to the sensitivity of individual areas (Champy). In two cases of congenital athyrosis with thyroid gland rudiments at the base of the tongue, Lotmar found further developmental inhibitions in the cerebrum of one of them, and more developmental inhibitions in the cerebellum of the other. There could be no other explanation than that the low level of thyroid gland function just happened to coincide with the chronologically differing development of intrinsic cortical formations in the cerebrum and the cerebellum. In any case, this example demonstrates quite clearly that a dissociation also occurs in congenital athyrosis, even if it is less obvious.

Apart from that, we know from W. Schulze's experiments that premature excision of the thyroid gland in amphibian larvae is able to interrupt the harmony of development, so that some organs abandon their development while others remain uninfluenced. First and foremost among the former are the ectodermal and endodermal organs, with the exception of the thymus, hypophysis, and pineal gland, while the mesodermal organs experience no inhibition.

Thus, in cretinism we have to take into consideration a *temporally-differing severe* hypothyrosis, as pointed out particularly by Wagner von Jauregg and Gamper. It is conceivable for example that the hypothyrosis has a particularly strong effect during foetal life, with brain development especially suffering. This involves the crucial differentiations being implemented at this time. Then, when thyroid gland function improves after birth, skeletal growth, maturation of the generative glands, and skin development come into action relatively well, thereby explaining satisfactorily the dissociation between mental and physical disorders. In other cases the situation is reversed, with cretins developing as dwarfs with reasonable mental faculties.

Furthermore, *dysthyrosis*, as yet still unproven, might explain the dissociation to some extent; and, finally, one of us (Wegelin) has pointed out the individually differing, genotypic predisposition that impacts both on cretins and normal people and, to a lesser extent, even on athyroids. Admittedly, this latter attempt at explanation is rejected by Gamper, who observes that the span between individual subgroups of cretinism in one endemic region, and even within a single family, is too great to be satisfactorily explained by an individually differing sensitivity. We concede that such differences within the same family are occasionally very strong, and can even involve non-identical twins (Flinker), with the result that only the first of the above hypotheses can be applied. However, genotypic predisposition could still offer a satisfactory explanation for smaller differences without cretinism itself being genotypically inherited. We will elaborate further on this major problem.

The idea of *different threshold values* is interesting as an attempt at explanation in the sense of a working hypothesis. At that time Gley and Pézard established the "all or nothing" law for the sex glands. We (de Quervain) have pointed out for years that the same can be applied only conditionally to thyroid glands, and that between the "nothing" and the number of glands that can perform "all," there are a series of steps that can be recognised as hypofunction. In their later work, Gley and Pézard themselves also narrowed the validity of this law for the sex glands, and demonstrated experimentally that for the various functional expressions of the secretion there are also different 'graduated' threshold values (*seuils differentiels*). In 1925 Gley transposed this idea to the endocrine activity of the thyroid gland, and at the same time adopted our previously expressed suspicion of a plurality of secretion.

In *pure hypothyroidism of incomplete athyroids* (dystopic thyroaplasia) dissociation of the clinical appearances can be explained satisfactorily by assuming staggered threshold values in a single secretion. For the interpretation of the far more pronounced dissociation in the cretinism pattern you might also come up with the same explanation. However, the explanation might be greatly simplified by assuming a plurality of secretions, which would be present in inadequate quantities and simultaneously in varying mixtures among cretins (a theoretical possibility that we (de Quervain) have designated as composite dysthyroidism), or which in normal mixing might present varying stimulus thresholds.

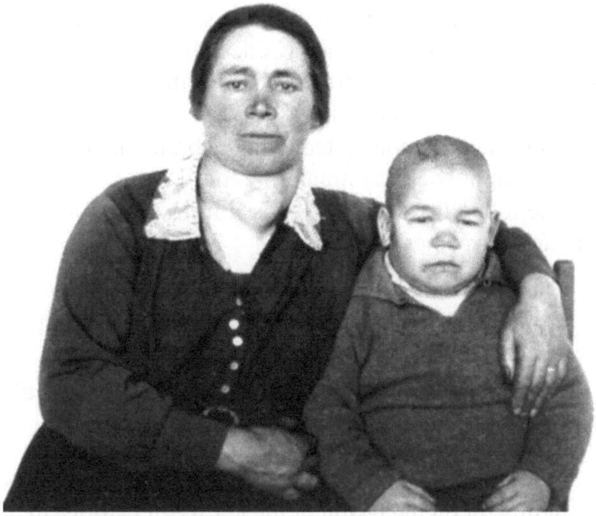

Fig. 120 A 12-year-old cretin boy without goitre, with an atrophic thyroid gland, with his goitrous non-cretin mother (cf. Figs. 11 and 57)

We have emphasised all along that, for the time being, we regard these ideas merely as possible interpretations. The further we advance in our knowledge of endocrine processes, the more we must convince ourselves that in reality our simple, schematic representations constitute only the framework of far more complex processes. The path of progress leads through the acquisition of carefully observed, factual data. Evaluation of the data requires working hypotheses. These hypotheses are useful only so long as they are not similarly converted into a 'theory' which is then to be bowled over by the very next experimental results.

Were we to use one or other of these remedial hypotheses, neither proven nor refuted, to explain the still-unclear dissociations in the cretinism pattern, we would resolve most of the remaining difficulties, such as the lack of parallels between the somatic and the intellectual anomalies of various cretins, the varying behaviour of myxœdema, the finer differences in the psyche etc. However, we must still examine the other possible explanations suggested by our scheme.

A significant path leads via the *parent*: NAB.

Since the beginning of the study of cretinism, authors have written much about the question: whether it is *inherited*, and right up until recent times they have given different answers. It is definite that, in the great majority of cases, *mothers* of cretin children suffer *from endemic goitre*. Arguing over percentages is of little value, since many mothers with deep-set goitre regard themselves as goitre-free, nor are they designated as goitrous in the statistical records. Thus, the percentages published in the statistics remain less than real. More uncommonly, the father is found to be suffering from goitre, but we must remember that, in the areas of severe endemic disease, the frequency of goitre among men is almost as high as among women. Usually therefore, the thyroid gland of neither parent would be normal. In exceptional cases, and more often among the mothers, there are signs of a cretinous disposition – even unmistakable first and second grade cretinism.

A second fact is that, within the same family, often several children are cretins, with no rhyme or reason, alongside individual euthyroid – though possibly goitrous – siblings. Alongside goitre-free cretins there are often those with goitre, in the same family (cf. Figs. 13 and 14).

As Lotmar demonstrated with the brain, the beginning of cretinous degeneration extends right back to intrauterine life.

The following theoretical possibilities exist for the prenatal emergence of cretinism and for its heritability:

1. The child is under the influence of the same exogenous disadvantage as the mother. His or her thyroid gland will, like that of the mother, be selectively affected by this malignancy, though perhaps in a different form (e.g., euthyroid goitre of the mother; cretinous thyroid gland atrophy in the child). *Heritability = 0.*
2. The cytoplasm of the female ovum is damaged by the noxious agent of goitre. The development of the embryo is directly impaired by the noxious agent, and indirectly by the lesion of the germ cell cytoplasm, without involving any alteration of the genes. *Individual and paraphoric* (Greek *paraphorein*; used geologically of two lamina being moved past each other) *damage to the embryo without actual heritability.*
3. The parental genes are damaged by the noxious agent of goitre. *Genotypic (idioplastic) mutative inheritance.*
4. There exists a geno(idio)typically-inherited *predisposition* to the illness through the noxious agent of goitre in the sense of a *racial or familial predisposition* (or – immunity!?)

Decision over *which of the four possibilities is pending in goitre and cretinism* can be made only on the basis of a substantial, carefully-assembled body of facts.

A primary, undisputed fact is *goitre and cretinism's dependence on 'place'*. We have known of this ever since the first historical references on goitre and cretinism, and it has been give valuable numerical confirmation from the very recent work of Dieterle and Eugster. The result of these studies shows that the inhabitants of the eight villages, re-examined after an interval of 20 years, were just as goitrous or goitre-free as they were at the first examination. The goitre incidence had occasionally even remained within groups of houses or individual houses and preferred the ground floor of particular houses. Documentation of *family trees* (Eugster), furthermore, demonstrates that mothers from goitre-free villages who shifted to a goitre-village produced goitrous offspring there, while conversely mothers who emigrated from a goitre-village to a goitre-free village, after the first child, gave birth to goitre-free children there.

Any influence of *inbreeding* on the frequency of goitre could not be established. The *local* influence was therefore the determining factor for the appearance of goitre among the children, both among the immigrants and the emigrants, and the mother's influence was expressed only for a short time, i.e., only for the first child born in a goitre-free region.

Dieterle and Eugster's investigations relate primarily to endemic goitre, but do consider cretinism in the same manner, making them valid for all endemic thyropathies. Incidentally, statistical compilations and graphs from 1843 demonstrate the local correlation of endemic goitre and cretinism in the regions examined by Dieterle and Eugster.

Among 99 Allgäu cretins, Schwalber found only one offspring of a marriage of relatives, and accordingly rejected inbreeding as being of relevant, aetiological moment in the incidence of cretinism. In contrast, Finkbeiner – with no supporting data – regarded inbreeding as important.

The most complete genetic surveys so far, conducted by Eugster and also audited by Lenz, demonstrate once again the *overarching prominence of the location factor*, and leave a certain leeway for *a rapidly decaying plasmatic (paraphore) transmission of the goitre disease through the mother*. On the other hand, they offer no clues about the participation of the *gene* in so-called goitre heredity – on the contrary they make it seem unlikely. The inheritable transfer of endemic goitre is therefore limited, insofar as evidence is available, to the aforementioned points 1 and 2, both of which fall within the ambit of *exogenous* influences.

Even when we have to reject a genotypic transmission of goitre and cretinism (the third possibility, above) on the grounds of fact, two questions remain that are related to this point:

(a) Is it conceivable that an exogenous cause, constantly renewed through generations, finally leads to *mutative*, i.e., *genotypic* alterations, as J. Bauer assumes in his *Status degenerativus*? This opinion is shared also by Jaensch, Höpfner and their co-workers and, as we shall see, also formed the foundation of prophylaxis. Bauer's *Status degenerativus* stands in opposition to the notion of mutation posited by de Vries, and transposed, by O Nägeli in particular, to human pathology. He seeks to build a bridge between the Lamarckian inheritance of acquired characteristics and de Vries' mutation. Whether such a bridge is sustainable remains to be proven. What we know so far of endemic thyropathy does not give us any clues for assuming such a mutative alteration.
(b) Does the noxious agent of goitre encourage the development of genotypically inheritable diseases that are not tied to one place, for example chondrodystrophy, Down's syndrome, harelip, etc.? The possibility of such an influence cannot theoretically be denied. However, supporting data for the greater frequency of more certain hereditary damage in the area of endemic goitre is not yet available. The general information from Eggenberger that, since the introduction of iodized cooking salt prophylaxis in the Appenzell canton, malformations have become less common is interesting, but so far we lack any possibility of comparative data. The same is true of Flinker's account of the occurrence of malformation in the endemic region. There is at least reference to the observations on the Berne autopsy material (Wegelin, p.127). Eggenberger's statement that since iodized cooking salt prophylaxis, cases of debility have dropped from 3.7‰ to 0.6‰ has been undermined by Wieland, an extensive critic. Incidentally, this is not a case of a genotypically-qualified phenomenon but of a lesion that could easily have arisen through exogenous influences on the mother's germ plasma and on the embryo. The greater frequency of hernias, cardiac disorders and adenoid proliferation

needs further investigation in the Berne endemic region (Lauener). This can occur through the thyroid gland, but can also be based on direct influence from the noxious agent of goitre – it does not need to be inherited.

Before the iodine prophylaxis, the increase in stature of the school pupils in the city of Berne (whose goitre incidence in 1919 was still very high in our opinion) had nothing to do with endemic thyropathy interfering with the genotype. In any case it contradicts the fateful linking of cumulatively genetic biological processes, which Jaensch also assumes for Switzerland as being a goitre country. The prime moment of explanation comes with the consideration of the hygienic lifestyle of youth: sport, and life in the open air and sunshine. The increase in stature is even more pronounced after iodine prophylaxis in schools. In evaluating the increase in stature it has to be borne in mind that the assessment in Europe had been made decades ago. Therefore it could only be ascribed in part to the thyroid gland because after the iodine upgrade growth rate would have accelerated (e.g., in the Appenzell canton according to Eggenberger).

We now come to the *fourth* of the above possibilities: Is there a greater or lesser *strength of resistance against the noxious agent of goitre* and, if so, how do we explain it? Are we dealing with congenital or inherited characteristics of certain population groups or certain races? Pfaundler, at least earlier, seemed to assume a defining moment of inheritance in the predisposition. Pfister regards the immigrant Javanese as less predisposed to goitre than the Malay inhabitants of Sumatra, which, according to a personal communication from Surbek in Bandung, is not always the case. So far we lack compelling reasons for assuming a racial predisposition extending across generations – or immunity against endemic thyropathy. The explanation of family trees, intimated by K.H. Bauer, with the existence of a familial susceptibility, is still controversial.

From the examination of capillary patterns, undertaken so far mainly in schools, no definite conclusions can be drawn that answer the question of heritability.

Gamper's cases of the impact of a cretin father, which could support an inherited factor, are not faultless, since in one case the mother was goitrous, and in the second case, although the mother did not present any symptoms of cretinism, she apparently lived in an endemic region (nothing is said about the mother's goitre).

Studies of twins are the easiest standard for the genotypic influence of goitre susceptibility. The one familiar before 1934 had been compiled by von Verschuer. Among 114 pairs of monozygote twins, six were non-conforming cases; among 74 pairs of non-identical twins on the other hand, there were 30. Eugster (pers. comm.), based on the study of 511 pairs of twins, came to the conclusion that it is not the susceptibility that is hereditarily influenced but the process and pathological form of the goitre. Compared with the data in the literature, the non-identical twins appeared to have a significantly higher conformity, as a consequence of the *duration of observation* (103 pairs).

We can summarise the current knowledge of the question as follows.

Endemic thyropathy is not an *inherited disease in the narrower sense, but can, rather, be a co-determined measure of inheritance, up to a certain level, of the manner of reaction to the exogenous noxious agent.*

For the *exogenous influence on the embryo* we have to leave the possibility open that this does not act exclusively *via the thyroid gland*, but that the embryo can also be *directly* damaged by the noxious agent of goitre. If we subscribe to the possibility of an extrathyroidal site of attack, this allows the further possibility that this noxious agent, as actually observed in a small number of cases, intensely damages the embryo without leaving behind any clinically severe signs on the progenitors.

If we take this line of thought a step further, i.e., beyond the moment of birth, then in our schematic representation we come to the path NB, i.e., postnatal damage to the whole organism of the cretin directly through the noxious agent of goitre, without detouring via the parent. This possibility can be theoretically conceded without further ado, but it still has certain limitations. From numerous observations, we know that adults coming into a goitrous area can acquire goitre. However, they do not acquire cretinism (Dieterle and Eugster), not even in the form of cretinism with goitre, and with more or less normal skeletal structure. Even for this latter form of thyropathy, the prerequisite is for the effect of the noxious agent to start at least in early childhood, even when the function of the damaged gland still extends to attainment of normal body size. The likelihood of in utero onset of thyroid gland damage (Lotmar's investigations) persuades us, prompted by Maffei and others, to place most weight on the *prenatal* emergence of cretinism.

Which symptoms of cretinism should be distributed along the paths NAB and NB (Fig. 116)? Since disorders arising potentially along these paths are much more difficult to uncover than those arising along the endocrine path NCB (which can be tested clinically and experimentally), we shall assign anything inexplicable on the endocrine path to the paths NAB and NB. These may be a few or many according to one's view of thyroid gland endocrinology. The more the knowledge of this advances, the sharper will be the outline of what does *not* belong to it. This leads us to the discussion of the path NDB, i.e., the *collaboration with other endocrine glands*.

Pighini's experiments are interesting. For example, by using very different substances (fluorine, boron, selenium, tellurium, butyric acid, propionic acid, oleic acid, hydrazine, paraphenylenediamine, guanidinoacetic acid, histamine and choline), Pighini has been able to produce not only degenerative changes and subsequent epithelial proliferations in the thyroid gland, but also degenerations in the thymus, the suprarenal glands and the gonads. In cretinism, however, the alterations found in the other endocrine glands do not have the character of a degeneration produced by the effect of poison, but are partly limitations in development, and partly premature involution. First of all, however, the alteration in the *hypophysis* cannot be one of the disorders coordinated by thyroid gland atrophy, because in virtually every case we are dealing with a purely proliferating process, a hyperplasia. That this hyperplasia is a consequence of inadequate thyroid gland function follows from its consistency with the hypophyseal findings in thyroaplasia and, above all, in experimental athyrosis. The findings in the endocrine glands of cretins do not support *simultaneous* damage; but in their totality allow themselves to be interpreted only as *consequent states and conforming phenomena* of the hypothyrosis.

The same applies, perhaps to an even greater extent, to the rest of the organ systems, the skeleton and skin in particular. So far at least, we know of no externally acting noxious agent that could cause disorders of bone growth in a manner analogous to that of cretinism, whereas there is total consistency with the growth restrictions in the absence of a thyroid gland. Not even the avitaminoses (which would be the easiest to compare, also influencing the thyroid gland according to MacCarrison) bring about skeletal alterations in a direct manner peculiar to cretinism. It is similarly very unlikely that the myxœdema of the skin has a direct external cause, independent of the thyroid gland.

The question still remains theoretically open, because, with the investigations so far, not all the possibilities have been exhausted. In this sense, we could include Gamper's concession of a twofold interpretation of cretinism, but not in the way that it might produce any *evidence* of a direct, postnatal effect of the noxious agent for goitre on the whole organism including the extrathyroidal endocrine system.

One non-thyroidal disorder occupies a special place, namely the co-partnership of parathyroidism in the *nervous cretinism* described in Indians by MacCarrison. However, this disease pattern alone, not observed in other cretin areas, is different from endemic cretinism, and therefore cannot be introduced as evidence for the multi-glandular cause of it. Neither from the anatomical nor from the clinical point of view does its disease pattern contain unequivocal features of an otherwise-endocrine disorder. For that reason, it cannot be explained by any other endocrine gland. This is also true of the rest of the phenomena still unsatisfactorily explained in cretinism. Since Finkbeiner appears to set particular store by the inadequate function of the gonads, it is emphasised that genital infantilism and cretinism are two totally different things, and that, in the former, the premature involution phenomena, e.g., in the thymus and skin, are completely absent, as is myxœdema and the intellectual characteristics of cretinism. In addition, the inadequate development of the testicles in the endemic area of Berne is no more common than in the goitre-free areas (Diamantopoulos) and, finally, that underdevelopment is incomparably more severe in genital infantilism and in hypophyseal *Typus adiposogenitalis* than among cretins, as anybody familiar with both disease patterns (cf. Figs. 51 and 57) knows.

Of course, as we have seen, different endocrine glands are anatomically altered among cretins, especially the hypophysis, the thymus and the gonads, and therefore their functions also deviate from the norm. However, the disorders of these glands show no autonomy compared with the thyroid gland; rather, everything pleads for their anatomical and functional alteration being dependent on the thyroid gland.

As for the *central nervous system*, Lotmar's investigations have very greatly increased the probability of there being a *thyrogenic* disorder, since in principle the same alterations are found in the brain as in thyroaplasia.

The behaviour of the *auditory system* in many cretins still remains unexplained. Interim contrasts that cannot easily be bridged on the endocrine path exist between cretinism and pure hypothyrosis. However, it is again pointed out that the difference is not absolute – the auditory system can be completely normal in the cretin. Admittedly, the syntropism between cretinism and hearing disorders is beyond doubt since, of the 118 cretins in Wydler's series, 47 were deaf-mutes in the sense just described, while 36 were hard of hearing. Equally important clinically is the so-called invariable speech difficulty which we cannot fully explain from the hearing disorders, and which we did not observe in this form in the above-mentioned (Fig. 119) case of non-cretinous partial thyroaplasia, nor in our cases of myxœdema and *cachexia thyreopriva* in adults. You could very easily be tempted to assume a direct effect of the noxious agent of goitre on the paths NB or NAB.

The *conclusion on pathogenesis* can be expressed as follows.

What we know with certainty of the development of endemic cretinism points to an intrauterine beginning and a foetal-period effect, continuing into extrauterine life to a varying degree and with a varying rate of damage and functional disorder of the thyroid gland through the noxious agent of goitre. A direct, parallel injury to the whole organism caused by the noxious agent of goitre, and a parallel co-participation of other endocrine glands is possible, but so far there are no hard facts, anatomically, clinically, or experimentally. So far we lack a positive explanation of any kind for the peripheral disorder of the auditory system. The same is true of the increased frequency of cardiac disorders, hernias, adenoid growths, and possibly also actual malformations occurring within the endemic region.

Also, it must be pointed out for the future that we will reach a complete solution of the problem if we do not unilaterally single out the goitre-free, dwarf cretins, as has happened so often in the past, but only if we encompass endemic thyropathy in its entirety and in all its forms, in the study.

Chapter 9
Prophylaxis and Treatment of Cretinism

Control of goitre and of cretinism, i.e., endemic thyropathy with its consequences and related phenomena, is today occasionally grouped under the title of *racial hygiene*. A word of interpretation is essential here. Goitre and cretinism appear in all races wherever the required environmental conditions exist. There is as yet no known race that might be considered secure against endemic thyropathy. Control of the latter is therefore not a question of racial hygiene, but a question of hygiene *per se*. If you want to define this more precisely, you would have to call it 'population hygiene'. The misnomer of the label 'racial hygiene' crops up particularly in countries inhabited by *different* 'races', such as the Bukowina studied by Flinker. In the *Alps*, representatives of the Nordic, Alpine and Mediterranean populations all participate in suffering from goitre. The designation 'racial hygiene' would have justification in goitre only if you follow Siemens in describing as race the 'permanent, surviving body of population'.

Restriction of cretinism to areas of severe goitre led to people discussing and tackling prophylaxis always for goitre *and* cretinism together, for just on 100 years, without having any accurate insight into the connection between the two evils.

Book upon book has been written on this subject, but we have still not achieved our goal. The starting point for any prophylaxis should theoretically be *knowledge of the aetiology*. Among the several dozen presumed causes of goitre, one has resounded increasingly during the first half century of the study of goitre study, or has at least come to the fore – the *inadequacy of hygienic living conditions*, which was palpable in some goitrous regions. This perception is supported by the observation that cretinism is less common in livelier, big towns than in small villages removed from centres of commerce; and goitre visibly retreated before the advance of a culture associated with greater cleanliness. Therefore the call went out to establish hygienically-improved living conditions. Through such improvements it was hoped to be able to explain the albeit modest decline in cretinism in particular areas, e.g. for Valais at the 1841 congress in Lyon, and the experts were probably not wrong in this. In 1844 Maffei and Roesch demanded drainage of the lowlands, valleys, and sinkholes where cretinism occurs; proper building regulations, particularly construction on elevations rather than in depressions, and not near water; foundations of ground floor dwellings with a 3–4 ft high basement; ensuring ventilation

J. Dennison et al., *Endemic Cretinism*,
DOI 10.1007/978-1-4614-0281-7_9, © Springer Science+Business Media, LLC 2011

and lighting in the houses and their surroundings – building for the sun! There is also the need of ensuring good drinking water and good diet. Their suggestions for domestic hygiene have been proven correct by the very recent studies by Dieterle and Eugster. More goitres arise on ground floors, and in damp houses without a cellar, than on higher floors provided with light and air. Dieterle and Eugster never found cretins in a new house.

Perhaps soil radioactivity (emphasised by Lang) plays the role of a localised factor. The radioactivity is brought about by the weathering of rock outcrops, and is particularly strong in goitre regions.

Of course we all know of living situations with the greatest filth imaginable where goitre is not endemic and cretinism is unknown. On the other hand both goitre and cretinism can be endemic in areas where the level of cleanliness is satisfactory and occasionally even of a relatively high standard. However, if we look at the situation at ground level, we see that the uncleanliness in the huts and dwellings of goitre-free populations is usually connected to a life predominantly lived in the open air and sunlight, or on the seashore with its abundant iodine. In the valleys, on the other hand, where goitre and cretinism are endemic, people spend a good part of their lives in the damp air of closed dwellings, especially during the long winters, and the occupants' efforts at relative cleanliness are no substitute for being in the open air and sunshine. What has been done to improve living conditions has undoubtedly had a beneficial effect, and we are justified in saying that cretinism is retreating before the railway and the automobile. Success is not yet, however, so complete that it renders the quest for *another prophylactic pathway* superfluous. In the iodine deficiency theory submitted by Boussingault, Prevost and Chatin and extended by Chatin with the developing research methodologies in the middle of the last century, people believed that they would find a way, even without the knowledge of thyroid gland function. A substantial half century elapsed before Hunziker, Bayard and Eggenberger reawakened that theory – this time based on our knowledge of thyroid gland physiology and iodine turnover in the body. We expect that our readers are familiar with Eggenberger's 1927 lucidly compiled history of the iodine deficiency theory, and its transformation into the practice of prophylaxis.

Compared with this, the notion of an *infectious genesis* of goitre and cretinism recedes into the background. Evidence for the existence of a specific goitre germ that infiltrates the body is also still missing. Folley's *Spirillum*, extensively referred to by Eggenberger, has proven itself to be a peculiar artefact (Doerr and others); while Houda's *Micrococcus*, following investigations in our clinic by Dr von Jacobi, has come to be recognised as an apathogenic, white *Staphylococcus* that had landed in the study material from out of the ambient air of the operating theatre. On the other hand, the idea of an inanimate, chemical or physical contagion or a multiplicity of such contagions has not lasted, and since 1850 the assumption of an *unknown noxious agent of goitre* has remained the principal front-runner in the iodine deficiency theory and remains so today.

We have taken a major step forward in the last 20 years, thanks to the systematic investigations of MacCarrison, who presented his final summated results at the second international goitre conference in 1933. He demonstrated that, in animals, an *excess* of particular substances in the food (certain fats, lime, specific goitre-producing substances in vegetables like cabbage) stimulates the thyroid gland to increased growth; while, on the other hand, the *lack* of important substances, such as certain vitamins, phosphates and certain goitre-adverse substances like iodine, has the same effect. Lack of cleanliness could also be added to the toxic nature of these goitre-producing conditions. Various substances act in a *goitre-restricting* manner, including thymol and bromine, but the most consistent is *iodine in small doses*. Even though the situation in humans may not be directly comparable with that of our study animals, through MacCarrison's experiments our knowledge is placed on a firmer footing than before, and the initial, purely empirical iodine prophylaxis has attained an experimental foundation.

Of course, this has still not eliminated the contrast between the theory of the noxious agent of goitre as a positive element and that of iodine deficiency as a negative factor; it has simply created a bridge between the two for iodine prophylaxis. For this reason we must return briefly to the theoretical problem.

Let us set aside for the moment those goitrous niduses identified in places with a good iodine supply. We can envisage that in such places thyroid gland function faces particularly great problems that can only be resolved with the help of a great excess of iodine. Our major difficulty lies in explaining an early-childhood (in odd cases possibly even primary) thyroid gland atrophy with severe signs of degeneration in cretins without goitre. Such a variation is not simply a compensatory process as offered by the physiological iodine deficiency theory. Even where a hyperplastic phase has gone before, you would have difficulty explaining such a sudden transition into the most severe atrophy – i.e., into the opposite of a compensation – if it were not a directly damaging feature affecting the cells. Such a sudden switch of a compensation is unknown in other pathology. Also MacCarrison's inferences for severe cases amount to an assumption of a toxic epithelial lesion.

Does iodine raise the resistance of the thyroid gland epithelium, rendering it immune to poison, or does it increase the toxicity of the substances in question?

The role that we ascribe to iodine is, on the one hand, a *physiological* one: restoration of the thyroid gland without compensatory hypertrophy coping with the goitre-producing toxins; on the other hand it is, so to speak, a *micropharmacological* role: neutralisation, rendering all goitre-causing toxins, or a number of them, harmless without detouring via thyroid gland function. The former explanation is without doubt a specious one, and MacCarrison's explanations give it a foundation insofar as he personally mentions the elevated demands on thyroid gland function as a result of certain nutritional disturbances as being among the causes of goitre.

In reality, the views are less far apart than often outlined in polemic writings. Even as little as there is a well-defined demarcation between physiological and pathological events, just as little can such a demarcation be established between a physiological and a micro-pharmacological effect. – Are we dealing with 'physiological' or 'micropharmacological' when we empower an organ to correct its task under aggravated external conditions?

Whatever answer you give to this question, you are, in a sense, doing just that.

It would be equally pointless to give up the testing of iodine prophylaxis of goitre because of the difficulty of this definition – as senseless as it would be to wait, patiently withholding tetanus prophylaxis through serum until its method of action has been clarified down to the last detail. The *advancement of a goitre-combating influence* has just as much right in the system of goitre prophylaxis as the *combat of goitre-promoting features*, especially when we are dealing with a substance whose daily supply amounts anyway to merely 0.1 mg, a basic condition of our physical and mental development. Ten years ago, we still stood before an unknown with regard to iodine effect. Today, we can learn from 10 years of experience in various places, that iodine supplementation within the physiological range using cooking salt actually promises to a certain extent to stem endemic thyropathy and its consequences.

Of particular importance for the prophylaxis of cretinism is Wegelin's discovery that the newborns of mothers who received iodized cooking salt during their pregnancy presented a normal or colloid histological thyroid gland picture, and that, in the Appenzell canton, the weight of the neonatal thyroid gland reduced from an average 8 g to 1.9 g, likewise with the histological picture becoming normal (Eggenberger). The experiences of Muggia in the province of Sondrio are an example of the favourable effect of iodine supply. Therefore, we must also assume for humans a favourable influence of the foetus through the improvement of the iodine supply to the mother, as has been established for several years in domestic animals in the United States. It is to be hoped that corresponding investigations will be undertaken on a larger scale. Nevertheless, we can already say that that besides the general improvement in hygienic living conditions, the revaluation of iodine supply to 1–2 γ per kg body weight – approximately 60–120 γ per day – is the right way for pregnant mothers. Even though perhaps not every noxious agent of goitre can be combated, at least we are dealing with those whose greatest impact can lead to endemic cretinism.

We have already mentioned Dieterle and Eugster's investigations on the improvement of general hygiene. According to them, domestic hygiene is to come first and foremost. The unfavourable influence of damp ground floors without a basement is beyond doubt. On the other hand, we know from T. von Fellenberg's research that the goitre-free villages studied by Dieterle and Eugster have a better natural iodine supply than do the neighbouring goitre villages. Has the iodine compensated for the effect of unfavourable living conditions there? This must be resolved by widened investigations. For the moment, Dieterle and Eugster's discoveries have already pointed out that both paths of prophylaxis will have to be trodden.

It cannot be denied that postnatal *iodine supply before and during school age* can also achieve a certain importance for the prophylaxis of cretinism. The broad elimination of goitre in Berne schools, admittedly using somewhat over-physiological iodine dosages – 150–450 γ per day justifies this assumption even though any damage *in utero* can no longer be totally reversed. As decades of experience and the histological investigations of recent years have shown, the principal damage has in fact already appeared during intrauterine life; therefore *iodine supplement for the pregnant mother* and, in practice, the whole population, must *remain the main means of prophylaxis*. That systematic improvement of iodine supply through cooking salt administered within the physiological range carries no disadvantages (despite iodine hypersensitivity of the thyroid gland in goitrous regions right through to very rare, partly questionable cases) has been demonstrated by the experiences of about 40% of the Swiss population who have been administered iodized cooking salt up to 5 mg per 1 kg. It is quite different right now in the United States of America, where the usual iodine supplement in cooking salt exceeds the physiological requirement about 20–40 times, and thus in pronounced goitre regions can, and indeed must, lead to the Jod-Basedow phenomenon among adults. If you want to test the general iodine revaluation of food from here on, you need not compromise it with too high iodine dosages as was the case around 1860 in several French *départements*. You have to come to terms with the fact that as a rule *adult* goitre is not eliminated at physiological iodine dosage. Larger doses usually do not achieve this either, nor do the 'huge doses of iodine' claimed by Jaensch for older children and adults; nor does endocrine substitution therapy. Daily iodine doses of 1 mg or more, administered in endemic regions over an extended period of time, will cause more harm than good in adults and adolescents.

Hoepner and Jaensch have recently declared *sterilisation legislation* as essential to more certain rehabilitation of the goitre regions; thereby cases of particular inferiority can be prevented from procreation. The idea is not new in the form of a marriage ban. Roesch, who attributed a greater role to inheritance than did his co-worker Maffei, says that marriages between two cretins should not be sanctioned, even when the level of cretinism in both is only small. He would permit marriage between a cretin and a non-cretinous individual only when the level of cretinism of one is very minimal and, preferably, when the male is the well-organised, lively, and intellectually sound partner.

Since then our perceptions have deepened, indeed in the direction of Maffei's views – he emphasizes repeatedly that cretinism is not an inheritable illness, not an inherited disease.

For full cretins we need no sterilisation law – nature by itself takes care of the necessity or prevents the undesired. We might emotionally prevent half-cretins from procreation because they would not be capable of looking after and bringing up their possibly normal children. Such a measure would not eliminate cretinism, for we know that the *majority of cretins do not come from half-cretin parents*, but from goitrous mothers who are usually not especially inferior at all, but just as normally created, physically and mentally, as their village companions who, by chance, did not produce cretins. We also know that the same mothers, who bring into the world goitrous and perhaps future cretin children in a goitre-village, will have goitre-free children in a goitre-free area. To sterilise all goitrous mothers because they could give birth to cretins would mean exterminating the population in favour of a new population that might dispense the same fate. Precisely because the endemic thyropathy is localised, it will not be influenced by sterilisation. You must therefore strike the latter off the measures expedient to the sanitization of a goitre region – as long as there is no proof that cretinism among the children of half-cretins is more common within the same environment than among the children of euthyroid goitrous mothers. For the foreseeable future, the prevention of propagation of half-cretins would be a purely fiscal measure in favour of the community, which has to be financially liable for the raising of children of socially-inferior parents.

Less promising than the prophylaxis of cretinism is the *treatment of individual cretins*, to which we shall now move.

The very understandable attempt to retrieve as much as possible for child cretins through *hygienic living conditions* and *education* was very enthusiastically undertaken by Dr. Guggenbühl in the middle of the last century, at his cretin institution on the Abendberg, near Interlaken. As can be appreciated based on our current knowledge, the successes of this internationally known institute were quite modest, apart from the fact that as a result of inadequacy of the diagnosis, not only cretins were included, but also cases of feeble-mindedness from other causes.

With the failure of Guggenbühl's attempt, the accurate basic idea was not lost. On the contrary, it has been carried forward for years in classes for the mentally retarded. In the severely afflicted endemic regions, alongside other forms of mental disability, these classes always boast fairly numerous cases of first and second grade cretinism, and fulfil a necessary function. Admittedly, we should be under no great illusions, as the educational abilities of cretins are bounded by limits. Apart from the usual clinical signs, microangioscopy is important as a diagnostic tool for orientating therapy at school age, admittedly with the reservations that we have made elsewhere, and particularly with the reservation of an extensive trial in the endemic region.

From the moment when the significance of cretinism as a hypothyrosis appeared on the scene, the way was open for an attempt at a *substitution treatment*. This was brought closer when the results from *Cachexia thyreopriva postoperativa* proved quite pleasing and, at an even higher level, from adult spontaneous myxœdema. First under consideration was the *implantation of functionally capable thyroid gland tissue*, based on the animal experiments of von Eiselsberg, Cristiani, and others. This had modest success, since in most cases the implanted glands decayed after a little time. Also, when people carried out the experiment, not with larger pieces of gland as at the start, but using thin strips, according to Voronoff, our observations were that the results did not exceed a temporary influence of the condition.

It must, however, be added that most experiments that we know about were carried out on congenital athyroid individuals, and not on cretins. In *adult* athyroid and cretin individuals, the condition has been established somatically from that point in such a way that any developmental leeway cannot be recovered. In children, either the cretinism is not diagnosed until later, or somebody has accepted the malady to be so obvious that the child has not once been taken to the physician before school age. Consequently, the number of cretin children treated by implantation is small. In spite of all the attempts by Kocher, Payr and others to guarantee favourable conditions to the transplant, the *site of implantation* does not seem to be of crucial importance. In terms of Voronoff's methodology, we have usually selected the thyroid gland as the site.

What we ourselves have observed entitles us, together with the experiences of others (see also E. Bircher), to the conclusion that implantation therapy in cretinism is not called upon to play a major role. From odd observations the most we could think of would be stimulation of the sparse thyroid gland tissue still present.

Substitution therapy by means of *orally* introduced *thyroid gland preparations* is far simpler to carry out. Wagner von Jauregg inaugurated extensive use of this therapy in cretinism, and it was then adopted, with higher doses, by Scholz. The initial gland sandwich of fresh thyroid gland was soon replaced by the administration of dried thyroid gland tissue and later by extracts of various kinds. Wagner von Jauregg began the treatment with a daily maximum 0.3 g of thyroid gland tissue and not exceeding 0.6 g; Scholz increased the dose to 1 g and, in accurately observed cases, up to 2.5 g. These experiments were carried out over several years on youthful cretins, excluding severe cases, in Steiermark. From Gamper's detailed, collated experiences and from our own observations, we have to conclude that oral substitution therapy does indeed favourably influence body growth, allowing the myxœdema to regress, and exerting a certain influence on mental alertness, in a similar manner to that seen in the treatment of congenital athyrosis and hypothyrosis. By this parallel observation, the specific character of the treatment and thereby the thyroprivic origin of the symptoms that have been ameliorated are proven up to a point. The limitation is based on the inability to exclude a *non-specific* effect of the thyroid gland preparation, especially on body growth. We have to interpret in this sense the widely varying improvements that many authors want to achieve with thyroid gland therapy in the feeble-mindedness of Down's syndrome.

The influence of thyroid gland treatment is also clearly present where it extends, not so rapidly, beyond the bounds of a non-specific effect, as occasionally in myxœdema and in growth disorders of congenital hypothyroid individuals. On the other hand, however, it is longer lasting (Wagner von Jauregg), and continues after treatment terminates. Something similar had also been observed in cases with a positive outcome after implantation, paralleling Voronoff's experiences in implantation of sexual glands. The result of the implantation only remained, or was at least longer lasting, where the organ to be replaced was still present at least partially. Whether it is a case of temporary relief or a stimulus remains to be seen. The implanted tissue might, even when it is finally reabsorbed, act as a long-lasting stimulus on the glandular tissue that is available in insufficient quantity or quality. As we have seen, the cretin always possesses some thyroid gland tissue still capable of functioning, and the possibility exists that this might be enhanced in functioning by long-duration substitution therapy. In dwarf cretins, with atrophic thyroid glands, the results appear to be better than in goitrous 'thyrogenic idiots' (Galli-Valerio).

According to every observer, pronounced mental defects and pronounced hearing difficulty or deaf-mutism are *not* influenced. Eysselt did find improvements in milder deafness.

From what has been said, the *whole outcome* is also widely varied in *oral substitution therapy*. This is not surprising, even when we assign hypothyrosis to the principal role in the pathogenesis of cretinism. The more fully the pathology of cretinism is studied, the more the impression is confirmed that the most severe or impervious cerebral disorders extend back to the earliest period of brain development; hence they are not reversible by employing substitution therapy several years later. The prognosis might be unfavourable even when substitution therapy is employed before school age, i.e., at a time when the diagnosis of cretinism has frequently still not been confirmed. Thus, we can have even less expectation of a therapy for cretinism in *adults*. Nevertheless, an attempt might be made where myxœdema, the easiest to influence, has stretched into adulthood. Of course, the situation among cretins in this regard is not the same as 40 years ago in *postoperative myxœdema*. Then, in the usually fully grown body and normally developed brain, the entire thyroid gland and vestiges were stripped at one fell swoop. Substitution therapy, which was not instituted until a decade after the last total excision, could then perform in full capacity. However, it was imperative that the thyroid gland preparations were prescribed long-term. As soon as patients suspended this, their condition deteriorated once more. In this regard, the adult cretin finds himself in a totally different situation. His thyroid gland defect is not total, but it has set in before birth. Therapy comes far too late and, accordingly, the patient's subjective needs are very small. The cretin has become physically and mentally attuned to the partial failure of the function of this important gland and has no subjective experience of it. He is therefore optimistic, whereas the person who has postoperatively become athyroid remembers his previous condition, experiences the difference, is disposed to depression, and desires treatment.

One final question must still be posed: does substitution therapy in any of its current forms offer *full* replacement of the failed gland's function? Its successes in acquired myxœdema, where the gland has been damaged by inflammation, have led to this idea springing up. However, the observation is not clear cut, due to the presence of an albeit temporarily defective gland. Neither does the criterion lie with the congenitally athyroid, because there, as with cretinism, the brain has suffered actually irreversible damage very early in development. More useful in assessing the question would be cases ranging from congenital *incomplete* thyroaplasia to low-grade infantile myxœdema. One such case (Fig. 119) that we followed up for years also gives rise to doubt. The result of an instant and subsequently used thyroid gland therapy in postoperative myxœdema would be really vital. In Kocher's cases, unfortunately, the substitution therapy could be instituted only 10 years after surgery as we said and, from our impression, the successes (cf. the Wölfli case published by Wegelin) were indeed quite pronounced, but not radical. In this regard, the same is true of an observation of a higher-grade case from our clinic suitable to be a 'control'.

From the other extreme, a man who had previously been mentally and vocationally normal had undergone apparently very radical surgery for a goitre 12 years earlier. After the operation he showed increasing signs of classic myxœdema. After he had been taking thyroid gland preparations irregularly since the operation, we saw him with a typical medium-grade myxœdema, a basal metabolic rate of –45%, and a vocational activity as a cobbler ruling out mental and physical torpor. In spite of our using thyroid gland medication (synthetic thyroxin) right up to the onset of signs of intoxication, bringing the basal metabolic rate back to –7%, we were unsuccessful in enabling the man to return to normal work.

Summing up our own experiences in this area, we must answer the above question with *no*. No form of substitution therapy proves capable of fully-valid replacement of the thyroid gland in its various spheres of effect. The Homunculus problem is not resolved even in this seemingly simply stated area. From the literature, I know of only *one* observational series that could respond to me – the cases of extremely severe Basedow where Sudeck removed the entire thyroid gland, and shielded the loss by thyroid gland medication. This substitution therapy was said to have fully alleviated the illness. How it will behave long-term remains to be seen. However, it should be noted that at the ages of these female patients the body's requirement for thyroid gland secretion is no longer as high as during their growing age, and consequently a malfunction is more easily masked, particularly when no greater demands are made of its capacity to function.

If you reflect on these various instances, you will easily convince yourself that the inadequate successes of thyroid gland therapy cannot be offered as evidence against the hypothyroid character of the most severe signs of endemic cretinism. We had as little success among congenitally athyroid individuals, who represent the classic example of thyroid gland breakdown, as we did among congenital cretins, in undoing the prenatal and early-postnatal onset of developmental disorders of the brain, and rendering the patient a normal member of human society, even when several months of thyroxin treatment allow the recovery of just as many years in skeletal development.

However, this is not to say that thyroid gland therapy should not be attempted. Today, the administration of thyroid gland tablets[1] to juvenile cretins is like a reflex action, at least here in Switzerland, possibly to such an extent that this therapy should be tried even where there is only a remote possibility of thyroid gland inadequacy. Yet even now, we are accustomed not to extend our expectations of success too far. In other words, substitution therapy successes are not so great that they would in any way restrict striving for an effective prophylaxis.

A final point is whether mild cretinism at school age can be influenced by *iodine treatment*. In Swiss schools generally, 1–3 mg potassium iodide or sodium iodide is administered per week, or 0.005 iodostarin + 0.001 g sodium iodide. The goitre control is very favourable. Extensive research is still lacking to show how far the boundaries of hypothyrosis are positively influenced, based on reliable comparative studies. Furthermore, what we said about iodine prophylaxis earlier, when we discussed the dosage, also applies here.

1 Goitre Surgery in Cretins

In the endemic region, the surgeon is often placed in the situation of having to undertake a goitre procedure on a cretin because of breathing difficulty. We can list more than 200 such interventions in our clinic over 15 years. The need must be established, as with euthyroid goitre sufferers, for the cretin too has the right to

[1]As well as other equally commendable thyroid gland preparations, we especially use Thyracrine prepared according to Oswald's recipe, adjusted to 0.15 mg iodine per tablet, which corresponds to 0.05 g thyroglobulin.

breathe freely, and he would think, if he could: '*primum vivere, deinde philosophare*' [Aristotle – live first, philosophise later]. Following surgery, he proves himself to be extremely grateful for the help given, and recommends – by gestures should he be deaf-mute – surgery to his not yet operated-upon companions in the institute.

In the great majority of cases, the operation can be carried out without difficulty under local anaesthesia, and the patient, convinced of the necessity of the intervention, generally behaves just as calmly as would a euthyroid goitrous individual. General anaesthesia is necessary only for children and the odd particularly unruly adult cretin.

The intervention differs from an euthyroid goitre operation purely technically, in that the goitre, even when it lies deeply, can be shelled out relatively easily because the tissues are loose. The blood vessels, however, as already mentioned, are usually very well developed, and in powerful male cretins we occasionally encounter thyroid arteries of 7–9 mm calibre, with correspondingly developed veins. Thus, for the surgery to run smoothly, it is doubly worthwhile to ligate the arterial trunk, particularly the inferior thyroid arteries, right at the start of the procedure. We ligate usually only the more anterior branch of the superior thyroid artery. We must especially remember to preserve as much relatively usable tissue as possible; this is found mainly at the upper pole and on the posterior surface of the gland, i.e., the area supplied by the more posterior branch of the superior thyroid artery. Since we are usually dealing with multi-glandular, parenchymatous goitre, enucleation will be applied as extensively as possible, especially in juvenile cretins. If you are convinced that only more remnant tissue is present, largely non-functional, and incapable of development, you will be driven by necessity to retain several nodules not compromising the trachea. However, among younger cretins you will then have to anticipate a recurrence. In this case, supplementary iodine treatment is desirable. In older cretins we also proceed conservatively, although with less trepidation than with younger individuals. Thus, we use enucleation resection more often, and, in small-nodular conglomerate goitre, we have even repetitively undertaken a proper horseshoe resection. When conserving too much tissue we have also experienced a relapse in adult cretins.

Postoperative healing proceeds just as smoothly as among non-cretins, and we have not seen pulmonary complications any more frequently than in non-cretins. This observation on the healing tendency applies also to other surgical procedures undertaken on cretins, such as hernia operations and occasional gastrointestinal tract intervention due to benign and malignant diseases.

The follow-up undertaken by Chaitan on our cretins who had undergone goitre surgery showed that in a good 60% of cases the ability of the post-surgical patients to function and be useful was just as good as before surgery; even better in around 23% of cases; and poorer in only 16% on account of a possible increase of signs of insufficiency.

It is self-evident that radiography should always be employed when establishing the need for intervention, in profile as well when necessary. Occasionally you may discover an intrathoracic portion of the goitre that might escape a summary – or even a careful clinical examination. That, among the respiratory difficulties of cretins, the possibility of a cardiac, pulmonary or renal origin should be considered needs hardly be emphasised.

2 Goitre and Cancer

In conclusion we should remember that goitre prophylaxis and the related control of cretinism were also associated with cancer control. Bayard (1919) was first to express the idea that hypothyroid conditions predisposed the individual to cancer. This idea was reiterated by Hunziker, and special emphasis was given to cancer of the digestive system. In 1924 Stiner established that in all goitre-free, or relatively goitre-free, Swiss cantons, with one exception, cancer of the digestive organs regressed significantly more than in the markedly goitrous areas. However, in Stiner's opinion, that is not a direct, causal relationship. For him, the connecting link is dental caries which, like goitre in his opinion, arises from vitamin-deficient food, and which, for its part, favours the onset of cancer in the digestive organs.

Percy Stocks followed the connection between the frequency of goitre and the occurrence of cancer statistically, and in the bigger cities of England and the United States of America he found a positive relationship between childhood thyroid gland enlargement and cancer mortality.

At first glance the thoughts of Bayard, Hunziker, Eggenberger and the perception of a lower resistance of cretinous hypothyroid individuals to causative agents of cancer undoubtedly have something captivating about them. However, if you go into the question in depth, certain thoughts arise. For example, the Neuenburger and Bernese Jura stand out for their pronounced freedom from goitre. There, school-age goitre usually regresses spontaneously after puberty. Endemic cretinism is unknown. Goitre was found in only 1% of the recruits examined. Against this, cancer mortality rate is medium (10–15 deaths annually per 10,000 inhabitants) according to Swiss Health Department statistics (Stiner). In the Bernese midlands and the Emmental on the other hand, goitre and, in some places also cretinism, is very common – 15% goitre among the recruits – while cancer mortality amounts to merely 5–10 per 10,000 inhabitants. Wallis has, from time immemorial, been known for its cretins, even though these have declined in numbers in recent times. However, cancer frequency is lower there than in most areas of Switzerland. The regions most heavily beset by cancer do not stand out for particular frequency of cretinism.

Finally, in our alms houses, where several hundred adult cretins are looked after until they die, cancer death is an exception. The most common causes of death are debility due to old age, circulatory diseases and tuberculosis (only in one institution).

Among the cancer material in our surgical clinic, which lies in the centre of the endemic region, only exceptionally do we find cretins.

Thus, if you follow up the problem in particular detail, you can at least identify no prevalence of cancer mortality among cretins. In our institutions, most cretins turned out to be well within the ‘cancer age’. Wegelin’s pathological-anatomical findings, cited above, similarly do not support a particular predisposition of cretins to malignant tumours. There is therefore no evidence so far of goitre and cretinism supporting cancer development. Endemic thyropathy is a good culture medium solely for cancer of the *thyroid gland*, but this is a case of a predisposition restricted to a particular *organ*; it is not a question of general cancer tendency. Through the control of endemic goitre, we will therefore merely stem the *struma maligna* but, in all probability, we will not reduce general cancer morbidity.

Appendix A
Cretinism Revisited: The View from 2010

Endemic cretinism includes two syndromes: a more common neurological disorder with brain damage, deaf mutism, squint and spastic paresis of the legs and a less common syndrome of severe hypothyroidism, growth retardation and less severe mental defect. Both conditions are due to dietary iodine deficiency and can be prevented by correction of iodine deficiency before pregnancy. Endemic cretinism is now included in the spectrum of the effects of iodine deficiency in a population termed the 'iodine deficiency disorders (IDD)', which also includes a wide range of lesser degrees of cognitive defect which can be prevented by the correction of iodine deficiency. Iodine deficiency is now recognised by the World Health Organization (WHO) as the most common preventable cause of brain damage with in excess of 2 billion at risk from 130 countries. A global United Nations (UN) program of prevention has achieved 68% household usage of iodized salt by the year 2000 compared with less than 20% before 1990.

In contrast with endemic cretinism the condition of sporadic cretinism occurs all over the world without any relation to iodine deficiency. It is usually found with evidence of a misplaced or absent thyroid or with goitre due to congenital defect in the biosynthesis of thyroid hormones causing clinical hypothyroidism (Hetzel 1989).

After the early descriptions from the seventeenth to twentieth centuries the problem of endemic cretinism was mostly forgotten until later in the twentieth century because these subjects were often confined to remote areas which limited access for scientific study. It was in the 1960s that the problem was rediscovered in various parts of the world – in Latin America (Brazil); Africa (the then Zaire, now Republic of the Congo); The People's Republic of China; Indonesia; and Papua New Guinea (Pharoah et al. 1980).

Questions were raised about the relation of iodine deficiency to cretinism in Europe (Switzerland and Northern Italy) because of the apparent spontaneous disappearance of cretinism in the absence of programs for the correction of iodine deficiency with iodized salt (Costa et al. 1964). These observations raised the question as to whether iodine deficiency was the cause of cretinism.

J. Dennison et al., *Endemic Cretinism*,
DOI 10.1007/978-1-4614-0281-7,

A.1 Studies in Papua New Guinea

In Papua New Guinea (PNG) studies were carried out in the Highlands in collaboration with the Public Health Department of the Territory (then under Australian administration) where a severe problem of goitre and cretinism had been identified. Advantage was taken of the availability of iodized oil 'Lipiodol' (a preparation of iodine in poppyseed oil long used in radiology as a contrast medium) for the correction of iodine deficiency in the remote Highlands where distribution of iodized salt was difficult to achieve. A single injection of iodized oil was shown to correct severe iodine deficiency in subjects in the Highlands for up to 5 years depending on the dosage (Buttfield and Hetzel 1967).

Subsequently the prevention of cretinism and stillbirths was demonstrated by the administration of iodized oil before pregnancy in a randomized controlled trial in the Western Highlands of New Guinea (Pharoah et al. 1971). This finding was subsequently accepted as definitive (*The Lancet* Editorial 1972). A mass injection program, with iodized oil was carried out in the Highlands, from 1971.

Wide experience in all parts of the world indicates that cretinism disappears in a population when iodine deficiency is corrected. The apparent spontaneous disappearance in Europe is now attributed to 'silent' correction of iodine deficiency by gradual dietary diversification associated with social and economic development (Burgi et al. 1990).

A.1.1 The Clinical Features of Endemic Cretinism

An agreed definition of endemic cretinism was adopted by the Pan American Health Organization (PAHO) in 1986 (Dunn et al.), with later confirmation in 1994 (WHO/UNICEF/ICCIDD). The definition consists of three major features:

1. Epidemiology: It is associated with endemic goitre and severe iodine deficiency.
2. Clinical manifestations: These comprise mental deficiency, together with either:
   (i) A predominant neurological syndrome including defects of hearing and speech and characteristic disorders of stance and gait of varying degree; or
   (ii) Predominant hypothyroidism and stunted growth.
   Although usually the neurological syndrome predominates in some areas a mixture of the two syndromes has been observed.
3. Prevention. In areas where adequate correction of iodine deficiency has been achieved, endemic cretinism has been prevented.

A.1.2 Clinical Manifestations

McCarrison reported the two types of endemic cretinism from the Karakoram Mountains (now Pakistan) in 1908. In addition to Europe (Switzerland and Italy) it

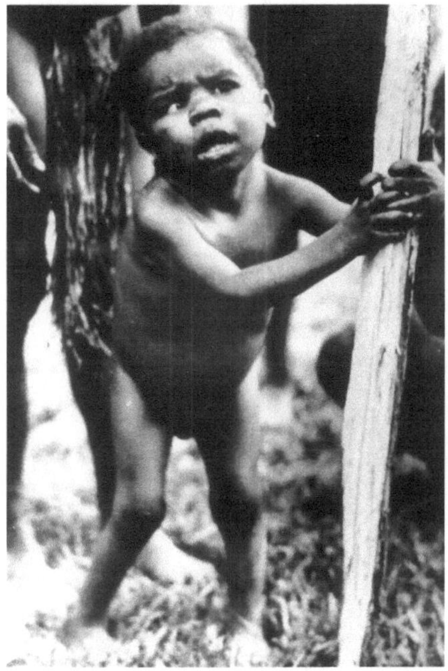

Fig. A1 Child with severe neurological cretinism associated with brain damage, squint, deaf mutism and ataxia, so that he is dependent on the stick he is holding (Papua New Guinea) (Reproduced from Hetzel (1989))

has been reported from South America (Argentina, Ecuador, Brazil); Africa (Democratic Republic of Congo); Oceania (New Guinea) and Asia (China, India, Nepal, Indonesia, Burma and Pakistan) (Pharoah et al. 1980; Zimmermann et al. 2008). The association of cretinism with severe iodine deficiency has been uniformly demonstrated.

The different features of the two types are summarized as follows:

1. Neurological Cretins: Worldwide this is the common type in areas of severe iodine deficiency (Hetzel 1989; Zimmermann et al. 2008) (Fig. A1). The obvious clinical features include mental retardation with the following neurological defects:
   (i) Defects of hearing and speech-most neurological cretins are deaf-mutes of varying degree.
   (ii) Squint.
   (iii) Predominant neurological signs: Impaired voluntary motor activity involving spastic diplegia or paresis of the lower limbs.
   (iv) Characteristic disorders of stance and gait of varying degree including spastic gait and ataxia with serious effects on standing and walking.

   Neurological cretins are usually euthyroid, but goitre and hypothyroidism can be seen in some cases. Urinary iodine levels are usually less than 20 μg/l compared to normal levels (100–150 μg/l) with a normal dietary intake.
2. Hypothyroid cretins: (McCarrison 1908; Hetzel 1989; Ma et al. 1989) (Fig. A2). Severe or long-standing hypothyroidism is predominant in this type with the

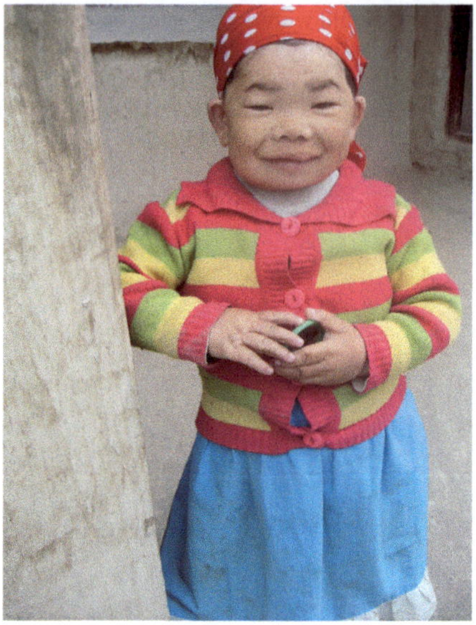

Fig. A2 Child with hypothyroid cretinism showing thickened features, dry skin and growth retardation (Xinjiang, China) (Personal photograph reproduced by kind permission of Prof.Chen Zu-Pei, China)

following features: dwarfism, myxoedema, dry swollen or thickened skin, sparseness of hair and nails, deep hoarse voice, sexual retardation, retarded maturation of body parts, skeletal retardation, weak abdominal muscles, inactive bowel function and delayed tendon reflexes. A typical feature is incomplete maturation of the face: wide-set eyes, saddle-nose deformity with retarded maturation of nasoorbital configurations, mandibular atrophy and thickened lips (Fig. A2).

The mental deficiency of neurological cretins is more severe than in the hypothyroid type (Ma et al. 1989; Zimmermann et al. 2008). They demonstrate difficulty in performing simple manual tasks, such as of simple dancing observed in southern Xinjiang of China. However, some hypothyroid cretins in the Republic of the Congo exhibit neurologic signs, such as spasticity of the lower limbs, jerky movements, Babinski sign and shifting gait (DeLong 1989). The prevalence of goitre in the hypothyroid type is much lower than in neurological cretinism. Lower or undetectable serum T_4, T_3 and very high levels of TSH are associated with low levels of urinary iodine usually in hypothyroid type (less than 20 μg/l) (Hetzel 1989; Zimmermann et al. 2008).

Hypothyroid endemic cretinism is found mainly in the Republic of the Congo; in Pakistan (in the Karakoram Mountains); and the western region of China (Xinjiang, Qinghai, Gansu Provinces and part of Inner Mongolia). The reasons for these geographic differences in the epidemiologic pattern of endemic cretinism are not known but cassava intake is a factor in the Republic of the Congo through the effect of thiocyanate in reducing iodine uptake by the thyroid (Delange et al. 1972).

Recently the emergence of neurological cretinism in some remote villages of the southern Xinjiang Region of China in 2006 was due to the failure of the local iodized salt program (Chen 2007). No new cretins had been born between 1970 and 1990, following the original iodine intervention.

A.1.3 Animal Models

Experimental studies of the effect of iodine deficiency studies on the sheep, the marmoset monkey and the rat have been particularly concerned with foetal brain development because of its relevance to the human problem of endemic cretinism and brain damage resulting from foetal iodine deficiency. These studies establish the significant effects of iodine deficiency in causing retardation of brain development in a variety of animal species including the primate (Hetzel and Mano 1989).

A.1.4 The Spectrum of Iodine Deficiency Disorders (IDD)

The results of these studies required a re-conceptualization of the main effect of iodine deficiency from the common lump in the neck (goitre) to a general effect on growth and development, including especially brain development.

The term IDD refers to all the effects of iodine deficiency on the growth and development of a human or animal population, which can be prevented by correction of the iodine deficiency. These include goitre, stillbirths, neonatal and other types of hypothyroidism but the most significant effect is that of foetal brain damage (Hetzel 1983). Effects on brain function occur from hypothyroidism in the foetus, the neonate, child or adult (Table A1).

A meta-analysis of recent research reported a total of 18 studies in which comparison was made between iodine deficient populations and suitable control populations with a similar social and cultural background (Bleichrodt and Born 1994). These studies revealed that the mean score for the iodine deficient group was 13.5 IQ points below that of the non-iodine deficient groups.

Social and economic effects result from iodine deficiency in both human and animal populations. In humans there is reduced school performance in children and reduced productivity in adults. Detailed calculations have been made of the economic costs of medical assessment and the treatment of goitre. In Germany where there has been much uncontrolled IDD, the costs of diagnosis have been estimated at US$250 million per year and the costs of treatment have been estimated at US$300 million per year. The cost of hours lost in working time for this medical care was calculated to be US$150 million. This makes a total of US$700 million (Pfannenstiel 1985).

There are also significant effects on all livestock with impaired reproduction in poultry, sheep, goats and cattle, with reduced wool growth and milk production and reduced rates of survival in offspring. Such effects indicate that correction of iodine deficiency has direct economic benefits. It has been calculated by the World Bank that each dollar dedicated to IDD prevention would yield a productivity gain of $28 (Pandav and Rao 1977; Levin et al. 1994).

Table A1 The spectrum of iodine deficiency disorders (IDD)

Fetus	Abortions
	Stillbirths
	Congenital anomalies
	Neurological cretinism:
	Mental deficiency, deaf mutism, spastic diplegia, squint
	Hypothyroid cretinism:
	Mental deficiency, dwarfism, hypothyroidism
	Psychomotor defects
Neonate	Increased perinatal mortality
	Neonatal hypothyroidism
	Retarded mental and physical development
Child & adolescent	Increased infant mortality
	Retarded mental and physical development
Adult	Goitre with its implications
	Iodine-induced hyperthyroidism (IIH)[a]
All ages	Goitre
	Hypothyroidism
	Impaired mental function
	Increased susceptibility to nuclear radiation

From Hetzel (1983, 1989)
[a]Transient following iodization minimised by reduced rate of increase in iodine intake [1]

A.1.5 The Global Program of Elimination of Brain Damage due to IDD

The global elimination program has developed through successful application of this knowledge at country level, mainly with the policy of universal salt iodization (USI), which required all salt for human and animal consumption to be iodized (WHO 1994).

The 1986 World Health Assembly (WHA) passed a resolution calling for the prevention and control of IDD with the use of iodized salt. This was followed by the WHA Resolution in 1990, calling for elimination of IDD by the year 2000 and a later Resolution in 1996, calling for sustainability of the program through systematic monitoring (Hetzel et al. 2004).

The International Council for Control of Iodine Deficiency Disorders (ICCIDD) recognised formally by WHO, has played an important role in bridging the gap between the research and its application in national programs. The ICCIDD now comprises more than 700 multidisciplinary professionals from over 100 countries with a majority from developing countries (Hetzel 2002). By 1990 a Global Action Plan for the elimination of IDD by the year 2000 was proposed by the ICCIDD and approved by the UN Subcommittee on Nutrition (SCN), which provided for actions at global, regional and national levels.

The endorsement of the Global Action Plan was followed by the adoption of the goal of elimination of IDD by 2000 by the World Summit for Children on September 30th 1990 at a special meeting at the United Nations, New York. This World Declaration (1990) was signed by 71 Heads of State and was subsequently signed by representatives of 88 other national governments. This Resolution provided unprecedented political support for 27 goals for the improvement of the health and education of children.

An informal global partnership following the World Summit developed for the common purpose of the virtual elimination of IDD. This partnership included the people and governments of the IDD affected countries, the salt industry of the affected countries; the bilateral aid agencies (such as Australia, Canada, Netherlands, Sweden); the international agencies, WHO, UNICEF, the World Bank; the ICCIDD and Kiwanis International. Subsequently the Micronutrient Initiative, the Global Network for the Sustained Elimination of Iodine Deficiency, the Global Alliance for Improved Nutrition (GAIN) and the Gates Foundation joined the global partnership with increased impact (Hetzel 2007; Gautam 2007).

The Director-General of WHO, Dr. Gro Brundtland has pointed out that the achievement of IDD elimination 'will be a major and total public health triumph ranking with small-pox and polio'. It will be a major global triumph in the elimination of a non-infectious disease (WHA 1999).

References

Abelin, I. (1930). Die Physiologie der Schilddrüse. In A. Bethe, G. von Bergmann, G. G. Embden, & A. Ellinger (Eds). *Handbuch der normalen und pathologischen Physiologie mit Berücksichtigung der experimentellen Pharmakologie, 16*, 94.

Ackermann, J. F. (1790). *Über die Kretinen, eine besondere Menschenabart in den Alpen*. Gotha: Ettinger.

Adlerkreutz, E. (1928). Orientierende Untersuchung über die Verbreitung des Kropfes in Finnland und über deren Zusammenhang mit dem Jodvorkommen im Wasser. *Acta Medica Scandinavica, 69*(1), 1–45.

Aeschbacher, S. (1905). Über den Einfluß krankhafter Zustände auf den Jod- und Phosphorgehalt der normalen Schilddrüse. *Mitteilungen aus den Grenzgebieten der Medizin und Chirurgie, 15*, 268–296.

Aeschlimann. (1933). Über die Verwertbarkeit der Phagocytose in der Diagnostik der Schilddrüsenerkrankungen. *Endokrinologie, 12*.

Alexander, G. (1908). Das Gehörorgan der Kretinen. *Anatomischer Teil. Archiv für Ohrenheilkunde, 78*, 54–128.

Allara, V. (1892). *Sulla causa del cretinesimo*. Milan: Studio Milano.

Anselmino, K. J. & Hoffmann, F. (1933). Darstellung, Eigenschaften und Vorkommen einer antithyreoiden Schutzsubstanz aus Blut und Geweben. *Klinische Wochenschrift, 12*(3), 99–102.

Arndt, H.-J. (1931). Der Kropf in Rußland. Eine morphogeographische Studie. *Ergebnisse der deutsch-russischen Rasseforschung* Jena: G. Fischer Verlag.

Aschoff, K. A. L. (1925). Über das Kropfproblem, besonders den Pubertätskropf in Baden. *Vorträge über Pathologie*. Jena.

Autenrieth, H. (1834). *Amtlicher Bericht über die Versammlung deutscher Naturforscher und Ärzte*. Stuttgart: Gesellschaft Deutscher Naturforscher und Ärzte.

Baillarger, J. G. F. (1873). *Rapport de la commission d'enquête sur le goître et le crétinisme en France*. Paris: Baillière et fils.

Ballet, G. & Enriquez, E. (1895). Corps thyroïde et maladie de Basedow. *Semaine médicale, 39*, 329.

Baló, J., Lovas, L., Bach, E. & Neufeld, L. (1935). Die antagonistische Wirkung eines neuen Pankreasextraktes auf die Thyroxinvergiftung. *Archiv für experimentelle Pathologie und Pharmakologie, 165*(1), 594–613.

Bauer, J. (1921). *Die konstitutionelle Disposition zu inneren Krankheiten*, 2. Aufl. Berlin: Julius Springer Verlag.

Bauer, J. (1927). *Innere sekretion, ihre physiologie, pathologie und klinik*. Berlin and Vienna: Julius Springer.

Bayard, O. (1919). *Beiträge zur Schilddrüsenfrage*. Basel: Schwabe.

Bayard, O. (1923). Über das Kropfproblem. *Schweizerische medizinische Wochenschrift, 53*, 703–707, 732–737.

J. Dennison et al., *Endemic Cretinism*,
DOI 10.1007/978-1-4614-0281-7, © Springer Science+Business Media, LLC 2011

Bayer. (1933). Kröpf und Kretinismus bei Hunden. *Prager Archiv für Tiermedizin und vergleichende Pathologie, 13.*

Bayon, G. P. (1903). *Beitrag zur Diagnose und Lehre vom Kretinismus.* Würzburg.

Bayon, G. P. (1904). Über angebliche verfrühte Synostose bei Kretinen und die hypothetischen Beziehungen der Chondrodystrophia foetalis zur Athyreosis. *Beiträge zur pathologischen Anatomie und zur allgemeinen Pathologie, 36,* 119. Jena: G. Fischer Verlag.

Bayon, G. P. (1904). Über das Zentralnervensystem der Kretinen. *Neurologisches Zentralblatt.* N° 8

Bayon, G. P. (1905). Hypophysis, Epiphysis und peripherische Nerven bei einem Fall von Kretinismus. *Neurologisches Zentralblatt.* N° 4.

Beitzke, H. (1912). Über die sog. Arthritis deformans atrophica. *Zeitschrift für Klinische Medizin, 74,* 215–29.

Bernard. (1892). *Die Kretine Pöhl.* Inaugural Dissertation, Würzburg.

Bernheim-Karrer, J. (1906). Über zwei atypische Myxödemfälle. *Jahresberichte über die Kinderheilkunde und physische Erziehung, 64.*

Bernheim-Karrer, J. (1924). Rhachitis und kongenitales Myxödem. *Jahresberichte über die Kinderheilkunde und physische Erziehung, 105.*

Betz. (1851). Zur pathologischen Anatomie des Kretinismus. *Beobachtungen über den Kretinismus,* vol. 2. Tübingen Bircher, E.

Bircher, H. (1883). *Der endemische Kröpf und seine Beziehungen zur Taubstummheit und zum Kretinismus.* Basel: Schwabe.

Bircher, H. (1890). Das Myxödem und diekretinische Degeneration. *Sammlung klinischer Vorträge* No. 357.

Bircher, H. (1896). Fortfall und Änderung der Schilddrüsenfunktion als Krankheitsursache. *Ergebnisse der allgemeinen Pathologie und pathologischen Anatomie, 1.*

Bircher, H. (1902). Die gestörte Schilddrüsenfunktion als Krankheitsursache. *Ergebnisse der allgemeinen Pathologie und pathologischen Anatomie, 8.*

Bircher, E. (1908). Zur Pathogenese der kretinischen Degeneration. *Beihefte zur Medizinischen Klinik, 4,* 6.

Bircher, E. (1908). Über eine der Coxa vara entsprechende Deformität der Schulter bei Kretinen. *Deutsche Zeitschrift für Chirurgie, 96.*

Bircher, E. (1909). *Die Entwicklung und der Bau des Kretinenskelets im Röntgenogramme; Atlas der normalen und pathologischen Anatomie in typischen Röntgenbildern.* Hamburg: Lucas Gräfe & Sillern.

Bircher, E. (1909). Zur Implantation von Schilddrüsengewebe bei Kretinen. *Deutsche Zeitschrift für Chirurgie, 98.*

Bircher, E. (1911). Fortfall und Änderung der Schilddrüsenfunktion als Krankheitsursache. *Ergebnisse der allgemeinen Pathologie und pathologischen Anatomie,15.*

Bircher, E. (1912). Ein Beitrag zur Kenntnis der Schilddrüse und Nebenschilddrüse bei Kretinoiden, Kretinen und endemisch Taubstummen. *Frankfurter Zeitschrift für Pathologie, 11.*

Bircher, E. (1925). Die kretinische Degeneration im Kanton Aargau. *Mitteilungen der Aargauischen Naturforschenden Gesellschaft, 17,* Bircher, H.

Bleichrodt, N., & Born, M. P. (1994). A metaanalysis of research on iodine and its relationship to cognitive development. In J. B. Stanbury (Ed.) *The damaged brain of iodine deficiency* (pp. 195–200). New York: Cognizant Communication Corporation.

Blum, F. (1932). Über Katechine. *Deutsche medizinische Wochenschrift, 58.*

Blum, F. (1933). Über die antithyreoidalen Eigenschaften des Blutes und das zugrunde liegende Katechin. *Schweizerische medizinische Wochenschrift, 63,* 777.

Bock, K.A. (1932). Über die Bedeutung atypischer Capillarbilder bei innersekretorischen Störungen. *Klinische Wochenschrift, 11*(3), 102–104.

Bommel van, L. B. (1930). *Struma Endemica en Cretinismus in Nederlandsch Oost-Indie: Meer in het Bijzonder in de Alaslanden.* Inaug.-Diss. Leiden: Rijks-Universiteit/ Eduard Ijdo.

Bourneville. (1903). Fin de l'histoire d'un idiot myxoedémateux. *Archives de Neurologie revue mensuelle des maladies nerveuses et mentales, 16,* N° 92.

Boyce, R. & Beadles, C.F. (1893). Enlargement of the hypophysis cerebri in myxoedema: with remarks upon hypertrophy of the hypophysis, associated with changes in the thyroid body. *Journal of Pathology and Bacteriology, 1*, 223–239.

Branovacky, M. (1926). Die biologische Wirksamkeit verschiedener Kröpfarten im Kaulquappenversuch. *Mitteilungen aus den Grenzgebieten der Medizin und Chirurgie, 39.*

Branovacky-Pelech. (1926). Über den funktionellen Wert der Langhansschen wuchernden Struma. *Mitteilungen aus den Grenzgebieten der Medizin und Chirurgie, 39*, 609–625.

Breus, C. & Kolisko, A. (1900). *Die pathologischen Beckenformen.* Leipzig & Vienna: Franz Deuticke.

Burghart & Blumenthal. (1902). Über eine spezifische Behandlung des Morbus Basedowii. *Internationale Beiträge zur inneren Medizin, 2*, 251.

Bürgi, H., Supersaxo, Z., & Selz, B. (1990). Iodine deficiency diseases in Switzerland one hundred years after Theodor Kocher's survey. A historical review with some new goitre prevalence data. *Acta Endocrinologica, 123*, 577–590.

Buttfield, I. H., & Hetzel, B. S (1967). Endemic goitre in Eastern New Guinea with special reference to the use of iodized oil in prophylaxis and treatment. *Bulletin of the World Health Organization, 36*, 243–262.

Campeanu, L. (1924). Problema gusii si cretinizmului in România si cercetâri biologice asupra glandei tiroide. *Editura Ardealului*, Cluj.

Carbonnières, L. R. de (1789). *Voyage dans les Pyrénées françaises et espagnoles.* Strasbourg.

Cerletti, U. (1923). Milan: Pubblicazioni dell'Istituto Sieroterapico Milanese.

Cerletti, U. & Perusini, G. (1906). A cretin dog and its thyroid apparatus. *Journal of Mental Pathology, 7.*

Cerletti, U. & Perusini, G. (1907). *L'endemia gozzo-cretinica nelle famiglie.* Rome: Tipografia operaia romana cooperativa.

Chaitan, S. (1924). Über die Beeinflussung des Kretinismus durch Entfernung von Kropfgewebe. *Schweizerische medizinische Wochenschrift.*

Champy, C. (1922). L'action de l'extrait thyroïdien sur la multiplication cellulaire. Caractère électif de cette action. *Archives de morphologie générale et expérimentale, 4*, 1–58.

Chen, Z. P. (2007). New cretins discovered in southern Xinjiang, China. *IDD Newsletter, 23*, 18.

Clerc, E. (1912). Die Schilddrüse im hohen Alter vom 50. Lebensjahr an aus der norddeutschen Ebene und Küstengegend sowie aus Bern. *Frankfurter Zeitschrift für Pathologie, 10*, 1–19.

Comte, L. (1898). Contribution à l'étude de l'hypophyse humaine et de ses relations avec le corps thyroïde. *Beiträge zur pathologischen Anatomie und zur allgemeinen Pathologie, 23.*

Coppola, A. (1926). *Un focolaio di endemia gozzo-cretinica in Sicilia. Studi neurologici dedicati a E. Tanzi.* Turin. (Cited by Gamper and Scharfetter).

Costa, A., Cottino, F., Mortara, M., & Vogliazzo, V. (1964). Endemic cretinism in Piedmont. *Panminerva medica Associazione medica italiana 6*, 250–259.

Coulon, W. de (1897). Über Thyreoidea und Hypophysis der Kretinen, sowie über die Thyreoidealreste bei Struma nodosa. *Virchows Archiv für pathologische Anatomie und Physiologie und für klinische Medizin, 147.*

Cristiani, H. (1901). Nouvelles experiences de greffe thyroïdienne chez les mammifères. *Journal de Physiologie et de Pathologie générale, 2*, 200–215.

Cristiani, H. (1904). De la greffe thyroïdienne chez l'homme. *Semaine médicale.*

Crookshank, F. G. (1917). Nervous cretinism. *The Lancet, 190*, 604–605.

Csépai, K. and Stamm, E. (1927). Beiträge zur Kenntnis der Beziehung zwischen Schilddrüse und Pancreas. *Münchener medizinische Wochenschrift.*

Csépai, K. and Stamm, E. (1928). Über die Insülinempfindlichkeit des menschlichen Organismus. *Wiener klinische Wochenschrift.*

Damerow. (1831). Der Kretinismus in anthropologischer Hinsicht. *Medizinische Zeitung Ver. Heilkunde Preußen 10.*

Dedichen. (1914). Untersuchungen aus einer Strumagegend über das Vorkommen von Morbus Basedowi, Myxödem und verwandten Zuständen im Verhältnis zur Häufigkeit und zur Verbreitung des gewöhnlichen Kropfes. In *Festschrift Herrn Dr. Heinrich Bircher.* Tübingen: H. Laupp.

Delange, F., Ermans, A. M., Vis, H. L., & Stanbury, J. B. (1972). Endemic cretinism in Idjwi Island (Kivu Lake, Republic of the Congo). *The Journal of Clinical Endocrinology and Metabolism, 34*, 1059–1066.

DeLong, G. R. (1989). Observations on the neurology of endemic cretinism. In G. R. DeLong, J. Robbins, & P. G. Condliffe (Eds) *Iodine and the Brain*, (pp. 231–238). New York: Plenum Press.

Demme, C. H. (1840). *Über endemischen Kretinismus*. Rektoratsrede Bern 1840.

Dexler, E. (1909). Über endemischen Kretinismus bei Tieren. *Berliner tierärztliche Wochenschrift*, p. 375.

Diamantopoulos, S. (1921). Über die Hypoplasie der Hoden in der Entwicklungsperiode. *Zeitschrift für Konstitutionslehre, 8*, 117–153.

Dieterle, T. (1906). Die Athyreosis unter besonderer Berücksichtigung der dabei auftretenden Skeletveränderungen. *Virchows Archiv für pathologische Anatomie und Physiologie und für klinische Medizin, 184*, 56–124.

Dieterle, T. (1906). Über endemischen Kretinismus und dessen Zusammenhang mit anderen Formen von Entwicklungsstörung. *Jahresberichte über die Kinderheilkunde und physische Erziehung, 64*, 465. 576–599.

Dieterle, T., & Eugster, J. (1934). Über den Verlauf der Kropfendemie in einigen Schweizer Dörfern nach 20 Jahren. *Archiv für Hygiene, 111*, 136.

Dieterle, T., Hirschfeld L., & Klinger, R. (1913). Epidemiologische Untersuchungen über den endemischen Kröpf. *Archiv für Hygiene, 81*, 128–178.

Dieterle, T., Hirschfeld L., & Klinger, R. (1913). Studien über den endemischen Kröpf. *Münchener medizinische Wochenschrift, 60*(33), 1813.

Diviak, R., & Wagner von Jauregg, J. (1918). Über die Entstehung des endemischen Kretinismus nach Beobachtungen in den ersten Lebensjahren. *Wiener klinische Wochenschrift, 31*(6), 149–62.

Doepfner, W. (1911). Beiträge zur Kenntnis des Meckelschen Divertikels. *Deutsche Zeitschrift für Chirurgie, 109*, 396.

Dubois, E. F. (1926). Vergleichende Untersuchungen über den biologischen Wert des Kretinenkropfes. *Mitteilungen aus den Grenzgebieten der Medizin und Chirurgie, 39*.

Dunn, J. T., Pretell, E.A., Daza, C.H., & Viteri, F.E. (Eds). (1986). Towards the eradication of endemic goiter, cretinism and iodine deficiency. *Pan American Health Organization Science Publication* No.502 (p. 373). Washington, D.C.

Eerland, L. D. (1932). Het Kropvragstuk in de residentie Kediri. Voordrachten over gezwellen: Bosscha-dag. *Geneeskundig Tijdschrift voor Nederlandsch–Indië, 72*, 1299–1302.

Eggenberger, H. (1928). Kröpf und Kretinismus. In M. Hirsch (Ed.) *Handbuch der inneren Sekretion* vol.3, 648. Leipzig: Kabitzsch.

Eggenberger, H. (1933). Die Jodmangeltheorie und ihre Erfolge. Second International Goitre Conference in Berne.

Eiselberg, A. F. von (1901). Die Erkrankungen der Schilddrüse. *Deutsche Zeitschrift für Chirurgie, 38*. Stuttgart: F. Enke.

Erdheim, J. (1904). 1. Über Schilddrüsenaplasie. 2. Geschwülste des Ductus thyreoglossus. 3. Über einige menschliche Kiemenderivate. *Beiträge zur pathologischen Anatomie und zur allgemeinen Pathologie, 35*, 366.

Eugster, J. (1934). Zur Erblichkeitsfrage der endemischen Struma, First Part. *Archiv der Julius Klaus-Stiftung für Vererbungsforschung, Sozialanthropologie und Rassenhygiene, 9*, 275.

Eugster, J. (1935). Zur Erblichkeitsfrage der endemischen Struma. Second Part. *Archiv der Julius Klaus-Stiftung für Vererbungsforschung, Sozialanthropologie und Rassenhygiene, 10*, 101.

Eugster, J. (1935). Neue Gesichtspunkte in der Prophylaxe gegen den endemischen Kröpf und Kretinismus. *Therapie der Gegenwart 3.*

Eulenburg, H. & Marfels, F. (1857). *Zur pathologischen Anatomie des Kretinismus*. Wetzlar: G. Rathgeber.

Ewald, C. A. (1896). Die Erkrankungen der Schilddrüse, Myxödem und Kretinismus. *Handbuch der speciellen Pathologie und Therapie, 22*(1). Vienna: Nothnagel.

Eysselt von Klimpely, A. (1910). Weitere Erfolge und Erfahrungen bei der Behandlung des endemischen Kretinismus mit Schilddrüsensubstanz. *Wiener medizinische Wochenschrift*, 7–14.

Fabre, J. P. A. (1857). *Traité du goitre et du cretinisme, et des rapports qui existent entre ces deux affections*. Paris.

Feldmann, E. (1927). Der endemische Kröpf der norddeutschen Tiefebene. *Bericht über die Internationale Kropfkonferenz in Bern 24–26 August 1927*. Berne: Verlag Hans Huber.

Ferrus, G. M. A. (1851). *Mémoire sur le Goitre et le Cretinisme*. Paris: Baillière.

Finkbeiner, E. (1918). Kretinismus im Noilengebiet. *Korrespondenzblatt für Schweizer Ärzte, 19/20.*

Finkbeiner, E. (1922). Kretinismus und endemische Ossifikationsstörungen. *Medizinische Klinik*

Finkbeiner, E. (1923). *Die kretinische Entartung*. Berlin: Julius Springer.

Finkbeiner, E. (1924). Neuere Gesichtspunkte in der Lehre vom Kretinismus. *Klinische Wochenschrift, 3*(13), 517–520.

Flinker, A. (1910). Über Kretinismus unter den Juden. *Wiener klinische Wochenschrift*, 1871.

Flinker, A. (1911). Über Körperproportionen der Kretinen. *Wiener klinische Wochenschrift, 6.*

Flinker, A. (1911). Zur Pathogenese des Kretinismus. *Wiener klinische Wochenschrift, 18.*

Flinker, A. (1911). Zur Frage der Kontaktinfektion des Kretinismus. *Wiener klinische Wochenschrift, 51.*

Flinker, A. (1930). *Studien über Kretinismus*. Leipzig & Vienna: Franz Deuticke.

Fodéré, F.-E. (1796). *Über den Kröpf und Kretinismus. Für Ärzte und Philosophen.* (trans. Lindemann). Berlin.

Folley, (1927). *Kröpfe und Infektionen*. International Goitre Conference, Berne.

Fonio, A. & Scheurer, G. (1931). Über die Wirkung des Thyroxins und des Jodes in einer dem Jodgehalt des Thyroxins entsprechenden Dosierung auf einige Abschnitte des Stoffwechsels, auf das Blut usw. bei endemischen Kretinen. *Mitteilungen aus den Grenzgebieten der Medizin und Chirurgie, 42*, 467.

Galli-Valerio, B. (1927). *L'étiologie et l'épidemiologie de l'endémie thyroïdienne*. International Goitre Conference. Berne.

Gamper, E. & Scharfetter, H. (1928). Das Myxödem und der endemische Kretinismus. *Bumkes Handbuch der Geisteskrankheiten, 10*. Berlin: Julius Springer.

Gautam, K. C. (2007). Global Progress in Addressing Iodine Deficiency through Universal Salt Iodization: The Makings of a Global Public Health Success Story — The Second Decade (1995–2007). *UN SCN News 35*, 12–18.

Gehri, G. (1930). Gibt es bei Schilddrüsenkranken ein pathognomonisch charakteristisches Capillarbild? *Schweizerische medizinische Wochenschrift.*

Getzowa, S. (1905). Über die Thyreoidea von Kretinen und Idioten. *Virchows Archiv für pathologische Anatomie und Physiologie und für klinische Medizin, 180*(1), 51–98.

Gilpin, A. (1934). Über die sogenannten Zellknospen in den Schilddrüsenarterien. *Virchows Archiv für pathologische Anatomie und Physiologie und für klinische Medizin, 293*(2), 257–271.

Gley, E. (1926). *Travaux du laboratoire de Collège de France*. vol. 1-10.

Gley, E. (1926). *Les grands problèmes de l'endocrinologie*. Paris.

Gley, E. (1929). La thyroïde, les progres de l'endocrinologie et la biologie générale. *Endokrinologie, 5.*

Goyanes, J. (1918). Sobre un foco de bocio y cretinismo endemico en los valles altos del Alberche y el Tormes, *El Siglo Médico, 65.*

Graham, A. (1916). A study of the physiological activity of adenomata of the thyroid gland, in relation to their iodine content, äs evidenced by feeding experiments on tadpoles. *Journal of Experimental Medicine, 24*(4), 345–359.

Grundler, & Nauwerck, (1884). Zur Kachexia strumipriva. *Bruns Beiträge zur klinischen Chirurgie, 1.*

Guggenbühl, J. J. (1853). Die Kretinenheilanstalt auf dem Abendberg. Berne and St. Gallen.

Guggisberg, H. (1925). Die Struma des Neugeborenen. *Zeitschrift für menschliche Vererbungs- und Konstitutionslehre, 11*, 280.

Gull, W. W. (1873). On a cretinoid state supervening in adult life in women. *Transactions of the Clinical Society of London. 7*, 180–185.

H'Doubler, F. T. (1922). Über den respiratorischen Gaswechsel bei der Struma vasculosa im Kindesalter und nach Implantation von Kropfgewebe bei Kretinen. *Schweizerische medizinische Wochenschrift, 52,* 926.

Habermann, J. (1904). Zur Lehre der Ohrenerkrankungen infolge von Kretinismus. *European Archives of Oto-Rhino-Laryngology, 63*(1–2), 100–112. doi: 10.1007/BF01834433

Habermann, J. (1909). Zur Lehre der Ohrenerkrankungen infolge von Kretinismus. *European Archives of Oto-Rhino-Laryngology, 79*(1–2), 23–42. doi: 10.1007/BF01962711

Haller, A. von (1772). Abhandlung über den Roche-Wind. *Sammlung kleiner Hallerischer Schriften* Third Part. Berne.

Hammar, J. A. (1929). Die Menschenthymus in Gesundheit und Krankheit, Part II. Das Organ unter anormalen Haltnissen. *Zeitschrift für mikroskopische-anatomische Zellforschung. Suppl.16.*

Hanau. (1891). Demonstration mikroskopischer Präparate von Atrophie der Schilddrüse bei Kretinismus, nebst Bemerkungen über das Verhältnis von Kretinismus zum Myxödem. *Proceedings of the Tenth International Medical Congress*. Berlin.

Hansemann, D. von (1908). Demonstration eines kretinischen Schakals. *Berliner klinische Wochenschrift 2,* 2005.

Hara, Y. (1923). Untersuchungen über die pathologische Physiologie des Kropfes mittelst der Asherschen Methode der Empfindlichkeit der Ratte gegen Sauerstoffmangel. *Mitteilungen aus den Grenzgebieten der Medizin und Chirurgie, 36,* 537.

Haumann, W. (1927). Osteopathia cretinosa scapulae nebst einem Beitrag zum Humerus varus cretinosus. *Bruns Beiträge zur klinischen Chirurgie, 140,* 136.

Hercus, C. E., Benson, W. N., & Carter C. L. (1925). Endemic goitre in New Zealand and its relation to the soil-iodine. *Journal of Hygiene, 24,* 321–330.

Hetzel, B. S. (1983). Iodine Deficiency Disorders (IDD) and their eradication. *The Lancet, 2,* 1126–1129.

Hetzel, B. S. (1989). *The story of iodine deficiency, an international challenge in nutrition* (pp. 36–51). New Delhi: Oxford University Press.

Hetzel, B. S. (2002). Eliminating iodine deficiency disorders — the role of the International Council in the global partnership. Round Table Discussion. *Bulletin of the World Health Organization, 80*(5), 410–417.

Hetzel, B. S. (2007). Global Progress in Addressing Iodine Deficiency through USI: The Makings of a Global Public Health Success Story —The First Decade (1985–1995). *UN SCN News 35,* 5–11.

Hetzel, B. S., & Mano, M. (1989). A Review of experimental studies of iodine deficiency during foetal development. *The Journal of Nutrition, 119,* 145–151.

Hetzel, B. S., Delange, F., Dunn, J., Ling, J., Mannar, V., & Pandav, C. (Eds). (2004). *Towards the global elimination of brain damage due to iodine deficiency*. New Delhi: Oxford University Press.

Heyn, F. (1906). Ein Beitrag zur Lehre vom Myxödem. *Archiv für Psychiatrie, 41,* 49.

Hintzsche, E. (1931). Untersuchungen an Stützgeweben III. Über Umbildungen im jungen menschlichen Hyalinknorpel. *Zeitschrift für mikroskopische-anatomische Forschung, 25,* 320–361.

Hirsch, A. (1883). *Handbuch der historisch-geographischen Pathologie*, vol. 2. Stuttgart: F Encke.

Hirschfelder, (1935). *Das Hand- und Knieskelet von Kretinen und Athyreoten im Röntgenbild.* Berne: Dissertation.

His, W. (1861). Zur Kasuistik des Kretinismus. *Virchows Archiv für pathologische Anatomie und Physiologie und für klinische Medizin, 22.*

Hitzig, T. (1894). Beiträge zur Histologie und Histogenese der Struma. *Archiv für klinische Chirurgie, 47,* 464.

Hoepfner, R. (1932). Prophylaktische Absichten bei Schilddrüsenstörungen. *Psychiatriatrische -neurologische Wochenschrift.*

Höjer, J. A. (1929). Untersuchungen über den endemischen Kröpf in Schweden. *Zeitschrift für Hygiene, 110,* 239–255.

Höjer, J. A. (1931). Kropfstudien V. Die Verbreitung des endemischen Kropfes in Schweden. *Svenska Läkarsällskapets Handlingar, 57*, 1–104.
Horsley, V. A. H. (1891). Die Funktion der Schilddrüse. Festschrift zu Virchows 70. Geburtstag. *Internat. Beiträge zur wissenschaftlichen Medizin.*
Hotz, G. (1921). Zur Kropffrage. *Schweizerische medizinische Wochenschrift, 51*, 1153–1155.
Hotz, G. (1922). Über endemische Struma, Kretinismus und ihre Prophylaxe. *Klinische Wochenschrift, 1*(42), 136.
Houda, E. O. (1932). The etiology of endemic goiter. *Journal of Clinical Medicine and Surgery, 39.*
Hunziker-Shild, H. (1915). *Der Kröpf, eine Anpassung an jodarme Nahrung.* Berne: Verlag A. Franke.
Hunziker-Shild, H. (1918). Vom Kröpf in der Schweiz. *Korrespondenzblätter für Schweizer Ärzte, 48*, 220–235. 247–261.
Hunziker-Shild, H. (1924). *Die Prophylaxe der großen Schilddrüse.* Berne & Leipzig: E. Bircher.
Iphofen, A. (1817). *Der Kretinismus.* Dresden.
Isenschmidt, R. (1910). Zur Kenntnis der menschlichen Schilddrüse im Kindesalter. *Frankfurter Zeitschrift für Pathologie, 5*, 205.
Isenschmidt, R. (1919). Histologische Veränderungen im Zentralnervensystem bei Schilddrüsenmangel. *Frankfurter Zeitschrift für Pathologie, 21*, 321–336.
Jackson, A. S. (1926). *Goiter and Other Diseases of the Thyroid Gland.* New York: P.B. Hoeber Inc.
Jackson, A. S. (1934). Cretinism in the United States. *Transactions of the American Association for the Study of Goiter.* Cleveland
Jacobi, M. (1933). Beitrag zur Kenntnis eines angeblichen Kropferregers. *Schweizerische medizinische Wochenschrift, 63*(32), 784.
Jadassohn, J. (1906). *Verhandlung des deutschen dermatologischen Gesellschaft, 9*, 451.
Jaensch, W. (1930). Die Hautcapillarmikroskopie am Lebenden. *Handbuch der biologischen Arbeitsmethoden, 9.* Berlin: Urban & Schwartzenburg pp. 866–940.
Jaensch, W., & Gundermann, O. (1934). Klinische Rassenhygiene und Eugenik. *Veröffentlichungen aus dem Gebiete der Medizinalverwaltung, 43*(l).
Josselin de Jong de, R. (1925). Über Kröpf in den Niederlanden. *Beiträge zur pathologischen Anatomie und zur allgemeinen Pathologie, 73.*
Justus, (1913). *Beitrag zu dem Vorkommen und die geographische Verbreitung des Kropfes in der Provinz Ostpreußen.* Inaugural Dissertation. Königsberg.
Kaufmann, E. (1931). Probleme der Schilddrüsenpathologie. Festrede 1912. *Lehrbuch der speziellen pathologischen Anatomie,* l. Berlin & Leipzig: G. Reimer.
Kerzmann, (1921). *Vergleichende Untersuchungen über die Häufigkeit des Kropfes im Kindesalter im Neuenburger Jura und in der Stadt Bern.* Inaugural Dissertation. Berne.
Kind, E. (1918). Blutbefunde bei endemischem Kretinismus. *Mitteilungen aus den Grenzgebieten der Medizin und Chirurgie, 30.*
Klar, R. (1914). Demonstrationen. Arthropathia deformans coxae juvenilis. *Münchener medizinische Wochenschrift, 11*,1589.
Klebs, E. (1874). Beobachtungen und Versuche über Kretinismus. *Archiv für experimentelle Pathologie 2.*
Klebs, E. (1876). Zur Verbreitung des Kretinismus in Böhmen. *Prague medizinische Wochenschrift*
Klebs, E. (1877). *Studien über die Verbreitung des Kretinismus in Österreich, sowie über die Ursache der Kröpfbildung.* Prague.
Klose, H., & Hellwig, A. (1923). Bau und Funktion der kindlichen Schilddrüsenhyperplasie. *Archiv für klinische Chirurgie, 124*, 347.
Knaggs, R. L. (1928). Cretinism. *The British Journal of Surgery, 16*, 370–400.
Kocher, T. (1883). Über Kropfexstirpation und ihre Folgen. *Archiv für klinische Chirurgie, 29*, 254–337.
Kocher, T. (1889). Vorkommen und Verteilung des Kropfes im Kanton Bern. *Archiv für klinische Chirurgie, 29.*

Kocher, T. (1892). Zur Verhütung des Kretinismus und kretinoiden Zuständen nach neuen Forschungen. *Deutsche Zeitschrift für Chirurgie, 34*, 556–626.
Kocher, T. (1908). Über Schilddrüsentransplantation. *Archiv für klinische Chirurgie, 87*, 1.
Kocher, T. (1912). Das Blutbild bei Cachexia thyreopriva (Myxödem, kretinoide Zustände). *Archiv für klinische Chirurgie, 99*, 280.
Kocher, T. (1914). Über die Bedingungen erfolgreicher Schilddrüsentransplantation beim Menschen. *Archiv für klinische Chirurgie, 105*, 832.
Korownikow (1932). Zur Charakteristik des endemischen Kretinismus in Pamir. *Archiv für innere Medizin, 22*.
Köstl, F. (1856). *Der endemische Kretinismus als Gegenstand der öffentlichen Fürsorge*. Memoir in honour of the Minister of the Interior. Vienna: Government Printer.
Kottmann, K. (1920). Kolloidchemische Untersuchungen über Schilddrüsenprobleme. *Schweizerische medizinische Wochenschrift, 50*(30), 644.
Krämer, C. (1910). *Über die Rückbildungsvorgänge in den Schilddrüsenadenomen (Struma nodosa)*. Dissertation, Freiburg im Breslau
Kranz, P. (1914). Innere Sekretion in Beziehung zur Kieferbildung und Zahnentwicklung. *Deutsche Zahnheilkunde in Vorträgen, 32*, 1–104.
Kraus, E. (1916). Zur Kenntnis der Übergangszeiten des menschlichen Gehirnanhangs mit besonderer Berücksichtigung der Befunde bei der progressiven Paralyse. *Beiträge zur pathologischen Anatomie und zur allgemeinen Pathologie, 62*.
Kraus, R. (1919). El problema de la etiologia y patogenia del bocio endémico y del cretinismo. *Revista del Instituto de Bacteriologia* Buenos Aires. (Cited, 1921, *Zentralblatt für allgemeine Pathologie und pathologische Anatomie, 31*(9).
Kraus, E. (1929). Zur Frage der Funktion endokriner Organe in der Foetalzeit. *Endokrinologie, 5*, 133–137.
Kraus, R., Rosenbusch, F., & Maggio, C. (1917). Kröpf, Kretinismus und die Krankheit von Chagas. *Wiener klinische Wochenschrift, 35*(28), 942–45.
Kurz, H. (1927). Über die Refraktion bei Schwachsinnigen. Ein weiterer Beitrag zur Refraktionsfrage. *Graefe's Archive for Clinical and Experimental Ophthalmology, 118*, 500.
Kutschera, A. von (1909). Das Größenwachstum bei Schilddrüsenbehandlung des endemischen Kretinismus. *Wiener klinische Wochenschrift, 22*, 771.
Kutschera, A. von (1910). Die Übertragung des Kretinismus vom Menschen auf das Tier. *Wiener klinische Wochenschrift, 8*, 1593.
Kutschera, A. von (1911). *Der endemische Kretinismus, seine Ursachen und seine Behandlung*. Vienna: Alfred Holder.
Kutschera, A. von (1912). Zur Frage der Kontaktinfektion des Kretinismus. *Wiener klinische Wochenschrift*, 1764.
Kutschera, A. von (1913). Gegen die Wasser — ätiologie des Kropfes und des Kretinismus. *Münchener medizinische Wochenschrift.*
Kutschera, A. von (1914). Ätiologie des Kropfes und des Kretinismus. *Prague medizinische Wochenschrift.*
Kutschera, A. von (1926). Kröpf und Kretinismus, endemische Dystrophie. *Wiener klinische Wochenschrift.*
Kux, E. (1935). Drosselvorrichtungen (Zellknospen, Polster) in den Arterien der Schilddrüse. *Virchows Archiv für Pathologische Anatomie und Physiologie und für klinische Medizin, 294*, 358–364.
Lang, T. (1922). Mikroskopische Befunde bei juveniler Arthritis deformans nebst vergleichenden Untersuchungen über- die Femurkopfepiphyse mit besonderer Berücksichtigung der Fovea. *Virchows Archiv für Pathologische Anatomie und Physiologie und für Klinische Medizin, 239*, 76–144.
Lang, T. (1932). Ergebnisse einer ersten Messungsserie zur Frage des Zusammenhanges zwischen Radioaktivität und Kröpf. *Zeitschrift für die gesamte Neurologie und Psychiatrie, 141*.
Lang, T. (1933). Ergebnisse einer zweiten Messungsserie zur Frage des Zusammenhanges zwischen Radioaktivität und Kröpf. *Zeitschrift für die gesamte Neurologie und Psychiatrie, 144*.

Lang, T. (1934). Versuche zur experimentellen Erzeugung des endemischen Kropfes bei weißen Ratten. *Zeitschrift für experimentelle Medizin, 95*(1), 378–396.

Lang, T. (1934). Ergebnisse einer dritten Messungserie zur Frage des Zusammenhanges zwischen Radioaktivität und Kröpf. *Zeitschrift für die gesamte Neurologie und Psychiatrie, 149.*

Lang, T. (1935). Ergebnisse einer vierten Messungserie zur Frage des Zusammenhanges zwischen Radioaktivität und Kröpf. *Zeitschrift für die gesamte Neurologie und Psychiatrie, 152*(1), 107–125.

Langhans, T. (1892). Über Veränderungen in den peripheren Nerven bei Cachexia strumipriva des Menschen und Affen, sowie bei Kretinen. *Virchows Archiv für Pathologische Anatomie und Physiologie und für klinische Medizin, 128.*

Langhans, T. (1897). Anatomische Beiträge zur Kenntnis der Kretinen. *Virchows Archiv für Pathologische Anatomie und Physiologie und für klinische Medizin, 149*, 155–187.

Lanz, O. (1899). Ein Vorschlag zur diätetischen Behandlung Basedowkranker. *Korrespondenzblätter für Schweizer Ärzte 23.*

Larson, J. A. (1920). Further evidence on the functional correlation of the hypophysis and the thyroid. *The American Journal of Physiology, 53*(1), 89–100.

Lauener, P. Ein Beitrag zur Begründung der Notwendigkeit einer planmäßigen Kröpfbekämpfung (unpublished).

Lauterburg, W. (1930). Über Insulinshock beim Kretin. *Mitteilungen aus den Grenzgebieten der Medizin und Chirurgie, 41*, 715.

Läwen, A. (1910). Zur Kenntnis der Wachstumsstörungen am Kretinenskelett. *Deutsche Zeitschrift für Chirurgie, 101*, 454–466.

Leichtenstern, O. (1894). Über Myxödem und Entfettungskuren mit Schilddrusenfütterung. *Deutsche medizinische Wochenschrift, 50.*

Lendvay, B. (1887). *Der Kretinismus auf der Insel Schutt.* Preßburg: Translated by Wartner.

Lenz, F. (1927). *Menschliche Erblichkeitslehre*, 3 rd edition. Munich.

Levin, H. M., Pollitt, E., Galloway, R., & McGuire, J. (1994). In *Enriching lives: overcoming vitamin and mineral malnutrition in developing countries*. Washington D.C.: The World Bank.

Lombroso, C. (1859). Ricerche sul cretinismo in Lombardia. *Gazzetta medica lombarda.*

Looser, E. (1929). Über die Ossifikationsstörungen bei Kretinismus. *Verhandlungen der Deutschen Gesellschaft für Pathologie, 24*, 352–360.

Looser, E. (1929). Die Kretinenhüfte. *Schweizerische medizinische Wochenschrift, 10*, 1258.

Lotmar, F. (1929). Histopathologische Befunde in Gehirnen von kongenitalem Myxödem (Thyreoaplasie). *Zeitschrift für die gesamte Neurologie und Psychiatrie, 119*, 491–513.

Lotmar, F. (1931). Entwicklungsstörungen in der Kleinhirnrinde beim endemischen Kretinismus. *Zeitschrift für die gesamte Neurologie und Psychiatrie, 136*(1), 412–435.

Lotmar, F. (1933). Histopathologische Befunde in Gehirnen von endemischem Kretinismus, Thyreoaplasie und Kachexia thyreopriva. *Zeitschrift für die gesamte Neurologie und Psychiatrie, 146*(1), 1–53.

Luchsinger, (1932). Die Verwertung der Capillarmikroskopie in der Otologie. *Schweizerische medizinische Wochenschrift, 189.*

Ma, T., Wang, Y. Y., Wang, D., Chen, Z. P., & Chi, S.P. (1989). Neuropsychological studies in iodine deficiency areas in China. In G. R. DeLong, J. Robbins, & P. G. Condliffe (Eds) *Iodine and the Brain*, (pp. 259–268). New York: Plenum Press.

Maffei, K. (1844). *Der Kretinismus in den norischen Alpen*. Erlangen.

Malacarne, V. (1789). *Sui gozzi e sulla stupidità che in alcuni paesi gli accompagna.* Turin 1789. (Cited by Scholz).

Manasse, P. (1909). Über kongenitale Taubstummheit und Struma. *Zeitschrift für Ohrenheilkunde und Krankheiten der Luftwege, 58*, 105–128.

Marañon, G. (1927). *El bocio y el cretinismo.* Madrid: Editorial Paez.

Marchand (1906). Über einen Fall von sporadischem Kretinismus und Myxödem mit fast totaler Aplasie der Schilddrüse. *Münchener medizinische Wochenschrift, 17*, 1440–1441.

Maresch, R. (1898). Kongenitaler Defekt der Schilddrüse bei einem 11-jährigen Mädchen. *Zeitschrift für Heilkunde, 19.*

Marimon, J. (1915). *Estudio quirúrgico del bocio*. Madrid.

Marine, D., & Kimball, O. P. (1917). The prevention of simple goiter in man. *Journal of Laboratory and Clinical Medicine, 3*, 40–48.

Marine, D., & Lenhart, C. H. (1923). Prevention and treatment of simple goiter. *Atlantic Medical Journal, 26*(3), 437–443.

Marthe (1873). *Quelques recherches sur le developpement du goïtre*. Inaugural Dissertation, Berne.

Mathez, C.-O. (1930). Contribution à l'étude du crétinisme et de l'épilepsie. *Schweizerische medizinische Wochenschrift*.

Mayer, O. (1910). Beiträge zur Kenntnis der endemischen Schwerhörigkeit und Taubstummheit. *Archiv für Ohrenheilkunde*, *83*.

McCallum, W. G., & Fabyan, M. (1907). On the anatomy of a myxoedematous idiot. *Johns Hopkins Hospital Bulletin, 18*, 341–345.

McCarrison, R. (1908). Observations on endemic cretinism in the Chitral and Gilgit valleys. *The Lancet, 2*, 1275–80.

McCarrison, R. (1913). *The Etiology of Endemic Goitre*. London: Bale.

McCarrison, R. (1914). Experimental researches on the etiology of endemic cretinism, congenital goitre and congenital parathyroid disease. *Indian Journal of Medical Research, 1*, 505–522.

McCarrison, R. (1914). Etiology of endemic cretinism, congenital goitre and congenital parathyroid diseases. *Lancet, 1*, 817–819.

McCarrison, R. (1917). *The Thyroid Gland in Health and Disease*. London: Baillière, Tindall & Cox.

McClendon, J. F. (1927). The distribution of iodine with special reference to goiter. *Physiological Reviews, 7*(2), 189–259.

Mendel, E. (1893). Ein Fall von Myxödem. *Deutsche medizinische Wochenschrift, 19*(2), 25–26. doi: 10.1055/s-0029-1205322

Mendel, E. (1895). Drei Fälle von geheiltem Myxödem. *Deutsche medizinische Wochenschrift, 21*(7), 101–103. doi: 10.1055/s-0029-1199666.

Meyer, M. (1933). Über einige für die Pathologie der Erkrankungen des Skeletsystems interessante Beobachtungen an der knöchernen Innenohrkapsel des Menschen. *Virchows Archiv für Pathologische Anatomie und Physiologie und für Klinische Medizin, 288*(1), 1–35.

Meyer-Ahrens, C. (1854). Die Verbreitung des Kretinismus in der Schweiz. *Schweizerischen Zeitschrift für Medizin, Chirurgie und Geburtshilfe, 1853*(4) & *1854*(1 & 2).

Meyerhofer, B. (1914). Kretinismus und Gebiß. *Ergebnisse der Zahnheilkunde, 4*(2), 144.

Michaud, L. (1906). Die Histogenese der Struma nodosa. *Virchows Archiv für Pathologische Anatomie und Physiologie und für Klinische Medizin, 186*(3), 422–477.

Miller, A. C. (1893). Case of myxoedema cured by iodine feeding. *Edinburgh Medical Journal, 39*.

Moebius, P. J. (1906). *Die Basedow'sche Krankheit*. Vienna: A. Holder.

Morel, B. A. (1864). Du goïtre et du crétinisme, étiologie, prophylaxie, traitement. *Archives de médecine générale*.

Muggia, G. (1929). L'endemia strumosa in Valtellina e l'opera di quel Comitato Provinciale per la lotta contro il gozzo. *Scritti biologici, 5*, 1–59.

Muggia, G. (1933). La tiroide in Valtellina otto anni dopo l'introduzione del sale jodurato. *Rassegna di studi psichiatrici, 22*.

Müller, B. (1913). Das Verhalten der Glandula thyreoideä im endemischen Kropfgebiet des Kantons Bern zu Schwangerschaft, Geburt und Wochenbett. *Zeitschrift für Geburtshilfe, 75*.

Müller, O. (1922). *Die Capillaren der menschlichen Körperoberfläche in gesunden und kranken Tagen*. Stuttgart: F. Enke.

Müller, P. (1880). Zur Frequenz und Ätiologie des allgemein verengten Beckens. *Archiv für Gynäkologie, 16*(2),155–173.

Murray, G. R. (1900). *Diseases of the thyroid gland*. London: H.K. Lewis.

Nager, F. R. (1921). Weitere Beiträge zur Anatomie der endemischen Hörstörung. *Zeitschrift für Ohrenheilkunde, 80*, 107–174.

Nager, F. R. (1934). Demonstration über die normale und pathologische Anatomie der Labyrinthkapsel. *Schweizerische medizinische Wochenschrift,154.*

Nager, F. R., & Meyer, M. (1932). *Die Erkrankungen des Knochensystems und ihre Erscheinungen an der Innenohrkapsel des Menschen.* Berlin: S. Karger.

Niderberger (1924). Das weiße Blutbild bei den verschiedenen funktionellen Zuständen der Schilddrüse. *Schweizerische medizinische Wochenschrift.*

Nièpce, B. (1851). *Traité du goïtre et du crétinisme.* Paris: J. B. Baillière.

Oldekop, M. P. (1858). Einiges über die Verbreitung des Kropfes in Rußland. *Medizinische Zeitung Rußlands, N° 8,* St. Petersburg (cited by Hirsch).

Oppikofer, E. (1921). Eine dem Kretinismus eigentümliche Veränderung im inneren Ohr. *Monatsschrift für Ohrenheilkunde und Laryngo-Rhinologie, 55,* 1519–1529.

Ottonello, P. (1925). Studio clinico ambientale di un focolaio di gozzo endemico in Sardegna. *Rassegna di Studi psichiatrici, 14.* (Cited by Gamper and Scharfetter).

Ottonello, P. (1927). Nuove indagini sulla distribuzione della endemia gozzigena in Sardegna. *Rivista di Patologia nervosa e mentale, 32.* (Cited by Gamper and Scharfetter).

Pandav, C. S., & Rao, A. R. (1977). *IDD in livestock: ecology and economics,* New Delhi: Oxford University Press.

Parhon, C. I., & Goldstein, M. (1925). *Traité d'endocrinologie. La glande thyroïde.* Jassy: Editura Viata Rominessca.

Pennacchietti, M. (1932). Osservazioni anatomopatologiche e patogenetiche su due casi di atiroidia congenita. *Archivio italiano di anatomia e istologia patologica, 3.*

Pereschiwkin. (1935). Der endemische Kröpf im Wanschtal. *Praxis, N° 6.*

Peucker. M. U. C. H. (1899). Über einen neuen Fall von kongenitalem Defekt der Schilddrüse mit vorhandenen Epithelkörperchen. *Zeitschrift für Heilkunde, 20,* 341–355.

Pfannenstiel, P. (1985). Direct and indirect costs caused by continuous iodine deficiency. In R. Hall, & J. Kobberling (Eds). *Thyroid disorders associated with iodine deficiency excess* (p. 447). New York: Raven Press.

Pfister, C. R. (1927). Statistische Beiträge zur Kropffrage. *Schweizerische medizinische Wochenschrift.*

Pfaundler, M. von (1924). Über die Entstehungsbedingungen von endemischem Kröpf und Kretinismus. *Jahresberichte über die Kinderheilkunde und physische Erziehung, 55,* 223.

Pharoah, P. O. D., Buttfield, I.H., & Hetzel, B. S. (1971). Neurological damage to the fetus resulting from severe iodine deficiency during pregnancy. *The Lancet, 1,* 308–310.

Pharoah, P. O. D., Delange, F., Fierro-Benitez, R., & Stanbury, J. B. (1980). In J. B. Stanbury & B. S. Hetzel (Eds) *Endemic goitre and endemic cretinism* (pp. 395–451). New York: Wiley.

Pick, E.P., & Pineles, F. (1910). Untersuchungen über die physiologisch wirksame Substanz der Schilddrüse. *Zeitschrift für experimentalische Pathologie und Therapie, 7,* 518–531.

Pighini, G. (1926). Ricerche sperimentali sulla tiroide in relazione älla etiologia del gozzo.-cretinismo. *Rivista sperimentale di freniatria e medicina legale delle alienazioni mentali, 50.*

Pineles, F. (1902). Ueber Thyreoaplasie und infantiles Myxoedem. *Wiener klinische Wochenschrift, 15,* 1129.

Pineles, F. (1904). Klinische und experimentelle Beiträge zur Physiologie der Schilddrüse und der Epithelkörperchen. *Mitteilungen aus den Grenzgebieten der Medizin und Chirurgie, 14.*

Quervain, F. de (1924). Crétinisme, Etats hypothyroïdiens et Système nerveux. *Schweizer Archiv für Neurologie und Psychiatrie, 14.*

Quervain, F. de (1924). Ist der Kretinismus ein anthropologisches Rückschlagsphänomen? *Die Naturwissenschaften, 13*(14), 277–284.

Quervain, F. de (1927). Die pathologische Physiologie der endemischen Thyreopathie. First International Goitre Conference. Berne: Hans Huber.

Quervain, F. de (1928). Über das Wesen der sog. Osteochondritis juvenilis des Hüftgelenks. *Schweizerische medizinische Wochenschrift, 1.*

Quervain, F. de, & Smith, W. E. (1928). The iodine content of blood in ordinary goiters and in cretinism. *Endocrinology, 28,* 177–189.

Quervain, F. de (1924). *Le Goitre.* Geneva: Atar; Paris: A. Maloine.

Quervain, F. de (1926). Rück- und Ausblicke in der Schilddrüsenpathologie. *Mitteilungen aus den Grenzgebieten der Medizin und Chirurgie, 39.*

Quervain, F. de (1935). Zur Begriffsbestimmung der endemischen Thyreopathie. *Schweizerische medizinische Wochenschrift, 1.*

Quervain, F. de (1935). Die wissenschaftlichen Grundlagen der Kropfprophylaxe. *Schweizerische medizinische Wochenschrift, 2.*

Quervain, F. de, & Abelin, I. (1932). Die experimentelle Prüfung der Schilddrüsenfunktion. In (E. Äberhaldin) *Handbuch der biologischen Arbeitsmethoden, Abt. VIII, Bd. l.* Berlin and Vienna: Urban & Schwartzenberg.

Quincke, H. (1900). Über Athyreosis im Kindesalter. *Deutsche medizinische Wochenschrift, 2,* 49–50, 805–807.

Reich (1923). Zur Klinik und Ätiologie der Perthes-Calvé-Leggschen Krankheit (Osteochondritis deformans juvenilis). *Schweizerische medizinische Wochenschrift, 2.*

Reverdin J., & Reverdin, A. (1883). Note sur 22 operations de goitre. *Revue médicale de la Suisse romande, 3,* 169–198.

Rieger, C. Beziehung zwischen Hirngewicht und Körpergröße. (Cited by Rössle and Roulet, p. 91).

Riquier, C. M. (1926). Un focolaio di gozzo-cretinismo individuate in Sardegna. Pavia, Relazione alla Direzione Generale, della Sanità Pubblica. (Cited by Gamper and Scharfetter).

Rocaz, C.-H.-F., & Cruchet, R. (1903). Myxoedème congénital. *Archives de Médicine des Enfants, 6,* 97.

Rogowitsch, N. (1889). Die Veränderungen der Hypophyse nach Entfernung der Schilddrüse. *Beiträge zur pathologischen Anatomie und zur allgemeinen Pathologie, 4,* 453–470.

Rösch, L. (1844). Untersuchungen über den Kretinismus in Württemberg. In Maffei K., & Rösch, L. (Eds), *Neue Untersuchungen über den Kretinismus oder die Entartung des Menschen in ihren verschiedenen Graden und Formen.* Erlangen.

Rössle, R. (1920). Über Myxödem bei totaler Thyreoaplasie. *Korrespondenzblatt der ärztlichen Vereins von Thüringen.* Jena, Sitzungsbericht der medizinischen. Gesellschaft, 4 Nov.

Rössle, R., & Roulet, F. (1932). Maß und Zahl in der Pathologie. *Pathologie und Klinik in Einzeldarstellungen* vol. 5. Berlin and Vienna: Julius Springer.

Roth, M. (1918). Coxitis deformans juvenilis. *Korrespondenzblatt der Schweizerischen Ärzte, 28,* 951.

Rüdin, E. (1932). Über Ursachen des endemischen Kropfes und Kretinismus. *Münchener medizinische Wochenschrift,* 1, 988–993.

Rupilius, K. (1934). Verschiedene Schwachsinnsformen mit besonderer Berücksichtigung des Kretinismus in Steiermark. *Wiener klinische Wochenschrift 2,* 1060.

Sägesser. M. (1933). Die Schutzfunktion des Organismus bei Thyreopathie. *Klinische Wochenschrift, 12*(17), 672.

Sägesser. M. (1932). Die Jonenverhältnisse beim Kröpf. *Mitteilungen aus den Grenzgebieten der Medizin und Chirurgie, 43.*

Sägesser. M. (1932). Jodfraktionen des Kropfes und funktionelle Wertigkeit. *Mitteilungen aus den Grenzgebieten der Medizin und Chirurgie, 43.*

Sägesser. M. (1932). Mineralstoffalkalität und Jodgehalt von Kropfgeweben. *Biochemische Zeitschrift, 254.*

Saint-Lager, J. (1867). *Études sur les causes du cretinisme et du goïtre endémique.* Paris: Bailliére.

Salvioni, C. (1898). Appunti etimologici e lessicali. *Zeitschrift für romanische Philologie, 23,* 514–532.

Sanderson-Damburg, E. (1911). Die Schilddrüsen vom 15.—25. Lebensjahr aus der norddeutschen Ebene und Küstengegend sowie aus Bern. *Frankfurter Zeitschrift für Pathologie, 6,* 312–334.

Sardinian Commission. (1848). *Rapport de la commission créé par S. M. le roi de Sardaigne pour étudier le cretinisme.* Turin.

Sattler, H. (1909). Basedow'sche Krankheit. In *Handbuch der Augenheilkunde von Graefe-Saemisch,* 2nd. ed., vol. 9, p.13). Leipzig: W. Engelmann.

Scabell, A. (1928). Zur Pathogenese der Osteochondritis dissecans bei endemischem Kretinismus. *Schweizerische medizinische Wochenschrift, 2.*

Schaer, H. (1928). Vergleichende Untersuchungen an Schilddrüsen zwischen dem 25. und 50. Lebensjahr. *Frankfurter Zeitschrift für Pathologie, 36*, 249–274.

Schenkel, K. (1931). Untersuchungen am Gebiß von Allgäuer Vollkretinen unter besonderer Berücksichtigung der Cariesfrage. *Zeitschrift für Konstitutionslehre, 16.*

Schiffner, K. T. Regelwidrigkeiten der Nerven bei Kretinen. *Medizinische Jahresberichte der österreichen Staat, 4*, 6. (Cited by Scholz).

Schilder, P. (1911). Über Mißbildungen der Schilddrüse. *Virchows Archiv für pathologische Anatomie und Physiologie und für klinische Medizin, 205*, 246.

Schilf, D. (1922). Die quantitativen Beziehungen der Nebennieren zum übrigen Körper. *Zeitschrift für Konstitutionslehre, 8*, 507.

Schlagenhaufer, F., & Wagner von Jauregg, J. (1910). *Beiträge zur Ätiologie und Pathologie des endemischen Kretinismus*. Leipzig & Vienna: Franz Deuticke.

Schlittler, E. (1917). Angeborene Taubstummheit mit negativem Befund im inneren Ohr. *Zeitschrift für Ohrenheilkunde und für Krankheiten der Luftweg, 75*, 309–323.

Schmidt, M. B. (1894). Über Zellknospen in den Arterien der Schilddrüse. *Virchows Archiv für pathologische Anatomie und Physiologie und für klinische Medizin, 137*, 330–347.

Scholz, W. (1906). *Klinische und anatomische Untersuchungen über den Kretinismus*. Berlin: Hirschwald.

Scholz, W. (1919). Kretinismus. In F. Kraus & T. Brugsch (Eds), *Spezielle Pathologie und Therapie innerer Krankheiten, 1*, 477. Berlin: Urban & Schwarzenburg.

Scholz, W., & Zingerle, H. (1906). Beitrag zur pathologischen Anatomie der Kretinengehirne. *Zeitschrift für Heilkunde, 27*, 97–111.

Scholz, W., & Zingerle, H. (1909). Über Gehirnveränderungen bei Kretinismus. *Zeitschrift für jugendliche Schwachsinn, 3.*

Schultz, A. (1921). Über einen Fall von Athyreosis congenita (Myxödem) mit besonderer Berücksichtigung der dabei beobachteten Muskel Veränderungen. *Virchows Archiv für pathologische Anatomie und Physiologie und für klinische Medizin, 232*, 302.

Schultze, W. H. (1914). Tödliche Menorrhagie in einem Falle von Thyreoaplasie mit Hauptzellenadenom der Hypophyse. *Virchows Archiv für pathologische Anatomie und Physiologie und für klinische Medizin, 216*(3), 443–452. doi: 10.1007/BF01993879

Schulze, W. (1924). Weitere Untersuchungen über die Wirkung inkretorischer Drüsensubstanzen auf die Morphologie. III. Über die Sprengung der Harmonie der Entwicklung. *Archiv für mikroskopische Anatomie und Entwicklungsmechanik, 101*, 338–381.

Schwalber, L. (1931). Untersuchungen über Herkunft der Vorfahren und Häufigkeit von Verwandtenehen in den Familien von Allgäuer Kretinen. *Zeitschrift für die gesamte Neurologie und Psychiatrie, 132*(1), 227–234. doi: 10.1007/BF02863846

Seemen, H. von (1928). Osteochondropathia cretinoidea (Osteoarthrosis hypothyreotica). *Langenbecks Archiv für klinische Chirurgie, 152*, 616–630.

Shein, B. (1933). Das Verhalten der Senkung der roten Blutkörperchen bei Funktionsstörungen der Schilddrüse. *Schweizerische medizinische Wochenschrift, 63*(21).

Siebenmann, F. (1906). Über die Funktion und die mikroskopische Anatomie des Gehörorgans bei totaler Aplasie der Schilddrüse. *Archiv für Ohren-, Nasen- und Kehlkopfheilkunde, 70*, 83–89.

Siebenthal, K. von (1921). *Über einen Fall von Thyreoaplasie (congenitales Myxödem).* Inaugural Dissertation, Zürich.

Siegert, F. (1901). Zur Pathologie der infantilen Myxidiotie und des sporadischen Kretinismus oder infantilen Myxödems der Autoren. *Jahrbuch für Kinderheilkunde und physische Erziehung, 53.*

Siegert, F. (1910). Myxödem im Kindesalter. *Ergebnisse der inneren Medizin und Kinderheilkunde, 6*, 601–654.

Siemens, H. W. (1924). Die Erblichkeitsfrage beim Kröpf. *Münchener medizinische Wochenschrift, 71*, 1789–1791.

Simons, L. (1933). *Een bijdrage tot de kennis van het endemisch kropgezwel en kretinisme in de Gajo en Alaslanden*. Inaugural Dissertation, Leiden.

Stahl, F. C. (1843). *Beitrag zur Pathologie des Idiotismus endemicus, genannt Kretinismus, in den Bezirken Sulzheim und Gerolzhofen in Unterfranken des Konigreichs Baiern*. Bonn.

Stahl, F. C. (1848). *Neue Beiträge zur Physiognomik und pathologischen Anatomie der Idiotia endemica (genannt Kretinismus)*. Erlangen: Ferdinand Enke.

Starlinger, W. (1929). Die zirkulierenden Eiweißkörper beim endemischen Kretinismus. *Archiv für clinische Chirurgie, 155* Statistics Austria, 1906.

Stefko, W. H., & Glagolewa, M. (1931). Die Nagelfalzcapillaren und die Schilddrüse der Mongolen. *Zeitschrift für Konstitutionslehre, 16*.

Stieda, H. (1890). Über das Verhalten der Hypophyse des Kaninchens nach Entfernung der Schilddrüse. *Zieglers Beiträge zur pathologischen Anatomie, 7*, 537.

Stiner, O. (1924). Der Krebs und die Frage seiner Beziehungen zum endemischen Kröpf. *Schweizerische medizinische Wochenschrift, 54*(27), 605.

Stoccada, F. (1916). Untersuchungen über die Synchondrosis spheno-occipitalis und den Ossifikationsprozeß bei Kretinismus und Athyreosis. *Zieglers Beiträge zur pathologischen Anatomie und zur allgemeinen Pathologie, 61*, 450–513.

Stocks, P. (1925). Some further notes on cancer and goitre distributions. *Biometrika* (Lond.) *17*, 159–165.

Stocks, P., & Karn, M. N. (1927). On the relation between the prevalence of thyroid enlargement in children and mortality from cancer and other diseases. *Annals of Eugenics, 3*, 395.

Streit (1932). Beitrag zur Frage des Calciumspiegels im Kretinenserum. *Mitteilungen aus den Grenzgebieten der Medizin und Chirurgie, 42*.

Surbek, K. (1916). Über die Verfettung der Skelettmuskulatur. *Frankfurter Zeitschrift für Pathologie, 19*, 447.

Taussig, S. (1912). *Kropf und Kretinismus. Eine epidemiologische Studie*. Jena: G. Fischer Verlag.

The Lancet Editorial. (1972). New light on endemic cretinism. *The Lancet, 2*, 1275–1280.

Thieme, O. (1842). *Der Cretinismus, eine Monographie*. Inaugural Dissertation. Weimar.

Thomas, E. (1912). Zur Einteilung der Myxödemformen. *Deutsche medizinische Wochenschrift, 38*(10), 461–462. doi: 10.1055/s-0029-1189351.

Troxler, I. P. V. (1833). Der Cretinismus und seine Formen, als endemische Menschenentartung in unserem Vaterlande. *Denkschriften der allgemeinen Schweizerischen Gesellschaft für die gesamten Naturwissenschaften, 1*(2), 175–199.

Veil, W. H., & Sturm, A. (1925). Beiträge zur Kenntnis des Jodstoff Wechsels. *Archiv für klinische Medizin, 147*, 166–223.

Verschuer, O. von (1934). *Erbpathologie*. Dresden & Leipzig: T. Steinkopff.

Virchow, R. L. K. (1856). Über die Kretinen-Physiognomie. *Verhandlungen der physikalisch-medizinische Gesellschaft Würzburg, 8*, 24.

Virchow, R. L. K. (1857). *Untersuchungen über die Entwicklung des Schädelgrundes*. Berlin: Reimer.

Virchow, R. L. K. (1858). Knochenwachstum und Schädelformen mit besonderer Rücksicht auf Kretinismus. *Virchows Archiv für pathologische Anatomie und Physiologie und für klinische Medizin, 13*, 323–357.

Virchow, R. L. K. (1862). Über den Kretinismus namentlich in Franken und über pathologische Schädelformen. *Gesammelte Abhandlungen zur wissenschaftlichen Medicin Hamm*.

Virchow, R. L. K. (1862). Über die Verbreitung des Cretinismus in Unterfranken. *Gesammelte Abhandlungen zur wissenschaftlichen Medicin Hamm*, 939–969.

Virchow, R. L. K. (1862). Zur Entwicklungsgeschichte des Cretinismus und der Schädeldifformitäten. *Gesammelte Abhandlungen zur wissenschaftlichen Medicin Hamm*, 969–997.

Virchow, R. L. K. (1883). Fötale Rachitis, Cretinismus und Zwergwuchs. *Virchows Archiv für pathologische Anatomie und Physiologie und für klinische Medizin, 94*, 183–184.

Virchow, R. L. K. (1912). Myxödem und Kretinismus. In *Aschaffenburgs Handbuch der Psychiatrie, Spez. Teil*, Section 2, First Half. Leipzig & Vienna: Franz Deuticke.

Voronoff, S. (1914). *Greffe de la glande thyroïde*. Paris: Académie de Médicine.

Vrolik, W. (1855). Verhandeling der Koninklijke akademie van Wetenschappen Amsterdam. *Schmidts Jahrbuch, 85.*

Wagner von Jauregg, J. (1900). Über endemischen und sporadischen Kretinismus und dessen Behandlung. *Wiener klinische Wochenschrift, 13*, 419–427.

Wälchli, E. (1922). Hypo- und Athyreosis und Blutbild. *Folia haematologica, 27*, 135.

Walder, E. (1926). Ein Beitrag zur Kottmannschen Reaktion. *Mitteilungen aus den Grenzgebieten der Medizin und Chirurgie, 39*, 626.

Wallmann, H. (1863). Lebensgeschichte und Leichenbefunde dreier Salzburger Idioten und einige Kulturgeschichtliche Bemerkungen über Land und Leute in Salzburg. *Zeitschrift der k. k. Gesellschaft der Ärzte in Wien*, 120–138.

Wangensteen, O. H. (1929). The blood supply of the thyroid gland with special reference to the vascular system of the cretin goiter. *The American Journal of the Medical Sciences, 178*(1), 133.

Wegelin, C. (1916). Über Ossifikationsstörungen beim endemischen Kretinismus und Kröpf. *Korrespondenzblätter für Schweizerische Ärzte, 20.*

Wegelin, C. (1925). Zur Kenntnis der Kachexia thyreopriva. *Virchows Archiv für pathologische Anatomie und Physiologie und für klinische Medizin, 254*(3), 689–709.

Wegelin, C. (1926). Schilddrüse. In F. Henke & O. Lubarsch (Eds) *Handbuch der speziellen pathologischen Anatomie und Histologie, 8.* Berlin: Julius Springer.

Wegelin, C. (1930). Der endemische Kretinismus. *Verhandlungen der Schweizerischen naturforschenden Gesellschaft St Gallen.*

Wegelin, C., & Abelin, J. (1921). Über die Wirksamkeit der menschlichen Schilddrüse im Froschlarvenversuch. *Archiv für experimentalische Pathologie,89*(5), 219–251.

Wegelin, C., & Abelin, J. (1924). Weitere Untersuchungen über die Wirksamkeit menschlicher Kröpfe im Kaulquappenversuch. *Archiv für experimentalische Pathologie, 105*(1), 137–168.

Weitz, W. (1925). Studien an eineiigen Zwillingen. *Zeitschrift für klinische Medizin, 101*, 115–127.

Wenzel, J., & Wenzel, K. (1802). *Über den Cretinismus*. Vienna: Schaumberg.

Werdt, F. von (1911). Über Lymphfollikelbildung in Strumen. *Frankforter Zeitschrift für Pathologie, 7*, 401–444.

Weygandt, W. (1904). Ueber Virchows Kretinentheorie. *Neurologisches Zentralblatt, 7–9.*

Weygandt, W. (1904). Weitere Beiträge zur Lehre vom Kretinismus. *Verhandlungen der physikalischmedizinischen Gesellschaft Würzburg, 37.*

Weygandt, W. (1904). Der heutige Stand der Lehre vom Kretinismus. *Sammlung zwangloser Abhandlungen aus dem Gebiete der Nerven- und Geisteskrankheiten, 4.*

WHO/UNICEF/ICCIDD. (1994). *Indicators for assessing iodine deficiency disorders and their elimination through salt iodization.* WHO/NUT/94.6 Geneva: WHO.

Wieland, H. (1923). Die Erkrankungen der Schilddrüse. In M. von Pfaundler & A. Schlossmann (Eds) *Handbuch der Kinderheilkunde*, (3 rd ed.) Leipzig: F.C.W. Vogel.

Wieland, H. (1926). Die Hypothyreosen im Kindesalter. In M. Hirsch (Ed.) *Handbuch der inneren Sekretion, 3.* Leipzig: Kabitzsch.

Willer, H. (1930). *Über die Ausbreitung und Anatomie der unterfränkischen Struma (unter Berücksichtigung des Kretinismus).* Jena: G. Fischer Verlag.

Wittneben, W. (1927). *Diskussionsbemerkungen zur Prophylaxe der endemischen Struma.* Berne: International Goitre Conference.

Woelz, E. (1921). Vergleichende Untersuchungen über die Häufigkeit der verschiedenen Kropfformen in Basel und in Bern. *Schweizerische medizinische Wochenschrift, 51*, 625.

World Declaration on the Survival, Protection and Development of Children (1990). *World Summit for Children.* New York: The United Nations.

World Health Assembly. (1999). Statement by the Director General of WHO. *WHA*/17. Geneva: WHO.

World Health Organization. (1994). *Iodine and health. A statement by the World Health Organization*, WHO/NUT/94.4 Geneva: WHO.

Wydler, A. (1926). *Die Histologie der Kretinenstruma, mit Berücksichtigung der Klinik des Kretinismus und der funktionellen Untersuchung*. Jena: G. Fischer Verlag.

Wyss R. von (1899). Beitrag zur Kenntnis der Entwicklung des Skelets von Kretinen und Kretinoiden. *Fortschritte auf dem Gebiete der Röntgenstrahlen, 3*, 18–27.

Ziegler, E. (1902). *Lehrbuch der allgemeinen pathologischen und speziellen pathologischen Anatomie*. Jena: G. Fischer Verlag.

Zimmermann, M. B., Jooste, P. L., & Pandav, C. S. (2008). Iodine-deficiency disorders. *The Lancet, 372*, 1251–1262.

Zingerle, H. (1930). Statistik kretinischer Entartungsmerkmale und deren Beeinflussung durch die neue Kropfprophylaxe. *Schweizerische Zeitschrift für Hygiene, 12*.

Zuckermann, H. (1913). Über einen Hypophysenbefund bei Schilddrüsenaplasie. *Frankfurter Zeitschrift für Pathologie, 14*(2), 1.

Index

J. Dennison et al., *Endemic Cretinism*,
DOI 10.1007/978-1-4614-0281-7, © Springer Science+Business Media, LLC 2011

MIX
Papier aus verantwortungsvollen Quellen
Paper from responsible sources
FSC® C105338

If you have any concerns about our products,
you can contact us on
ProductSafety@springernature.com

In case Publisher is established outside the EU,
the EU authorized representative is:
Springer Nature Customer Service Center GmbH
Europaplatz 3, 69115 Heidelberg, Germany

Printed by Libri Plureos GmbH
in Hamburg, Germany